Electrocardiography of Complex Arrhythmias

Editors

MOHAMMAD SHENASA
EDWARD P. GERSTENFELD

CARDIAC ELECTROPHYSIOLOGY CLINICS

www.cardiacEP.theclinics.com

Consulting Editors
RANJAN K. THAKUR
ANDREA NATALE

September 2014 • Volume 6 • Number 3

ELSEVIER

1600 John F. Kennedy Boulevard • Suite 1800 • Philadelphia, Pennsylvania, 19103-2899

http://www.theclinics.com

CARDIAC ELECTROPHYSIOLOGY CLINICS Volume 6, Number 3
September 2014 ISSN 1877-9182, ISBN-13: 978-0-323-31209-7

Editor: Adrianne Brigido
Developmental Editor: Barbara Cohen-Kligerman

Cardiac Electrophysiology Clinics (ISSN 1877-9182) is published quarterly by Elsevier Inc., 360 Park Avenue South, New York, NY 10010-1710. Months of issue are March, June, September, and December. Subscription prices are $200.00 per year for US individuals, $293.00 per year for US institutions, $105.00 per year for US students and residents, $225.00 per year for Canadian individuals, $331.00 per year for Canadian institutions, $285.00 per year for international individuals, $354.00 per year for international institutions and $150.00 per year for Canadian and foreign students/residents. To receive student/resident rate, orders must be accompanied by name of affilliated institution, date of term, and the signature of program/residency coordinator on institution letterhead. Orders will be billed at individual rate until proof of status is received. Foreign air speed delivery is included in all Clinics subscription prices. All prices are subject to change without notice. **POSTMASTER:** Send address changes to Cardiac Electrophysiology Clinics, Elsevier Health Sciences Division, Subscription Customer Service, 3251 Riverport Lane, Maryland Heights, MO 63043. **Customer Service: 1-800-654-2452 (US and Canada). From outside of the US and Canada, call 314-477-8871. Fax: 314-447-8029. E-mail: JournalsCustomerService-usa@elsevier.com (for print support); JournalsOnlineSupport-usa@elsevier.com (for online support).**

Reprints. For copies of 100 or more of articles in this publication, please contact the Commercial Reprints Department, Elsevier Inc., 360 Park Avenue South, New York, NY 10010-1710. Tel.: 212-633-3874; Fax: 212-633-3820; E-mail: reprints@elsevier.com.

Contributors

CONSULTING EDITORS

RANJAN K. THAKUR, MD, MPH, MBA, FHRS
Professor of Medicine and Director, Arrhythmia
Service, Thoracic and Cardiovascular Institute,
Sparrow Health System, Michigan State
University, Lansing, Michagan

ANDREA NATALE, MD, FACC, FHRS
Executive Medical Director, Texas Cardiac
Arrhythmia Institute, St. David's Medical
Center, Austin, Texas; Consulting Professor,
Division of Cardiology, Stanford University,
Palo Alto, California; Adjunct Professor of
Medicine, Heart and Vascular Center, Case
Western Reserve University, Cleveland, Ohio;
Director, Interventional Electrophysiology,
Scripps Clinic, San Diego, California; Senior
Clinical Director, EP Services, California Pacific
Medical Center, San Francisco, California

EDITORS

MOHAMMAD SHENASA, MD
Attending Physician, Department of
Cardiovascular Services, O'Conner Hospital,
Heart & Rhythm Medical Group, San Jose,
California

EDWARD P. GERSTENFELD, MD
Chief, Section of Cardiac Electrophysiology;
Melvin M. Scheinman Endowed Chair in
Cardiology, Cardiology Division; Professor of
Medicine, Department of Medicine, University
of California, San Francisco, San Francisco,
California

AUTHORS

AMIN AL-AHMAD, MD
Texas Cardiac Arrhythmia Institute, Austin,
Texas

HAMID ASSADI, MD
Heart & Rhythm Medical Group, San Jose,
California

NITISH BADHWAR, MBBS, FACC, FHRS
Associate Professor of Medicine, Director of
Cardiac Electrophysiology Training Program,
Section of Electrophysiology, Division of
Cardiology, University of California,
San Francisco, San Francisco, California

FRANK BOGUN, MD
Associate Professor, University of Michigan
Hospital, Ann Arbor, Michigan

MOHAMED BOUTJDIR, PhD
Professor of Physiology, State University of
New York, Downstate Medical Center,
Brooklyn, New York

NOEL G. BOYLE, MD, PhD
Professor of Medicine; Director, Cardiac EP
Labs and Fellowship Program, UCLA Cardiac
Arrhythmia Center, UCLA Health System,
David Geffen School of Medicine at UCLA,
Los Angeles, California

DAVID J. CALLANS, MD
Cardiovascular Division, Hospital of the
University of Pennsylvania; Professor of
Medicine, University of Pennsylvania,
Philadelphia, Pennsylvania

SHIH-LIN CHANG, MD, PhD
Division of Cardiology, Department of
Medicine, Taipei Veterans General Hospital,
National Yang-Ming University School of
Medicine, Taipei, Taiwan

SHIH-ANN CHEN, MD
Chief, Department of Medicine, Taipei
Veterans General Hospital; Professor of
Medicine, National Yang-Ming University
School of Medicine, Taipei, Taiwan

**KARIN K.M. CHIA, MBBS, PhD, FRACP,
FCSANZ**
Staff Cardiac Electrophysiologist, Senior
Lecturer, Department of Cardiology, Royal
Brisbane and Women's Hospital, University of
Queensland, Queensland, Australia

MITHILESH KUMAR DAS, MD
Associate Professor of Clinical Medicine,
Krannert Institute of Cardiology, Indiana
University Health; Chief, Cardiac Arrhythmia
Service, Roudebush Veterans Affairs Medical
Center, Indianapolis, Indiana

PEERAWUT DEEPRASERTKUL, MD
Department of Medicine, University of Texas
Medical Branch, Galveston, Texas

SANJAY DIXIT, MD
Associate Professor, University of
Pennsylvania School of Medicine; Director,
Cardiac Electrophysiology, Philadelphia VA
Medical Center, Philadelphia, Pennsylvania

SRIKANT DUGGIRALA, MD
Fellow, Section of Cardiac Electrophysiology,
University of California, San Francisco,
San Francisco, California

NABIL EL-SHERIF, MD
Professor of Medicine and Physiology, State
University of New York, Downstate Medical
Center; Chief, Cardiology Division, New York
Harbor VA Healthcare System, Brooklyn,
New York

KENNETH A. ELLENBOGEN, MD, FHRS
Kontos Professor of Medicine; Chair, Division
of Cardiology, Virginia Commonwealth
University Pauley Heart Center, Medical
College of Virginia/VCU School of Medicine,
Richmond, Virginia

EDWARD P. GERSTENFELD, MD
Chief, Section of Cardiac Electrophysiology;
Melvin M. Scheinman Endowed Chair in
Cardiology, Cardiology Division; Professor of
Medicine, Department of Medicine,
University of California, San Francisco,
San Francisco, California

DAVID HAMON, MD
Research Fellow, UCLA Cardiac Arrhythmia
Center, UCLA Health System, David Geffen
School of Medicine at UCLA, Los Angeles,
California

HARIS M. HAQQANI, MBBS(Hons), PhD
Department of Cardiology, The Prince Charles
Hospital; Senior Lecturer, School of Medicine,
University of Queensland, Chermside,
Brisbane, Australia

ROBERT M. HAYWARD, MD
Electrophysiology Fellow, Section of Cardiac
Electrophysiology, Division of Cardiology,
Department of Medicine, University of
California, San Francisco, San Francisco,
California

KURT S. HOFFMAYER, PharmD, MD
Division of Electrophysiology, Department of
Cardiology, University of Wisconsin, Madison,
Madison, Wisconsin

HENRY H. HSIA, MD, FACC, FHRS
Chief, Electrophysiology Service, VA-San
Francisco; Health Science Professor of
Medicine, University of California,
San Francisco, San Francisco, California

MOHAMMAD-REZA JAZAYERI, MD
Department of Cardiology, Bellin Health,
Green Bay, Wisconsin

JONATHAN M. KALMAN, MBBS, PhD
Department of Cardiology, The Royal
Melbourne Hospital, Melbourne; Department
of Medicine, University of Melbourne, Victoria,
Australia

VIKAS KALRA, MBBS
Krannert Institute of Cardiology, Indiana
University Health, Indianapolis, Indiana

PETER M. KISTLER, MBBS, PhD
Department of Medicine, University of
Melbourne, Victoria, Australia

LEILA LAROUSSI, MD, FRCPC
Cardiac Electrophysiology Fellow, University of California, San Francisco, San Francisco, California

RAKESH LATCHAMSETTY, MD
Clinical Lecturer, University of Michigan Hospital, Ann Arbor, Michigan

MARK S. LINK, MD
Professor of Medicine, Department of Medicine, The Cardiac Arrhythmia Center, Tufts Medical Center, Boston, Massachusetts

AMIT MEHROTRA, MD, MBA
Cardiovascular Division, Hospital of the University of Pennsylvania, Philadelphia, Pennsylvania

NILUBON METHACHITTIPHAN, MD
Department of Medicine, University of Texas Medical Branch, Galveston, Texas

GWILYM M. MORRIS, BmBCh, PhD
Department of Cardiology, The Royal Melbourne Hospital, Melbourne, Australia; Institute of Cardiovascular Sciences, University of Manchester, Manchester, United Kingdom

BRYAN OTTE, MA
Research Associate, Cardiology Research Program, New York Harbor VA Healthcare System, Brooklyn, New York

ROLAND PEDALINO, MD
Chief, Cardiology Section, Kings County Hospital, Brooklyn, New York

SAJIN PILAI, MD
Cardiac Telemetry Service, New York Harbor VA Healthcare System, Brooklyn, New York

ARCHANA RAJDEV, MD
Krannert Institute of Cardiology, Indiana University Health, Indianapolis, Indiana

MELVIN M. SCHEINMAN, MD
Professor of Medicine, Section of Electrophysiology, Division of Cardiology; Shorenstein Chair in Cardiology, University of California San Francisco Medical Center, San Francisco, California

HOSSEIN SHENASA, MD, MsC
Heart & Rhythm Medical Group; Attending Physician, Department of Cardiovascular Services, O'Connor Hospital, San Jose, California

MOHAMMAD SHENASA, MD
Attending Physician, Department of Cardiovascular Services, O'Connor Hospital, Heart & Rhythm Medical Group, San Jose, California

KALYANAM SHIVKUMAR, MD, PhD
Professor of Medicine and Radiological Sciences; Director, UCLA Cardiac Arrhythmia Center and Electrophysiology Programs, UCLA Health System, David Geffen School of Medicine at UCLA, Los Angeles, California

MONA SOLEIMANIEH, RN
Heart & Rhythm Medical Group, San Jose, California

STEVEN M. STEVENS, MD
Clinical Instructor, UCLA Cardiac Arrhythmia Center, UCLA Health System, David Geffen School of Medicine at UCLA, Los Angeles, California

ZIAN H. TSENG, MD, MAS
Associate Professor of Medicine in Residence, Section of Cardiac Electrophysiology, Division of Cardiology, Department of Medicine, University of California, San Francisco, San Francisco, California

GIOIA TURITTO, MD
Director, Electrophysiology Service, New York Methodist Hospital, Brooklyn, New York

PUGAZHENDHI VIJAYARAMAN, MD, FHRS, FACC
Director of Cardiac Electrophysiology, Geisinger Wyoming Valley Medical Center, Wilkes Barre; Fellowship Director, Cardiac Electrophysiology, Geisinger Heart Institute, Danville, Pennsylvania

RICKY YU, MD
Research Fellow, UCLA Cardiac Arrhythmia Center, UCLA Health System, David Geffen School of Medicine at UCLA, Los Angeles, California

Contents

> Concealed conduction (CC) occurs when an impulse penetrates a part of the conduction system but fails to complete its course. This partial penetration is untraceable on the surface ECG, so CC is recognizable only by its influence on subsequent impulses. Any cardiac electrical activities not directly detectable on the surface ECG could be considered as concealed. This article highlights various electrophysiologic (EP) concepts and phenomena that may represent the aftermath of CC or be linked to its genesis. EP characteristics and behavior of the atrioventricular conduction system relevant to CC are outlined, and the consequences of CC discussed.

> Ventricular arrhythmias in structurally normal hearts can be divided into idiopathic ventricular arrhythmia, in which there is no known ion mutation or genetic component, and inherited ion channelopathies, in which gene mutations causing ion-channel dysfunction play an important role in the mechanism of ventricular arrhythmia. Inherited channelopathies are long QT syndrome, short QT syndrome, Brugada syndrome, and catecholaminergic polymorphic ventricular tachycardia. Recognizing ECG patterns of these arrhythmias is important because they can cause sudden cardiac deaths that are preventable with defibrillator implantations.

> In this article, the electrophysiologic basis of the various electrocardiogram characteristics of torsades de pointes (TdP) arrhythmias in long QT syndrome (LQTS) is presented. The in vivo electrophysiologic mechanism of TdP in LQTS is described using, as a paradigm, the anthopleurin-A canine model. In LQTS, prolonged repolarization is associated with increased spatial dispersion of repolarization. Prolongation of repolarization also acts as a primary step for the generation of early afterdepolarizations. An electrophysiologic basis of the characteristic twisting QRS configuration of TdP is discussed. Also explained is the mechanism of the short-long cardiac sequence.

> Conduction slowing or block can occur in the atrioventricular (AV) node, the bundle of His, or both, and manifest as characteristic patterns in the electrocardiogram and

intracardiac electrogram. These patterns lead to differences in prognosis and therapy, depending on the location and severity of disease. In general, the prognosis is better when the level of block is above the AV node (supra-His), whereas block below the AV node (intra-His or infra-His) portends a higher risk of progression to complete heart block. Causes of AV block are numerous and recognition of the cause is essential, because many are easily treated.

Electrocardiographic Characteristics of Focal Atrial Tachycardias 459

Haris M. Haqqani, Gwilym M. Morris, Peter M. Kistler, and Jonathan M. Kalman

Focal atrial tachycardia (AT) is uncommon and characterized by centrifugal atrial activation from a point source. ATs are found clustering around well-defined sites of structural and electrophysiologic heterogeneity in both atria. Focal AT most often occurs in patients without structural heart disease. The P-wave morphology on the surface ECG provides a good guide to the site of origin. With electrophysiologic study, activation mapping efforts can begin in the region suggested by P-wave analysis. Catheter ablation is an effective therapy that can result in long-term cure in most patients with a low risk of complications.

Right and Left Atrial Macroreentrant Tachycardias 469

Shih-Lin Chang and Shih-Ann Chen

The incidence of macroreentrant atrial tachycardias is increasing. Surface ECGs provide important information in the management of macroreentrant atrial tachycardias. Atrial flutter (AFL) represents macroreentrant atrial tachycardia on surface ECG. Catheter ablation of the cavotricuspid isthmus can terminate typical AFL with a high success rate and a low rate of complications. Atypical AFL is more difficult to eradicate. Electroanatomic mapping and a transseptal approach are sometimes needed in catheter ablation of atypical AFL. Recognizing the location of macroreentrant tachycardia from the 12-lead ECG can facilitate the mapping of reentrant circuit, guide ablation, and help in understanding the tachycardia mechanism.

Paroxysmal Supraventricular Tachycardias: Atrioventricular Nodal Reentrant Tachycardia and Atrioventricular Reentrant Tachycardias 483

Mohammad Shenasa, Hossein Shenasa, Hamid Assadi, and Mona Soleimanieh

Atrioventricular nodal reentrant tachycardia (AVNRT) and atrioventricular reentrant tachycardia (AVRT) are the most common forms of paroxysmal supraventricular tachycardia. Both occur in otherwise healthy young individuals, most of them without significant structural heart disease. Both AVNRT and AVRT are A-V nodal–dependent tachycardias, and in AVNRT the reentry circuit is confined within the so-called compact atrioventricular node. In most cases the reentry loop uses the anterograde slow pathway and retrograde fast pathway designated as typical or common form of AVNRT. About 20% to 30% of the variant forms of AVNRT are diagnosed during intracardiac electrophysiologic studies.

Wide Complex Tachycardia 511

Mithilesh Kumar Das, Archana Rajdev, and Vikas Kalra

A patient with a wide complex tachycardia (WCT) needs immediate attention because it is often a life-threatening arrhythmia, especially in the presence of structural heart disease. A quick but careful evaluation of various ECG criteria points toward the accurate diagnosis. The quick and correct diagnosis helps not only in prompt treatment but also in the optimal long-term management of these patients. This review discusses the differential diagnosis of WCT using various ECG criteria, correlation with intracardiac findings during electrophysiology study, and its management in brief.

The diagnosis, definition, localization, and management of postinfarct ventricular tachycardia (VT) in the patient with coronary artery disease depends critically on the surface 12-lead ECG. A systematic analysis of both the sinus rhythm and tachycardia ECGs provides much information that is critical for further decision making. The 12-lead ECG is used to exclude the other differential diagnostic possibilities, outline the substrate for postinfarct VT, define the likely region of VT exit from the scar border, as well as allow for detailed intracardiac analysis using entrainment and pace mapping during catheter ablation procedures.

Recognizing the ECG features that localize the exit or focus of the ventricular tachycardia (VT) and intracardiac electrogram (EGM) characteristics that delineate the arrhythmia substrate is essential to the development of a successful ablation strategy. These ECG and EGM characteristics in patients with nonischemic cardiomyopathy are also useful to predict success and durability of the procedure. This article focuses on these pertinent ECG and EGM characteristics of VT in patients with nonischemic dilated cardiomyopathy which influences the management approach for the patient's arrhythmia.

Outflow tract ventricular tachycardias (VTs) constitute a subgroup of idiopathic VT. The mechanism underlying outflow tract VT is triggered activity. These arrhythmias arise from locations in the right or left ventricular outflow tracts, and as a result, they manifest electrocardiographic characteristics that are helpful in accurately localizing their focal site of origin (SOO). Pace mapping from locations in the outflow tract region can mimic the 12-lead electrocardiogram characteristics of these arrhythmias, and this can be used to develop diagnostic algorithms for localizing clinical tachycardias. Recognition of the SOO is critical for procedural planning and ablation of outflow tract VT.

Fascicular tachycardia is a reentrant ventricular tachycardia using the left fascicular conduction system with distinct ECG characteristics and clinical manifestations. Patients commonly present with exercise-induced palpitations and are often treated acutely with calcium channel blockers. Chronic management can be achieved either pharmacologically or by catheter ablation. The arrhythmia is usually found in patients without structural heart disease and has a favorable long-term prognosis.

Srikant Duggirala and Edward P. Gerstenfeld

Idiopathic premature ventricular contractions (PVCs) or ventricular tachycardia (VT) sometimes originate from unusual sites, including the tricuspid or mitral annulus, right or left ventricular papillary muscles, or coronary venous system. Patients with symptomatic PVCs/VT or worsening left ventricular function may undergo catheter ablation. Understanding typical electrocardiogram morphology of VT/PVCs can be useful for patient counseling and planning a mapping/ablation strategy. Electroanatomic three-dimensional mapping systems and intracardiac echocardiography are often useful for mapping these complex regions. Although the success rate of ablation is lower than for typical right ventricular outflow tract PVCs, careful mapping and ablation can often safely eliminate PVCs.

Kurt S. Hoffmayer and Melvin M. Scheinman

Ventricular arrhythmias in patients with arrhythmogenic right ventricular dysplasia/cardiomyopathy (ARVD/C) are common. Baseline sinus rhythm and ventricular arrhythmia electrocardiogram characteristics are described. Using the electrocardiogram to differentiate between ARVD/C and idiopathic right ventricular outflow tract ventricular tachycardia can be an invaluable tool in sinus rhythm as well as during ventricular arrhythmias (ventricular tachycardia or premature ventricular contractions) in helping differentiating the two disease states. Recent data distinguishing ventricular arrhythmias between ARVD/C and cardiac sarcoid are also discussed.

Steven M. Stevens, David Hamon, Ricky Yu, Kalyanam Shivkumar, and Noel G. Boyle

In this article, specific ECG criteria to diagnose epicardial ventricular arrhythmia are reviewed. Four general measurement criteria are used: (1) the pseudo-δ wave, (2) intrinsicoid deflection time, (3) the shortest RS complex, and (4) the QRS complex duration. Additional criteria, including precordial maximal deflection index, precordial pattern break, and analysis of the Q wave pattern in lead I and the inferior leads, were derived in populations of patients with nonischemic cardiomyopathy. Algorithms on how to approach patients with suspected epicardial ventricular tachycardia are reviewed. ECG findings suggestive of epicardial accessory pathways in Wolff-Parkinson-White syndrome are reviewed.

Amin Al-Ahmad, Mohammad Shenasa, Hossein Shenasa, and Mona Soleimanieh

Ventricular tachycardia (VT) and ventricular fibrillation (VF) storm (sometimes called "electrical storm") is a very challenging clinical problem. Management of VT storms is often empiric and typically depends on the identification of a cause or underlying pathophysiology that needs treatment. The ECG can often be useful in identification of a cause and initiating a plan of therapy. In this review the common associated pathophysiology and ECG findings are discussed as well as options for therapy.

Late after surgical repair of complex congenital heart disease, atrial arrhythmias are a major cause of morbidity, and ventricular arrhythmias and sudden cardiac death are a major cause of mortality. The 6 cases in this article highlight common challenges in the management of arrhythmias in the adult congenital heart disease population.

The electrocardiogram may be useful in evaluating patients with cardiac resynchronization therapy and in particular may help to determine the site of left ventricular pacing and whether a patient is likely to respond to cardiac resynchronization therapy. Other electrocardiographic features of a wide variety of pacing algorithms are discussed. Knowledge of these specific pacing algorithms may avoid unnecessary evaluation for pacing system malfunction. Many of these algorithms are carefully described in the manufacturers' manuals.

CARDIAC ELECTROPHYSIOLOGY CLINICS

FORTHCOMING ISSUES

December 2014
Cardiac Sodium Channel Disorders
Hugues Abriel, *Editor*

March 2015
Frontiers in Non-invasive Cardiac Mapping
Ashok Shah, Michel Haissaguerre, and
Meleze Hocini, *Editors*

June 2015
Arrythmias in Cardiomyopathies
Mohammad Shenasa, Martin Maron, and Mark
Link, *Editors*

RECENT ISSUES

June 2014
**Implantable Devices: Design, Manufacturing,
and Malfunction**
Kenneth A. Ellenbogen, and
Charles J. Love, *Editors*

March 2014
Stroke in Atrial Fibrillation
Samuel J. Asirvatham, Ranjan K. Thakur, and
Andrea Natale, *Editors*

December 2013
**Clinical and Electrophysiologic Management
of Syncope**
Antonio Raviele and Andrea Natale, *Editors*

ISSUES OF RELATED INTEREST

Cardiology Clinics May 2014 (Vol. 32, No. 2)
Pacemakers and Implantable Cardioverter Defibrillators
Theofanie Mela, *Editor*
Available at: http://www.cardiology.theclinics.com/

Heart Failure Clinics October 2013 (Vol. 9, No. 4)
Atrial Fibrillation in Heart Failure
Mark O'Neill, Andrew Grace, and Sanjiv M. Narayan, *Editors*
Available at: http://www.heartfailure.theclinics.com/

NOW AVAILABLE FOR YOUR iPhone and iPad

Foreword
Not Such a Trivial Pursuit

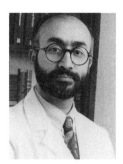

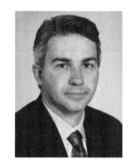

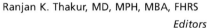

Ranjan K. Thakur, MD, MPH, MBA, FHRS   Andrea Natale, MD, FACC, FHRS

Editors

In cardiac electrophysiology we often face challenging cases that require deliberate application of electrophysiological principles to ascertain arrhythmia mechanisms and determine where ablation should be targeted. We initially acquire these skills from our teachers in the electrophysiology laboratory during fellowship training or going over complex tracings one-on-one.

A successful electrophysiology career requires that we continue practicing these skills as consultants, but we still need to keep learning and re-learning by discussing difficult cases with our colleagues and reading monographs like the one Drs Shenasa and Gerstenfeld have put together to illustrate the established core principles for electrocardiographic and electrophysiologic diagnosis of complex arrhythmias.

This issue of *Cardiac Electrophysiology Clinics* deals with important complex cases that electrophysiologists don't see every day; therefore, they could easily forget some important principles that may be critical. The reader will find articles written by thought leaders in specific arrhythmias, which summarize the known important principles in dealing with these arrhythmias. Some examples include articles on fascicular tachycardias, epicardial arrhythmias, arrhythmias in congenital heart disease, electrocardiographic analysis of paced rhythms and their correlation with intracardiac electrograms, electrocardiographic characteristics of ventricular tachycardias in right ventricular dysplasia, and so on.

These arrhythmias are not encountered routinely in clinical practice. For this reason, it is important to review and refresh our understanding of important principles in diagnosis and management of these arrhythmias periodically. We congratulate Drs Shenasa and Gerstenfeld for assembling a thoughtful table of contents that will be helpful for fellows in training as well as clinical electrophysiologists in practice. In addition, we congratulate them for assembling a formidable list of contributors who draw upon decades of study and research to illuminate these issues authoritatively.

Ranjan K. Thakur, MD, MPH, MBA, FHRS
Sparrow Thoracic and Cardiovascular Institute
Michigan State University
1200 East Michigan Avenue, Suite 580
Lansing, MI 48912, USA

Andrea Natale, MD, FACC, FHRS
Texas Cardiac Arrhythmia Institute
Center for Atrial Fibrillation at
St. David's Medical Center
1015 East 32nd Street, Suite 516
Austin, TX 78705, USA

E-mail addresses:
thakur@msu.edu (R.K. Thakur)
andrea.natale@stdavids.com (A. Natale)

http://dx.doi.org/10.1016/j.ccep.2014.06.002
1877-9182/14/$ – see front matter

Preface
Electrocardiography of Complex Arrhythmias

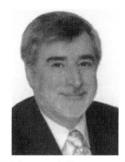 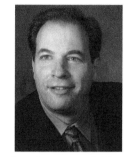

Mohammad Shenasa, MD   Edward P. Gerstenfeld, MD
Editors

This issue of *Cardiac Electrophysiology Clinics* is focused on electrocardiography (ECG) of complex arrhythmias. Intracardiac electrograms and mapping studies are utilized to confirm the ECG findings.

The ECG remains the first diagnostic test for evaluation and management of cardiac arrhythmias. As once said by Shlomo Stern, "the ECG is still the cardiologist's best friend."[1]

In the last two decades, several new forms of ventricular tachycardia have been described. We think it is incredible that more than a century after the first description of ECG, new ECG patterns are still being discovered. These new findings occur, in large part, because invasive electrophysiologists now often have the "answer" to the true origin of these arrhythmias, and then, can look back on the ECG for characteristic features that correlate with these intracardiac findings.

Likewise, new observations on a variety of supraventricular arrhythmias, atrioventricular conduction disturbances, and paced rhythms have been described.

We are pleased that a group of leading experts in the field have unanimously accepted our invitation to participate and provide their up-to-date state-of-the-art work on the subject. Articles in this issue describe well the correlation of arrhythmia mechanisms with their anatomic location and electrophysiological characteristics.

We are confident that this volume will be useful to cardiologists, electrophysiology fellows, and electrophysiologists as an important reference to better understand the correlation of ECG characteristics with intracardiac electrograms and mapping investigations.

Mohammad Shenasa, MD
Department of Cardiovascular Services
O'Conner Hospital
Heart and Rhythm Medical Group
105 N. Bascom Avenue, Suite 204
San Jose, CA 95128, USA

Edward P. Gerstenfeld, MD
Cardiac Electrophysiology
Cardiology Division, Department of Medicine
University of California, San Francisco
500 Parnassus Avenue, MUE-434, Box 1354
San Francisco, CA 94143-1354, USA

E-mail addresses:
mohammad.shenasa@gmail.com (M. Shenasa)
egerstenfeld@medicine.ucsf.edu (E.P. Gerstenfeld)

REFERENCE

1. Stern S. Electrocardiogram: still the cardiologist's best friend. Circulation 2006;113:753–6.

cardiacEP.theclinics.com

Concealed Conduction and Allied Concepts

Mohammad-Reza Jazayeri, MD

KEYWORDS

- Concealed conduction • Concealment • Aberrant ventricular conduction • Nonpropagated impulse
- Functional block • Transseptal conduction • Collision of impulses • Linking phenomenon

KEY POINTS

- Concealed conduction is a common electrocardiographic phenomenon whereby a series of events may occur as a result of incomplete propagation of an impulse.
- The occurrence, maintenance, and resolution (termination) of several events such as functional block and supraventricular tachycardias are linked to concealed conduction.
- This phenomenon should be suspected on the surface electrocardiogram when an event occurs unexpectedly.
- His-bundle electrocardiography and comprehensive electrophysiology may be needed to verify this phenomenon.

We should first endeavor to better understand the working of the heart in all its details, and the cause of a large variety of abnormalities. This will enable us, in a possibly still-distant future and based upon a clear insight and improved knowledge, to give relief to the suffering of our patients.[1]
— Willem Einthoven

INTRODUCTION

Concealed conduction (CC) is a common phenomenon that has fascinated both electrocardiographers and electrophysiologists for decades. This phenomenon occurs when an impulse penetrates a part of the conduction system but fails to complete its course. Partial penetration of the conduction system is untraceable on the surface electrocardiogram (ECG) and thus CC is recognizable only by its influence on the subsequent impulse(s). Therefore, incomplete or partial propagation of an impulse through a conduction pathway is the sine qua non of CC. The

electrophysiologic (EP) sequelae of CC could manifest as a simple block or a subsequent complex event. Intracardiac recordings and/or complex EP maneuvers may be needed for verification of such a cascade or elucidation of its underlying mechanism(s). Conceptually, any cardiac electrical activities that are not directly detectable on the surface ECG could be considered as concealed. The objective of this article is to highlight various EP concepts and phenomena that may represent the aftermath of CC or somehow be linked to its genesis. It is organized so as to first outline the normal EP characteristics and behavior of the atrioventricular (AV) conduction system that are relevant to CC, and then discuss the consequence(s) of CC on the fate of the subsequent impulse (event).

HISTORICAL BACKGROUND

The seminal and ingenious work of Willem Einthoven[1,2] leading to the development of the ECG in early 1900s has indebted all physicians, scientists, and especially patients who benefit from

The author has nothing to disclose.
Department of Cardiology, Bellin Health, 744 South Webster Avenue, Green Bay, WI 54305, USA
E-mail address: jazmo@bellin.org

Card Electrophysiol Clin 6 (2014) 377–418
http://dx.doi.org/10.1016/j.ccep.2014.06.001
1877-9182/14/$ – see front matter © 2014 Elsevier Inc. All rights reserved.

this invention. Langendorf[3] introduced the term CC to electrocardiography for the first time in 1948. However, others[4–7] had previously made observations on certain aspects of this concept, during animal experiments, as early as 1894, even a few years before the introduction of ECG. With the advent of intracardiac signal recording and stimulation techniques, extensive animal studies and clinical investigations were undertaken, and CC became a provocative concept being considered in both simple and complex arrhythmias.[8–14] Over the past 65 years, CC has gained popularity among both electrocardiographers and electrophysiologists for the analysis and interpretation of cardiac arrhythmias.

ECG AND EP MANIFESTATIONS

CC can occur during propagation of the antegrade or retrograde impulses by exhibiting conduction delay or conduction block. It should be borne in mind that the coupling interval between the blocked impulse and its subsequent (rather than preceding) impulse is a crucial determinant of whether CC would occur and, if so, how it would manifest.[15]

Concealment During Antegrade Conduction of Impulses

Premature atrial complex

- CC might occur at different sites along the AV conduction system depending on the prematurity of the blocked impulse and its preceding cycle length (CL).
- The effective refractory period (ERP) of the AV node is inversely related to its preceding input CL: the shorter the CL, the longer the ERP.[16,17]
- The His-Purkinje system (HPS) refractory period (RP) is directly related to its preceding input CL: the longer the CL, the longer the ERP.[16,17]
- In most blocked premature atrial complexes (PACs), the site of CC is in the AV node (**Fig. 1**).[11]
- CC of a blocked PAC exerts its impact on the subsequent atrial impulse as conduction delay (see **Fig. 1**D) or block (see **Fig. 1**E). In the latter case, several consecutive blocked PACs would manifest as repetitive CC (see **Fig. 1**E).[10]
- The PR-interval prolongation caused by CC mostly depends on the coupling interval between the blocked impulse and the subsequent impulse, and not on the prematurity of the former.[15]

- An impulse exerts greater conduction delay on a subsequent impulse if the former is fully propagated instead of being concealed.[15]
- Like most of the AV nodal EP properties, modulation of the autonomic nervous system may potentially enhance or hamper concealment in the AV node.[18]
- The concealment index has been proposed as a parameter for assessing the effect of pharmacologic agents on CC and, ultimately, their efficacy in controlling ventricular response in atrial tachyarrhythmias.[19,20]
- CC of a blocked premature atrial impulse (A2) may affect the retrograde AV nodal conduction of a subsequent ventricular impulse (VI) in individuals with intact ventriculoatrial (VA) conduction. In response to progressive shortening of the A2-VI coupling interval, the corresponding VA interval may exhibit a (1) progressively increasing (crescendo), (2) flat, or (3) discontinuous curve with a sudden jump before the onset of VA block.[21]
- The shortest A2-VI interval attainable in each individual represents the recovery of excitability of the retrograde AV node after antegrade concealment has occurred.[22–24] This parameter is markedly shorter in patients with AV nodal reentry (with sustained tachycardia or single echo beats) than those without.[22] This fact may have important implications in the genesis of antidromic reentrant tachycardia (ART) in patients with the Wolff-Parkinson-White syndrome.

Regular high-rate atrial impulses

Because the physiologic responses of the AV node and HPS to the incremental pacing or a sudden change of rate are different, each component is discussed separately.

1. AV Node
   - Normally, during incremental atrial pacing, the AV nodal conduction time (ie, AH interval) progressively increases as the pacing CL is shortened.
   - The initial AV nodal accommodation pattern in response to a sudden rate of acceleration[25] is 1 of the following:
     - Crescendo (increasing): Progressive prolongation of the AH interval until it reaches the steady state
     - Decrescendo (decreasing): Progressive shortening of the AH interval until it reaches the steady state
     - Instantaneous (flat): The AH remains constant and at the steady state

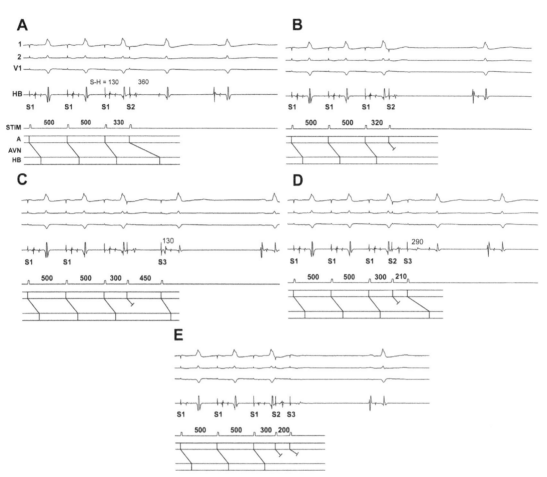

Fig. 1. Concealment during propagation of premature atrial impulses. Each panel depicts electrocardiogram (ECG) leads (1, 2, V1), intracardiac His bundle (HB) recording, and stimulation marker (STIM). Ladder diagrams are also shown for all panels. Premature atrial stimulation is performed at a basic drive cycle length of 500 milliseconds (ms). (*A*) At an S1-S2 coupling interval of 330 ms, the S2 is conducted with an AH interval (time between onset of first atrial deflection and His bundle deflection) of 360 ms. (*B*) On further shortening of the coupling interval to 320 ms, the S2 blocks in the atrioventricular node (AVN). The S1-S2 coupling interval is kept constant at 300 ms, and conduction of the S3 stimulus is scanned from a coupling interval of 450 ms to 200 ms (*C–E*), until it blocks in the AVN. Note that the AH prolongation of the S3 impulse (with S1-S3 interval of 510 ms, *D*) and its block (with S1-S3 interval of 500 ms, *E*) are due to the prior concealed conduction of the S2 impulse. Block of 2 consecutive premature (S2 and S3) impulses is termed repetitive concealed conduction (*E*). A, atrium.

- On further CL shortening the AV node reaches its maximum ability to conduct in a 1:1 fashion and then a periodic block, also known as the Wenckebach block (WB), ensues.[26]
- WB CL (usually in range of 300–600 milliseconds) is heavily influenced by the autonomic nervous system and the neurohumoral changes.[27–29]
- On further shortening of the CL, functional AV block of higher degrees (2:1, 3:1, and so forth), which tend to be more stable, will ensue (**Fig. 2**); this is when CC comes into play.[30]
- From the time that WB starts to occur until a stable higher-degree AV block is established, the AV node goes through a transition whereby the AV nodal conduction ratio may gradually progress from 6:5 to 4:3 and then to 3:2, before reaching a 2:1 ratio.[30]
- Occasionally a short-lasting run of alternating 3:2 and 2:1 conduction ratios may precede the occurrence of stable 2:1 ratio.[30,31]
- Another type of 2:1 behavior is when the AV (PR) intervals of the conducted beats progressively prolong until this period ends with a higher-degree block. This phenomenon is called alternate-beat Wenckebach periods (AWP) (**Fig. 3**).[32–36] Conversely, a less common situation is encountered when these (AV or PR) intervals of conducted 2:1 impulses progressively shorten until the

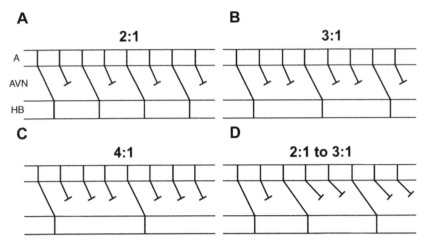

Fig. 2. (*A–D*) Various typical A:V ratios during rapid atrial impulses. These ladder diagrams represent the usual AV nodal responses to ultrarapid atrial impulses (ie, atrial tachycardia or flutter). A, atrium; AVN, atrioventricular node; HB, His bundle.

period ends with a lesser-degree AV block. This phenomenon is called reverse AWP (RAWP) (see **Fig. 3**).[37,38]

- Typically, a 2:1 conduction pattern occurs at a wider range of pacing CLs in comparison with that producing a WB.[30]
- The magnitude of concealment (ie, the difference between the AH intervals of 2:1 conducted beats and those produced by a 1:1 conduction pattern at exactly half the atrial rate) is fixed for the whole range of CLs demonstrating 2:1 conduction (**Fig. 4**).[30]
- During 2:1 AV conduction, the AV nodal refractoriness oscillates with dramatic

shortening of AV nodal ERP after the blocked beat and marked lengthening of that after the conducted beat. Moreover, the effect of CC is manifested not only by a prolonged conduction time of the subsequent conducted beat but also by a delayed recovery of the AV nodal excitability after the conducted beat.[39]

- Right ventricular pacing at CLs longer than the average ventricular CL during atrial tachyarrhythmias may completely or predominantly prevent the impulses from reaching the ventricles via the normal pathway (NP) by increasing the magnitude of CC (**Fig. 5**).[40]

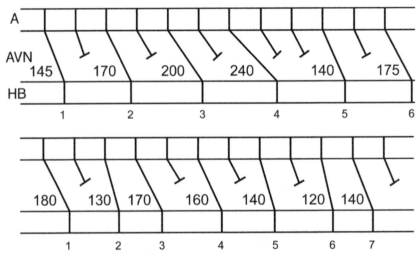

Fig. 3. Different forms of Wenckebach periodicity during 2:1 conduction. The top panel depicts the alternate-beat Wenckebach periods with progressive AV-interval prolongation of the conducted impulse (1–4) until a higher-degree block ensues. The lower panel demonstrates the reverse alternate-beat Wenckebach periods, in which the AV interval progressively shortens (3–6) until a lesser-degree block ensues. A, atrium; AVN, atrioventricular node; HB, His bundle.

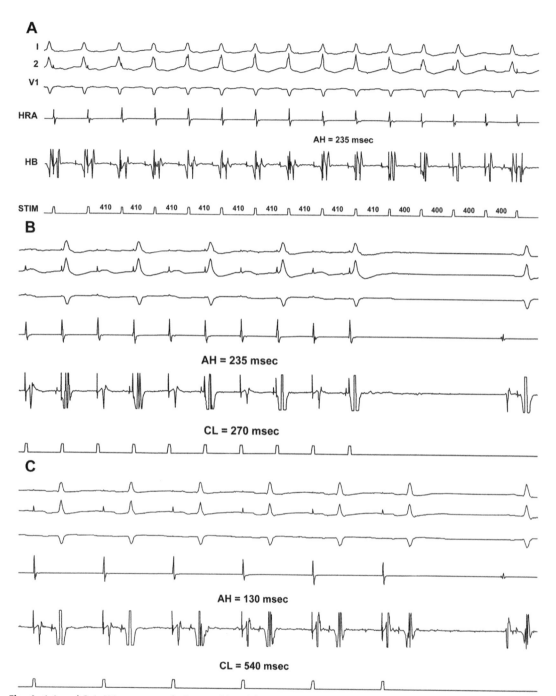

Fig. 4. 1:1 and 2:1 AV responses during rapid atrial rates. (*A*) A segment of AV conduction during incremental atrial pacing. Of note, on shortening of the pacing cycle length (CL) from 410 to 400 ms, the Wenckebach block occurs. (*B*) The terminal portion of a 2:1 response at pacing CL of 270 ms is demonstrated. Note that from the last atrial impulse, not being conducted, one could deduce that the atrial impulse in the middle of each R-R pair is the conducted one. (*C*) 1:1 AV conduction at a CL of twice that in *B*. The AH prolongation of the conducted beats in *B* (235 vs 130 ms in *C*) is due to "concealed conduction" of the blocked beats. HB, His bundle; HRA, high right atrial electrogram; STIM, stimulation marker.

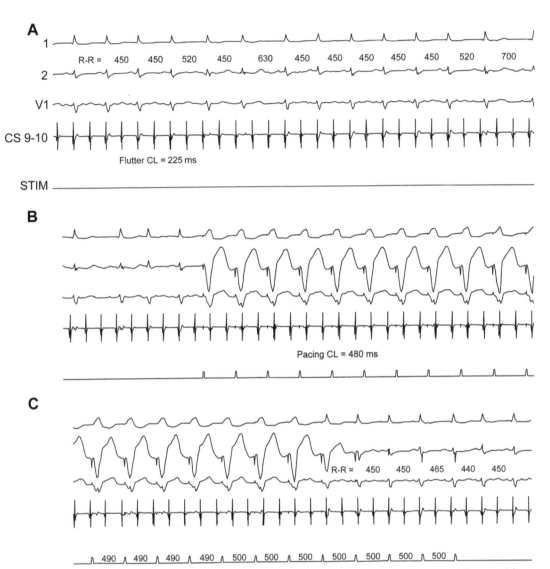

Fig. 5. Suppression of AV conduction by enhancement of concealment. (*A*) A segment of atrial flutter with variable ventricular response (R-R interval of 450–700 ms) is shown. Right ventricular pacing is done with a gradual increase in its cycle length (CL). (*B* and *C*) At pacing CLs (480–490 ms) longer than most R-R cycles, complete suppression of the antegrade conduction is noted, most likely because of the increased magnitude of AV nodal concealment caused by ventricular pacing. CS, coronary sinus electrogram; STIM, stimulation marker.

2. His-Purkinje system
- Normally, in response to incremental atrial pacing, the HPS conduction time (HV interval) and the QRS configuration remain unchanged during 1:1 conduction.
- Owing to the AV nodal conduction and refractoriness characteristics, the assessment of the HPS behavior during sudden atrial rate acceleration may be somewhat impeded.
- To impinge on the HPS refractoriness, the AV nodal functional refractory period must be shorter than the former.[41]

- In response to sudden atrial rate acceleration, functional 2:1 block in the HPS[42,43] (2:1 HPS-FB), functional bundle branch block (FBBB),[43,44] or functional fascicular block[43] may occur transiently or persistently. Ordinarily this is expected if the onset of rapid pacing is preceded by a long or short-to-long CL sequence.
- This phenomenon is more common in individuals with a rapidly conducting AV node at baseline or after administering atropine injection or isoproterenol infusion.[43]

- The antegrade refractory period of the bundle branches (BBs) shortens as the rate is increased.[45]
- The maintenance of 2:1 functional block (FB) is primarily due to a long-to-short activation CL, distal to the site of functional block.[42]
- The HV interval of the conducted beats during 2:1 HPS-FB is typically the same as that during sinus beats if the QRS configuration is unchanged.[42]
- Higher-degree HPS block greater than 2:1 (eg, 3:1, 4:1, and so forth) should be considered as pathologic.[17]
- The rare occurrence of successive blocks first in the HPS and then in the AV node during conduction of 2 consecutive beats, exhibiting a 3:1 block pattern, could still be functional.[46]
- The onset of 2:1 HPS-FB may be preceded or followed by 1 or more beats exhibiting FBBB.[43]
- FBBB may have normal or prolonged HV intervals. The latter is more common with functional left bundle branch block (FLBBB) or functional bifascicular block.[43,44]

3. ECG perspectives
- The entire spectrum of the AV nodal conduction in response to rapid atrial impulses may be divided into 4 patterns, namely, 1:1 conduction, Wenckebach periodicity, stable 2:1 (and less likely 3:1 or 4:1) conduction, and variable or unstable (AWB or RAWB) block.
- Atrial tachycardia and flutter with atrial CL less than 300 milliseconds are the most common arrhythmias that could potentially exhibit 1 or more of these patterns.
- In addition to the AV nodal intrinsic factors such as CC, refractoriness, and excitability; the extrinsic factors, such as the rate of atrial impulses, variations in the tone of the autonomic nervous system, use of drugs (eg, digitalis, AV nodal blocking agents, and antiarrhythmic agents, especially class Ic), and the presence or absence of AV nodal disease by exerting "facilitation or fatigue," play important roles in determining which patterns of conduction ultimately prevail.
- With regard to the relationship of the flutter waves (F) and the QRS complexes in 2:1 conduction pattern, it seems highly likely that first, the F wave closer to the midline between the 2 successive QRS complexes would be the conducted impulse; and second, the same F wave exhibits an F-R interval that is usually equal to or longer than the P-R interval during sinus beats.
- The occurrence of 2:1 conduction during typical AV nodal reentrant tachycardia (AVNRT)

in the EP laboratory is not uncommon. However, the HPS is the site of FB much more frequently than the AV nodal common pathway, below the distal turnaround point of the reentrant circuit.

Irregular high-rate atrial impulses

- Atrial fibrillation (AF), the most common sustained arrhythmia in man, by virtue of having disorganized atrial impulses at rates of greater than 400 beats/min, is the sole member of this group.
- The ventricular response during AF is typically characterized by irregular RR intervals. Although the exact reason for these irregularities is not well understood, several mechanisms, individually or in combination, may be implicated:
  - CC. Experimental studies in animals and humans have supported CC as being a major determinant of the ventricular rate during AF.[47–50]
  - The status of the autonomic nervous system.[47,51] Fluctuations of the autonomic tone may be profoundly affecting the EP principles governing the ventricular rate during AF.
  - AV nodal refractoriness and conductivity. These intrinsic AV nodal properties have been proposed as one of the best determinants of the mean ventricular rate during AF.[52]
  - Characteristics of the atrial impulses reaching the AV node. The degree of concealment in the AV node depends on the strength, form, number, direction, and sequence of the fibrillatory impulses approaching it.[53]
  - Functional interaction(s) between dual or multiple atrionodal pathways (inputs). Indirect evidence for supporting this hypothesis comes from the results of catheter ablation of the AV nodal slow pathway (SP) in patients with AV nodal reentry. These data clearly demonstrated that in patients with AV nodal reentry, a selective slow-pathway ablation may reduce the ventricular rate during induced AF, particularly after dual-pathway physiology is completely abolished or the AV nodal ERP is lengthened after ablation.[54,55]
- In the strict mathematical sense, the irregular ventricular response during AF is not considered as chaotic, because in a significant number of patients the beat-to-beat variation is somewhat predictable.[56]

- The concealment index may be a useful predictor of the magnitude of CC and irregularity of ventricular transmission during AF.[19]

ECG PERSPECTIVES PERTINENT TO ATRIAL FIBRILLATION

- Because repetitive CC is an expected AV nodal behavior in response to rapid and successive atrial impulses, the irregularity of the ventricular response during AF is predominantly caused by CC in the AV node rather than the HPS.
- Conversion of atrial tachycardia or flutter to AF is usually associated with a marked drop in ventricular rate, which is predominantly a manifestation of enhanced AV nodal CC during AF (**Fig. 6**).
- Ventricular pacing at relatively long CLs may suppress spontaneous short-cycle ventricular responses during AF; this is most likely related to the enhanced AV nodal concealment in response to ventricular pacing.
- Long-to-short CL variations in AV nodal outputs (ie, H-H intervals) during AF set the stage for the genesis of FBBB (the Ashman phenomenon).
- Persistence of FBBB during conduction of several successive beats is not uncommon in AF and is due to linking, a phenomenon addressed in more detail later in this article.

Concealment During Retrograde Conduction of Impulses

Normal behavior of the conduction system in response to premature stimulation and incremental pacing, pertinent to CC, are discussed before addressing any specific manifestations of CC. It is noteworthy that the bulk of published data has been obtained during right ventricular (RV) stimulation.

Premature ventricular impulse

1. His-Purkinje system[57–59]
   - At long premature coupling intervals (ie, >65% of the pacing drive), the premature ventricular impulse (PVI or V2) conducts to the His bundle (HB) via the right bundle (RB), and also turns around in the left bundle (LB) and collides with the same impulse reaching the LB transseptally (**Fig. 7A**). The corresponding HB potential is usually overlapped with and obscured by V2.
   - At shorter premature coupling intervals (ie, <50% of the pacing drive), the V2 usually blocks in the RB and traverses the septum to reach the LB. Thus, conduction of V2 to the HB is exclusively via the LB (see **Fig. 7B**). The longest coupling interval associated with the occurrence of RB block (the emergence of HB potential from V2) is defined as the relative refractory period (RRP) of the HPS.
   - On further shortening of the coupling interval, V2 would block in both RB and LB (ie, bilateral block), defined as the ERP of the HPS. At any certain basic drive CL, the HPS-ERP is approximately 50 to 150 milliseconds shorter than its RRP.
   - In patients with normal HPS, it would be highly unlikely that a single premature ventricular impulse (PVI) would block retrogradely in the HPS during sinus rhythm.
   - Couplets, triplets, or longer runs of consecutive PVIs, however, have a higher likelihood of retrograde conduction delay or block in the HPS.
   - The HPS refractoriness during long-to-short or short-to-long CL variations, undershoots or overshoots, respectively, the steady-state value that would be expected for a constant drive at the corresponding (short or long) CL.[17,60]
2. AV node[61,62]
   - At least 20% of individuals with normal AV conduction, at rest and in nonmedicated state, have no retrograde VA conduction, which is almost always due to the retrograde AV nodal block.
   - In the remaining individuals with intact VA conduction, the AV nodal conduction could fall into 1 of 3 categories:

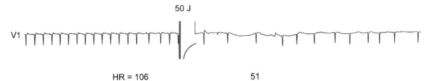

50 J

V1

HR = 106   51

Fig. 6. Different degrees of concealment during different atrial arrhythmias. A single synchronized transthoracic electrical countershock at 50 J converts atrial flutter to atrial fibrillation. Marked slowing of the ventricular rate (51 vs 106 beats/min) denotes a significant enhancement of the AV nodal concealed conduction during atrial fibrillation. HR, heart rate.

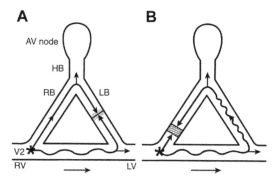

Fig. 7. Patterns of retrograde His bundle conduction during premature (V1-V2) ventricular stimulation. (*A*) At long V1-V2 intervals, the V2 impulse conducts to the His bundle (HB) via the right bundle (RB); it turns around in the left bundle (LB) and collides with the impulse entering the latter by way of the interventricular septum. (*B*) At shorter coupling intervals, the V2 blocks in the right bundle and conducts transseptally to the HB via the LB.

- ○ Short (fast pathway [FP]). The HA interval is 70 milliseconds or less.
- ○ Long (SP). The HA interval is 150 milliseconds or longer.
- ○ Intermediate. The HA interval is between 70 and 150 milliseconds.
- Retrograde AV nodal block in the presence of the fast category is uncommon during introduction of PVI. However, the response of the other 2 categories is unpredictable.

- These AV nodal characteristics are profoundly sensitive to the state of autonomic tone.[29]

Incremental ventricular pacing

1. His-Purkinje system[17,41,63]
   - Gradual shortening of the pacing CL down to 300 milliseconds does not usually show any discernible change in the VH interval (**Fig. 8**).
   - In contrast to a gradual CL shortening, the response of the HPS to a sudden rate of acceleration is somewhat unpredictable. During RV pacing at CLs ranging from 400 to 280 milliseconds, different HPS conduction patterns may be observed:
     - ○ 1:1 response with either no conduction delay or a short-lasting conduction delay followed by subsequent accommodation (ie, sudden VH shortening or normalization) (**Fig. 9**)
     - ○ 2:1 HPS block or 3:2 Wenckebach periodicity with subsequent accommodation or persistent block
     - ○ Persistent marked VH delay owing to linking phenomenon
   - In the presence of preexisting bundle branch block (BBB) during sinus rhythm, unexpected VH interval prolongation with pacing at relatively longer CLs from the ipsilateral ventricle would indicate the presence of bidirectional BBB.

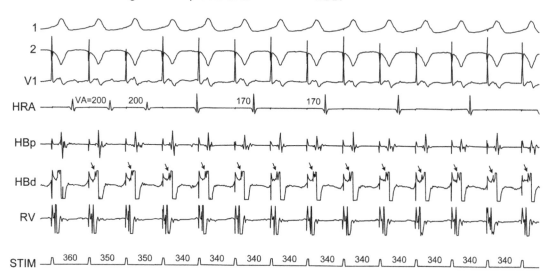

Fig. 8. Response of the normal pathway during incremental ventricular pacing. A segment of incremental right ventricular (RV) pacing at cycle lengths (CLs) of 360 to 340 ms is shown. A short VH interval (*arrows* point out the retrograde His bundle potentials) remains unchanged throughout this pacing episode. A brief period of Wenckebach block followed by 2:1 block in the ventriculoatrial (VA) pattern is due to the AV nodal behavior. Also, as a result of concealed conduction, the VA interval during 2:1 conduction is 170 ms, shorter than that during 1:1 conduction (200 ms) and markedly longer than 110 ms (not shown here) during RV pacing at 680 ms (doubling of pacing CL that resulted in 2:1 response). HBp and HBd, proximal and distal His bundle electrograms; HRA, high right atrial electrogram; STIM, stimulation marker.

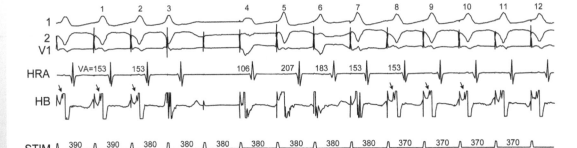

Fig. 9. Response of the normal pathway during sudden rate acceleration of ventricular pacing. Tracing is from the same patient shown in **Fig. 8**. During incremental right ventricular pacing at cycle lengths (CLs) of 390 to 370 ms, owing to a spontaneous premature ventricular impulse (#3), the pacing spike failed to capture. Consequently, a ventricular pause of more than 700 ms, with its previous and subsequent short cycles, created a short-long-short sequence. These sudden CL variations resulted in marked retrograde His-Purkinje system (HPS) conduction delay of impulse #5, as indicated by significant prolongation of its ventriculoatrial (VA) interval (207 vs 153 ms before the pause) and disappearance of the retrograde His bundle (HB) potential, compared with that during conduction of complexes 1 and 2, where the HB potentials (*arrows*) are inscribed in front of the corresponding ventricular electrograms. Of note, this HPS conduction delay lasts for 1 more beat (#6) before it accommodates and the VA interval returns to its steady-state magnitude. The morphology and timing of complexes 4 and 6 are slightly different than those of the other paced complexes, probably because these beats are also spontaneous premature ventricular impulses. HRA, high right atrial electrogram; STIM, stimulation marker.

2. AV Node[17,61]

- The AV node is almost always the site of block during incremental pacing when CL of pacing is longer than 300 milliseconds (see **Fig. 8**).
- In the presence of a short HA interval, minimal (10–20 milliseconds) VA prolongation may be seen, which is primarily due to an AV nodal delay.
- Most adults with intact VA conduction exhibit Wenckebach periodicity at pacing CLs of 400 to 700 milliseconds. Up to one-third of these individuals have their Wenckebach periodicity interrupted by a ventricular echo beat resulting from atypical AV nodal reentry, which is almost always a single-beat phenomenon.

3. ECG perspectives on the impact of retrograde CC on conduction of subsequent antegrade impulses

- Isolated ectopic junctional or ventricular beats are of 3 types[64–67]: escape, extrasystolic, and parasystolic. The escape beat occurs after a constant interval (or pause) from the preceding sinus (or supraventricular) beat when the latter fails to reach the AV junction or ventricles. The extrasystoles are premature impulses occurring at constant coupling intervals, whereas parasystoles are characterized by constant discharges independent of and asynchronous with the dominant rhythm. Any form of these beats can lead to CC if they fail to completely traverse the conduction system.

- If the occurrence of an extrasystole has no influence on the timing of the next sinus beat, it will be sandwiched between 2 sinus beats, and thus is termed interpolated extrasystole (**Fig. 10**).[66] It is apparent that in order for the junctional or ventricular extrasystolic impulses (JEI and VEI, respectively) to become interpolated, they must have no retrograde conduction. In other words, they tend to block in the AV node and set the stage for the development of CC.
- In the context of CC, the effect of both JEI and VEI is, for the most part, interchangeable. The HB has a shorter refractory period (RP) than the structures immediately adjacent to it (ie, AV node and the BBs). Therefore, JEI would be undetectable on the surface ECG if it blocks in both antegrade and retrograde directions (concealed JEI) (**Fig. 11**).[68]
- Manifestations of CC in response to appropriately timed JEI or VEI[69–84]:
  - PR interval prolongation (see **Figs. 10** and **11**; **Fig. 12**)
  - Pseudo–first-degree AV block (due to concealed JEI) (see **Fig. 11**)
  - Pseudo–second-degree AV block (due to concealed JEI)
  - Pseudo-BBB produced by extrasystoles arising in the BBs
  - Transient enhancement or resumption of conduction in the presence of first-degree, second-degree, or advanced AV block
  - Abrupt PR interval changes by shifting from a set of long to a set of short PR intervals or

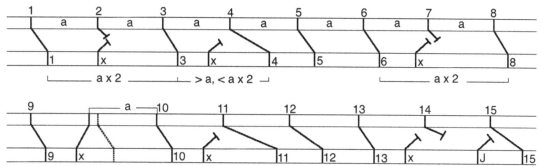

Fig. 10. Potential influences of ventricular extrasystoles on conduction of sinus beats. This ladder diagram represents several presumptive situations, in which a single (isolated) ventricular extrasystole (X) occurs during regular sinus rhythm (constant rate of a) with normal conduction (#1, 3, 5, 6, 8–10, and 13). Except for the fourth X, all the other X impulses are "interpolated" with no retrograde conduction to the atrium. The first X occurs simultaneously with the sinus impulse (#2). The retrograde concealment of the X in the conduction system completely blocks the sinus beat from reaching the ventricle. Most likely, the X would obscure the P wave and there would be a fully compensatory pause to follow. The second and third X impulses occur late in diastole and block retrogradely in the AV node, giving rise to concealed conduction. The subsequent sinus beats (#4 and #7) are conducted with either PR prolongation (#4) or (pseudo) second-degree AV block (#7). The fourth X conducts retrogradely to the atrium, which may or may not reset the subsequent sinus impulse (#10). The dotted line represents the anticipated timing of the sinus beat if the X had not occurred. The fifth X, after blocking retrogradely in the AV node, is followed by extra-long PR intervals of the subsequent 2 sinus beats (#11 and #12) (see Figure 1 in ref[79] and Figure VD8 in ref[80]). The alternative explanation for the latter situation is as follows. The sixth X blocks retrograde in the AV node. The subsequent sinus impulse (#14) is completely blocked and followed by a junctional escape beat (J), which in turn bocks retrogradely in the AV node and sets the stage for a prolonged PR interval of the subsequent sinus beat (#15).

vice versa in the presence of dual or multiple AV nodal pathways (**Fig. 13**)

- ○ Promoting double ventricular response (DVR) attributable to sequential conduction of the sinus beats over the FP and the SP in the presence of antegrade dual or multiple AV nodal pathways (**Fig. 14**)
- ○ Concealed reciprocation (reentry) in the presence of an AV junctional reentrant circuit[85–87]
- Occasionally ECG interpretation may be inconclusive and, therefore, an HB recording would be required to make the diagnosis accurately (**Fig. 15**).

CC During Collision of Antegrade and Retrograde Impulses

- Antegrade and retrograde impulses may penetrate a pathway simultaneously or sequentially. Depending on the timing of their arrival, collision of these opposing impulses may occur at different sites along the AV node–HPS axis.[88–91]
- This phenomenon may facilitate conduction and shorten the refractoriness of the corresponding tissue(s) in both antegrade and retrograde directions.[88,89,92]
- A likely mechanism of this phenomenon is the preexcitation of the conductive tissue that

would allow the recovery of its excitability to occur earlier than anticipated, a phenomenon also known as peeling back refractoriness (**Fig. 16**).[93] The second possibility is shortening of the RP of the tissue where the collision occurs. The third possible mechanism is the electronic summation,[94–96] a concept analogous to the Wedensky facilitation[97] in neurons.

- In the absence of VA conduction at baseline, collision of impulses may facilitate the retrograde conduction and allow the subsequent ventricular impulse to conduct to the atrium.[91]
- By the same token, in the presence of second-degree or more advanced AV block, an appropriately timed (spontaneous or induced) PVI may facilitate the antegrade propagation of the next atrial impulse temporarily, and thereby allow its conduction.[80]
- Simultaneous or sequential atrial and ventricular pacing may prevent or facilitate the development of AV junctional reentrant tachycardias.[98,99]

Transseptal CC

- Conduction of impulses across the interventricular septum (ie, transseptal conduction) occurs in certain situations detailed herein. This phenomenon, however, must be considered

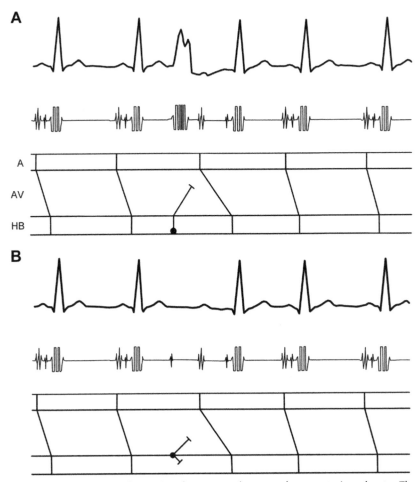

Fig. 11. The effect of ventricular and junctional extrasystoles on subsequent sinus beats. These computer-generated tracings represent surface ECG leads, His bundle electrograms, and ladder diagrams. (*A*) Ventricular extrasystole blocking retrogradely in the AV node (concealed conduction) with resultant PR prolongation of the subsequent sinus beat. (*B*) Similar situation created by a junctional extrasystole with bidirectional block. A, atrium; AV, atrioventricular; HB, His bundle.

"concealed" because there is no direct evidence on the surface ECG that would suggest its presence.

- Block of one BB during antegrade conduction will lead to the transseptal activation (also known as the retrograde invasion) of the same BB via the contralateral BB (**Fig. 17**).[100–102]
- This phenomenon has also been observed occasionally in the presence of pathologic BBB (**Fig. 18**),[103] but its repetitive and successive occurrence is essential for the maintenance of FBBB.
- As an obligatory component of the reentrant circuit, transseptal conduction plays a vital role in the following arrhythmias:
  o Orthodromic reentrant tachycardia (ORT) in the presence of antegrade BBB, ipsilateral to the accessory pathway (see **Fig. 17**)
  o ART in the presence of retrograde BBB, ipsilateral to the accessory pathway (**Fig. 19**)
  o BB reentrant ventricular tachycardia (BBR-VT) (**Fig. 20**)

Perpetuation of CC by Virtue of the Linking Phenomenon

- As already mentioned, retrograde activation of a blocked BB via its contralateral BB is the essence of FBBB maintenance. This dynamic process has been termed the linking phenomenon.[104]
- The EP utility of this concept has expanded beyond the elucidation of FBBB maintenance, to the extent that it embraces a broader range of situations in which FB is perpetuated.[105–107] In the context of CC, the following

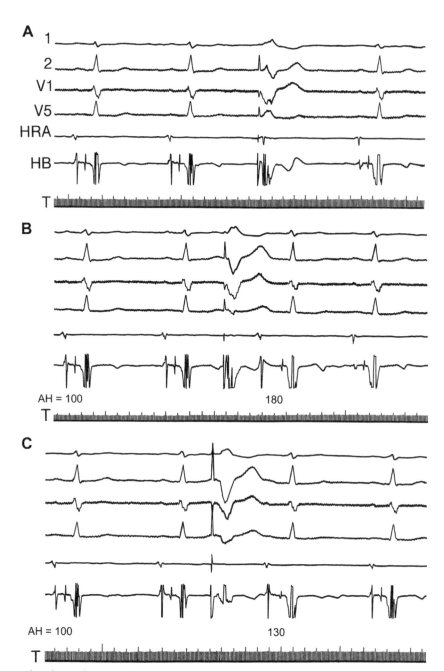

Fig. 12. Interpolated paced ventricular complexes. A single paced ventricular beat (PVB) is introduced during sinus rhythm at different timing. Note that the PVB has no retrograde conduction. (*A*) The PVB occurs late in diastole and obscures the sinus beat. (*B*) The PVB is introduced early in diastole and as a result of its concealed conduction to the AV node, the subsequent sinus beat is conducted with a prolonged AH interval (180 vs 100 ms during normal conduction). (*C*) The scenario is similar to that in *B*, but the PVB is even earlier in diastole than it is in *B*. Consequently, the ensuing concealment has a lesser impact on the subsequent AH interval (130 ms). It becomes apparent that there is an inverse relationship between the timing of the PVB, relative to the subsequent sinus beat, and the magnitude of AH (or PR) prolongation of that beat. HB, His bundle electrogram; HRA, high right atrial electrogram; T, timelines.

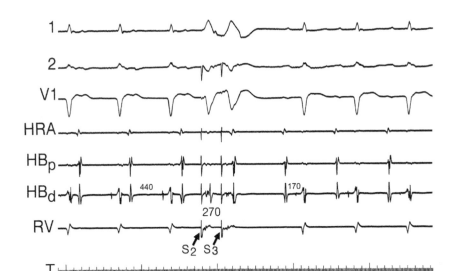

Fig. 13. Impact of concealed conduction on dual AV nodal pathways. Two paced ventricular beats (PVBs) (S2-S3) are introduced during sinus rhythm with a coupling interval of 270 ms. Note that there is no retrograde conduction for these 2 PVBs. This patient has dual AV nodal pathways with 2 sets (short and long) of PR intervals during sinus rhythm. The 2 conducted sinus beats on the left have long PR intervals (AH intervals of 440 ms), which are switched to the shorter PR interval (AH interval of 170 ms) by this ventricular couplet. This situation is due to concealed conduction of these PVBs in the AV node, which inhibited conduction in the slow pathway and facilitated conduction in its faster counterpart. Under the same circumstance, a shift of conduction from the short-PR to the long-PR set is also feasible (see Figure 86-26 in ref[84]). HBp and HBd, proximal and distal His bundle electrograms; HRA, high right atrial electrogram; RV, right ventricular electrogram; T, timelines.

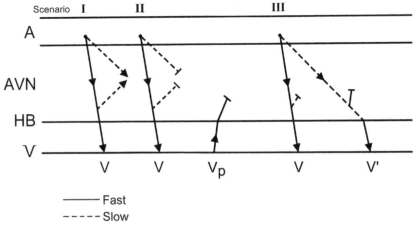

Fig. 14. Unmasking dual-pathway conduction by retrograde concealment. This ladder diagram depicts the presence of antegrade AV nodal fast (FP) and slow pathways (SP) during sinus rhythm. As shown in scenario I, each sinus beat completes its course over the FP and then enters the SP retrogradely. The latter impulse collides with the same sinus beat that has already entered the SP antegradely. Alternatively, the retrograde impulse reaching the SP via the FP blocks in the SP and makes it refractory for the same sinus impulse propagating over the SP antegradely (scenario II). Concealed conduction exerted by a premature ventricular (or junctional) impulse (Vp) could change such a relationship between the 2 pathways. As a result, there would be a new interplay between these pathways, so each sinus impulse would be conducted sequentially via both pathways (double ventricular response) with concealed retrograde penetration of their counterparts (scenario III). A, atrium; AVN, atrioventricular node; HB, His bundle.

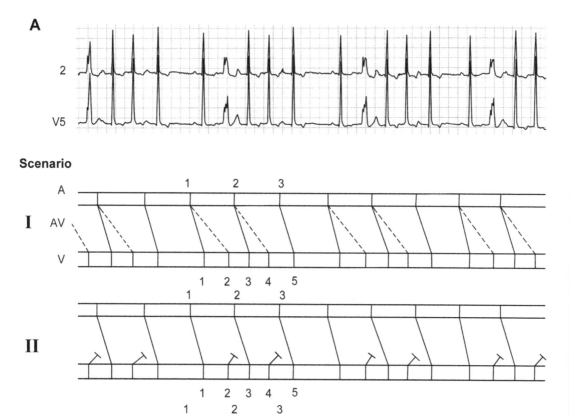

Fig. 15. (*A*) ECG diagnosis of double ventricular response. Top panel shows a pattern of group beating in 2 ECG leads (2 and V5). The bottom ladder diagrams represent 3 possible scenarios elucidating the potential underlying mechanism of this group beating. A close examination of ECG lead 2 shows regular sinus P waves. The QRS complexes outnumber the P waves 5 to 3 in each group. The second QRS complex in each group is consistently wider than the others. Because all groups are identical, the one that is numbered is commented on. In scenario I, the first and second sinus beats are conducted sequentially over both fast (FP) and slow pathways (SP), a phenomenon also known as double ventricular response (DVR). The second QRS complex exhibits FBBB because of its preceding long-to-short cycle length sequence. The third sinus impulse is conducted normally. In scenario II, the first, third, and fifth QRS complexes are normally conducted sinus beats. The second and fourth QRS complexes are extrasystoles, both arising from the atrioventricular (AV) junction with the second one exhibiting FBBB for the same reason outlined above. Alternatively, the second complex is a ventricular extrasystole and the fourth one is a junctional extrasystolic impulse. In scenario III, the first and third sinus beats are conducted normally with the second complex being a (junctional or ventricular) extrasystole, which in turn, by blocking retrogradely in the AV node, facilitates the genesis of a DVR. Panel *B*, using a His bundle electrogram, discloses the precise mechanism of this arrhythmia. (*B*) His bundle recording for accurate diagnosis of a double ventricular response. Recording obtained from the same patient shown in *A*. During an electrophysiologic study, the patient had spontaneous runs of nonsustained tachycardia, almost the same group beating that he had demonstrated earlier, but with less frequency. QRS complexes 1, 3, 7, and 8 are normally conducted sinus beats. QRS complex 2 is a conducted premature atrial complex (PAC) with functional left bundle branch block (FLBBB). QRS complexes 4 and 8 are junctional extrasystolic impulses (JEI) conducted with FLBBB. The HV intervals of these 2 complexes are slightly shorter than those during normally conducted sinus beats (30 vs 38 ms), indicating that they probably originated within the His bundle (HB) stem below the recording site. Sinus beat 5 following the first JEI is conducted sequentially over 2 antegrade AV nodal pathways, giving rise to a double ventricular response. It is now apparent that scenario III in *A* illustrates the correct mechanism of the group beating in this patient. Therefore, without an HB recording it would have been impossible to determine the exact mechanism of this group beating. HBp, HBm, and HBd, proximal, medial, and distal HB electrograms.

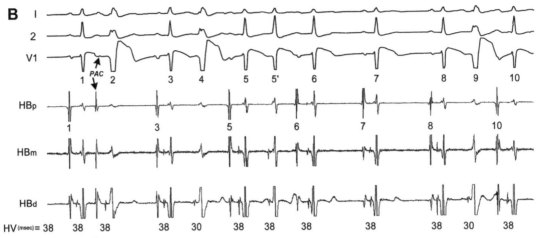

Fig. 15. (*continued*)

scenarios characterize known putative mechanisms operative in the perpetuation of FB:

1. Linking by "interference"[105] is a process whereby successive alternating antegrade and retrograde impulses block repeatedly and sequentially at a certain site and, therefore, render the site refractory for the upcoming impulse (**Fig. 21**). The classic example of this form is sustained FBBB (see **Fig. 17**; **Fig. 22**).
2. Linking by collision is a process whereby the opposing wavefronts repeatedly collide with each other in the circuit (see **Fig. 21**; **Fig. 23**). Two subsets are distinguishable:
   a. Simple collision: The opposing wavefronts are the "head" and "tail" of the same impulse entering the circuit from the opposite directions. A classic example is during RV pacing at relatively long CLs when the retrograde impulse via the RB reaches the LB and collides with same pacing impulse reaching the latter transseptally (see **Fig. 7A**).
   b. Complex collision[105]: The opposing impulses are typically a paced impulse colliding head-to-head with another impulse, which is either a circulating reentrant wavefront or a paced impulse introduced into the circuit during the previous cycle. Entrainment of the reentrant tachycardias[108–110] is the classic example of this form of linking phenomenon (**Fig. 24**).
3. Linking by fusion is a further situation in which pacing impulses fuse with the reentrant impulses at the periphery of the reentrant circuit without perturbing the reentrant process. Overdrive ventricular pacing during AVNRT at similar or slightly

shorter CLs is a typical example. The paced ventricular complexes may fuse with the reentrant impulses anywhere from the Purkinje network up to the AV nodal common pathway. Obviously this form of linking has no impact on the reentrant circuit as long as it remains beyond the boundaries of the circuit.

- Linking by complex collision is the only scenario whereby the reentrant process would ensue on cessation of pacing (**Figs. 25–28**).

Aberrant Ventricular Conduction

Development

1. Refractoriness
   - Aberrant ventricular conduction (VAb) occurs when a supraventricular impulse arrives at the HPS during its RP.[43,111–117] This phenomenon can occur in any portion of the intraventricular conduction system; namely, main HB, RB branch (RBB), and LB branch (LBB) or its fascicles.
   - VAb patterns are contingent on the RPs of different components of the HPS, which are all CL-dependent.
   - VAb may occur as a result of: (1) physiologic and reversible behavior (functional); (2) an acceleration-dependent (also known as tachycardia-dependent or rate-related) block; or (3) a fatigue phenomenon.
   - VAb caused by conduction delay or complete block in the BBs has similar electrocardiographic features, therefore the mechanism is not readily discerned by ECG or even EP studies. Thus, both terms of conduction delay or block may be used interchangeably in this situation.

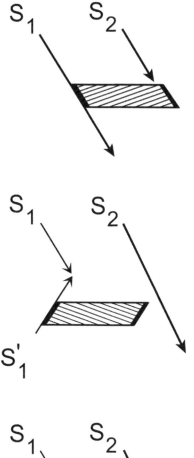

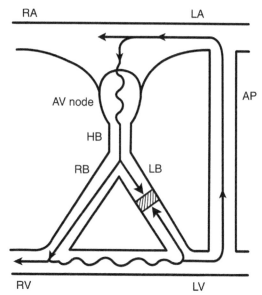

Fig. 17. Maintenance of functional bundle branch block by concealed transseptal conduction. This diagram shows the orthodromic reentrant tachycardia circuit in which there is a functional left bundle branch block (FLBBB). Retrograde activation of the LB via the right bundle (RB) maintains FLBBB for the subsequent cycles. AP, accessory pathway; AV, atrioventricular; HB, His bundle; LA, left atrium; LB, left bundle; LV, left ventricle; RA, right atrium; RV, right ventricle.

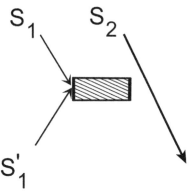

Fig. 16. Facilitation of conduction attributable to collision of antegrade and retrograde impulses. (*Top*) A premature (S1-S2) stimulation whereby the S2 encounters refractoriness (*hashed area*) of the tissue along the way. (*Middle*) Collision of antegrade and retrograde (S′$_1$) impulses with earlier activation of the tissue by S′$_1$ and, thus, earlier recovery of its excitability. This phenomenon, also known as peeling back refractoriness, permits the S2 to complete its course across the tissue. Similarly, collision of the opposing impulses (S$_1$ and S′$_1$), by shortening the tissue refractoriness, may allow the S2 to propagate (*bottom*).

- Because of the longer RBB-RP, functional right bundle branch block (FRBBB) is more common than FLBBB.
- VAb preceded by a long-to-short CL variation is known as the Ashman phenomenon.[118] Because of the higher prevalence of CL variations of the impulses arriving at the HPS during AF, the Ashman phenomenon (**Fig. 29**) is more common during AF than in any other supraventricular arrhythmia.

2. Retrograde concealment in the HPS.[43,116]

   a. *Immediate manifestation.* A retrograde block in the HPS may set the stage for the occurrence of FB during propagation of an appropriately timed subsequent supraventricular impulse (**Figs. 30 and 31**). Depending on the prematurity of the respective supraventricular impulse, functional fascicular block, FLBBB, or functional bilateral BB may ensue when the PVI originates in the right ventricle. It is reasonable to surmise that FRBBB occurs more often if the PVI originates in the left ventricle. In contrast to FB occurring during antegrade conduction, the site of the retrograde concealment is usually located more distally in the HPS.[43]

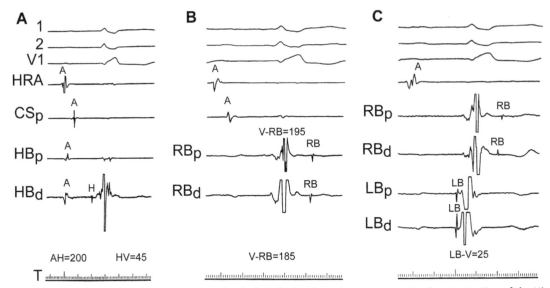

Fig. 18. Retrograde (transseptal) activation of right bundle (RB) branch during sinus rhythm. Activation of the His bundle (HB) and its bundle branches during sinus rhythm are shown. (A) Despite complete RB branch block, the HV interval is 45 ms. (B) RB activation occurs after ventricular activation with distal RB (RBd) being 10 ms earlier than the proximal RB (RBp), which indicates that the RB is activated retrogradely via the left bundle (LB). (C) LB activation occurs normally with an LB-V interval of 25 ms. CSp, proximal coronary sinus electrogram; HBp and HBd, proximal and distal HB electrograms; HRA, high right atrial electrogram; LBp and LBd, proximal and distal LB electrograms; T, timelines. (*From* Jazayeri MR, Deshpande SS, Sra JS, et al. Retrograde (transseptal) activation of right bundle branch during sinus rhythm. J Cardiovasc Electrophysiol 1993;4:280–7; with permission.)

b. *Delayed manifestation.* In this situation, the aftermath of the retrograde concealment is not immediately apparent in the subsequent beat, as it typically is in the classic form of CC. There are at least 2 scenarios that may fall into this category.

- First, the occurrence of alternating VAb patterns[119–121] during atrial bigeminy (ie, successive long-short-long cycles). These patterns are: RBBB alternating with no VAb, RBBB alternating with RBBB, RBBB alternating with LBBB, and bilateral BB alternating with bilateral BB. Concealed transseptal activation of the blocked BB via its contralateral BB plays a major role in displaying these patterns. For instance, in the most fascinating pattern where RBBB alternates with LBBB (**Fig. 32**), the first BB manifesting block is activated retrogradely via its contralateral BB. Thus, the CL of activation and hence the RP of the blocked BB (distal to the site of block) for the next cycle is shorter than those of the contralateral BB. The likelihood of the contralateral BB being the site of FBBB during conduction of the subsequent beat, ending the next short cycle, is therefore higher than that of the ipsilateral BB. Obviously several other factors may also be important in facilitating the occurrence of this phenomenon, including the prematurity of the impulses ending the short cycles, the long CLs separating every 2 successive short cycles, differential RPs of BBs, and the AV nodal functional RP.

- Second, the occurrence of FBBB in the second beat of SVT (SVT-2), when the first beat (SVT-1) is conducted with a narrow QRS complex and preceded by impulses originating in the ventricle.[122] The resultant FBBB in SVT-2 is usually of FRBBB type when SVT-1 is preceded by RV pacing (**Fig. 33**) and of FLBBB type when SVT-1 is preceded by a BB reentrant beat (**Fig. 34**). The mechanism of this phenomenon may be related to the temporal relationship of the retrograde CC in the BBs. Therefore, owing to its longest CL of activation and RP, the earliest site of CC is the most likely site of FB during propagation of SVT-2.

Maintenance

Once FBBB develops it may become persistent, at least for several cycles. Repetitive

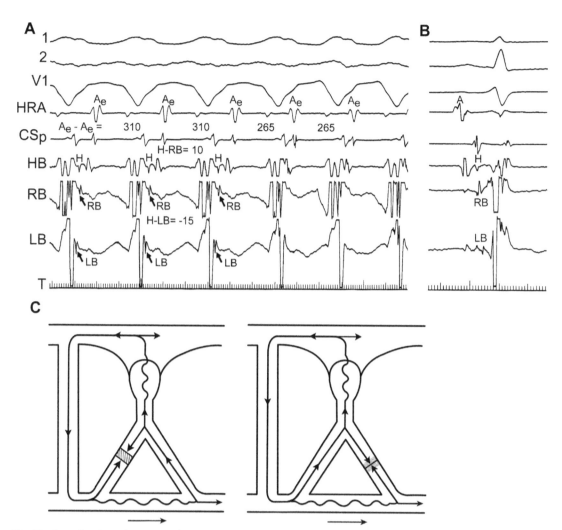

Fig. 19. Contribution of transseptal conduction during antidromic tachycardia. (*A*) A segment of true antidromic reentrant tachycardia (ART) using a right-sided accessory pathway (AP) antegradely and the normal pathway retrogradely. (*B*) A sinus beat. (*C*) The ART circuit. Note that at the beginning of the tracing in *A*, the cycle length (CL) of the tachycardia is 310 ms, which after 2 cycles decreases to 265 ms. The reason for this change in CL lies in the route of the retrograde activation. As shown in *C* (*left*), because of functional right bundle branch block (FRBBB), the retrograde impulse uses the left bundle (LB) to activate the His bundle (HB). The LB is activated before the HB (15 ms) and right bundle (RB) (25 ms). Once FRBBB resolves (*C*, *right*), the retrograde ventriculoatrial activation time, and consequently the ART-CL, shorten. CSp, proximal coronary sinus electrogram; HRA, high right atrial electrogram; T, timelines.

retrograde (transseptal) conduction of the distal portion of the blocked BB (ie, linking by interference) was proposed in humans[118] and subsequently shown by studies in laboratory animals[100] to be the mechanism of FBBB maintenance. Similarly, concealed retrograde interfascicular conduction may also maintain functional fascicular block (as an isolated FB or in combination with FRBBB) for several successive beats.[123]

Resolution

One or more of the following mechanisms may be operative in FBBB resolution.[43]

1. Spontaneous
   a. Migration of the site of the block. The site of FBBB may gradually migrate (ordinarily to more distal direction toward the Purkinje network[124]) until it reaches the point of a shorter effective refractory period. During

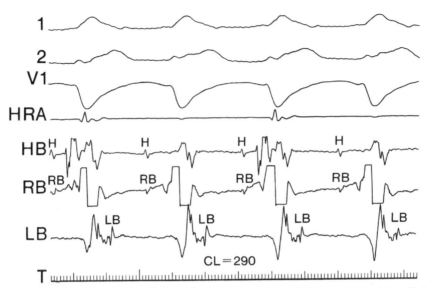

Fig. 20. Transseptal activation during bundle branch reentrant tachycardia. This sustained bundle branch reentrant tachycardia has a cycle length of 290 ms and left bundle branch block morphology. In addition to His bundle (HB) electrogram, both right bundle (RB) and left bundle (LB) potentials are also recorded. Note that the HB activation occurs after the LB potential and before the RB potential. This sequence of activation is typical for this type of bundle branch reentry whereby the LB is activated transseptally via the RB. CL, cycle length; HRA, high right atrial electrogram; T, timeline. (*From* Jazayeri MR, Deshpande S, Dhala A, et al. Transcatheter mapping and radiofrequency ablation of cardiac arrhythmias. Curr Probl Cardiol 1994;19:285–396; with permission.)

the course of distal migration, FLBBB may convert to functional left anterior fascicular block before its complete resolution. Functional bifascicular block (RBBB plus left anterior or posterior fascicular block) may resolve to either an isolated RBBB or an isolated fascicular block.

b. Accommodation.[63,117,125,126] The refractory period of the blocked BB (or fascicle) may gradually shorten over the course of several complexes until it permits the subsequent impulses to reach the distal HPS beyond the site of block (**Fig. 35**).

2. Mediated by premature impulses
   a. PVI. Introducing a PVI at the time that the HB is refractory may resolve FBBB without affecting the tachycardia CL (**Fig. 36**). Two possible explanations may be offered. First, the PVI may prematurely penetrate the BB retrogradely and by preexciting the site of block (or linking), resulting in earlier recovery of the BB excitability (ie, peeling back refractoriness) (see **Fig. 35**).[93] This process will allow propagation of the next antegrade impulse when the BB is no longer

refractory. Second, the PVI may block retrogradely at a site distal to the linking site with a shorter RP and therefore, by abolishing the linking phenomenon, terminate FBBB.[43] If the premature impulse is introduced early enough to conduct retrogradely and preexcite the atrium, prolongation of the AV nodal conduction time (ie, ArH interval) may allow the HPS to fully recover.

b. PAC. During propagation of an appropriately timed PAC, sufficient delay in the AV nodal conduction may result in complete recovery of the HPS.

DVR and CC

DVR is a phenomenon that has also been termed as "1:2 response." DVR is characterized with 2 sets of ventricular activation in response to a single atrial impulse; this could be a spontaneous phenomenon or laboratory-induced. DVR may develop in 3 distinct circumstances as follows.

1. A supraventricular beat, usually a premature (A2) impulse, is conducted sequentially over

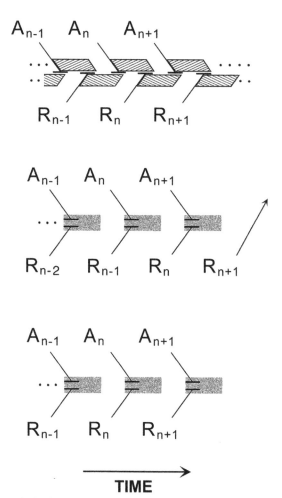

Fig. 21. Linking phenomenon (LP). These panels represent different forms of LP, which is the primary mechanism of maintaining functional block. (*Top*) A piece of conductive tissue being penetrated by a set of antegrade (A) and retrograde (R) successive (n−2, n−1, n, n+1, and so forth) impulses occurring in a sequential and alternating fashion. For LP to sustain, each blocked impulse must make the tissue refractory for the subsequent opposing impulse (*shaded areas*). This type of LP is therefore termed linking by interference. The middle and bottom panels represent another type of LP, whereby opposing impulses arrive at the tissue simultaneously and thus collide with each other (linking by collision).[105] (*Middle*) If the opposing impulses were from 2 successive cycles, cessation of 1 impulse would permit the unopposed impulse to propagate. This form of LP may be further subcategorized into a complex form of linking by collision. (*Bottom*) On the other hand, if the opposing impulses are generated from the same cycle, the LP may be subcategorized into a simple form of linking by collision. See **Fig. 23** for further details.

an accessory pathway (AP) and NP, generating V2 and V2′, respectively (**Fig. 37**).[43,127,128] The V2 impulse normally generates CC retrogradely in the NP that would not allow the A2 to give rise to the V2′ response. Therefore, for the DVR to occur, the retrograde concealment must at least partially resolve. Depending on the time interval between V2 and V2′, the V2′ impulse may propagate with a narrow

QRS complex or FBBB owing to the retrograde HPS CC generated by the V2 impulse. The V2′ impulse may, in turn, initiate ORT if the AP is fully recovered from its prior activation.

2. A supraventricular impulse is conducted sequentially over dual AV nodal pathways.[129] Once the initiating atrial impulse completes its course over the antegrade AV nodal FP, it

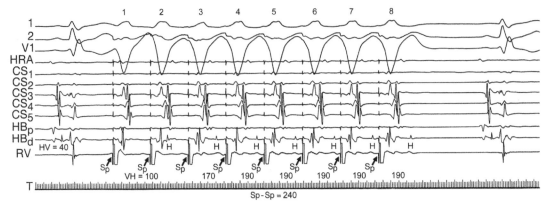

Fig. 22. Linking phenomenon for maintaining functional bundle branch block in the His-Purkinje system during rapid ventricular pacing. Tracings are from a patient with a concealed posteroseptal accessory pathway (AP). An 8-beat train of ventricular pacing at a cycle length (Sp-Sp) of 240 ms is introduced during sinus rhythm. A progressive VH interval prolongation (100–190 ms) is seen from the second to fourth paced complexes. Note that the retrograde ventriculoatrial (VA) conduction (paced complexes 2–8) is exclusively via the AP, as indicated by a constant VA interval despite progressive VH prolongation and the occurrence of His bundle (HB) potential subsequent to the atrial activation (from third to eighth complexes). The VH interval remains unchanged from the fourth to the eighth complexes. The paced ventricular impulses block retrogradely in both bundle branches, therefore by the time the atrial impulse (via the AP) turns around in the normal pathway, both bundle branches are still refractory from the retrograde concealment (the HB activation from the third to eighth complexes is via the atrioventricular node); this explains why the last paced complex does not initiate orthodromic reentrant tachycardia. The maintenance of this bilateral bundle branch block is due to linking by interference. CS, coronary sinus; HBp and HBd, proximal and distal HB electrograms; HRA, high right atrial electrogram; RV, right ventricular electrogram; Sp, pacing spike.

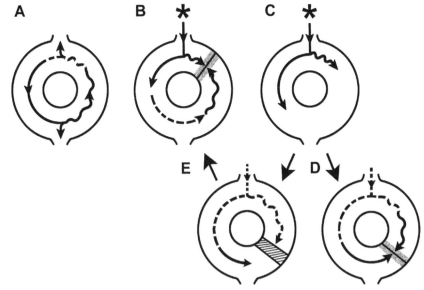

Fig. 23. Linking by collision. (*A*) Various situations occurring in a reentrant circuit. (*B*) Pacing during a reentrant tachycardia. The paced impulses (*asterisk*) propagate simultaneously in 2 directions. The impulse propagating in a clockwise direction collides (head-to-head) with the reentrant impulse (propagating in a counterclockwise direction). The paced impulse propagating in a counterclockwise direction, in turn, completes its course and collides with the subsequent clockwise (paced) impulse (linking by complex collision). Transient entrainment of a reentrant tachycardia by paced impulses is the classic example of this type of linking. If pacing is done in the absence of reentrant tachycardia (*C*), the resultant clockwise and counterclockwise impulses will persistently collide at a certain point in the reentrant circuit (*D*), as long as the pacing remains uninterrupted (linking by simple collision). In certain situations, a simple collision may convert into a complex collision as follows. A paced impulse (rotating in a clockwise direction in this example), by encountering refractoriness, may block at one site in the circuit (*E*). By the time the opposing impulse (rotating in a counterclockwise direction) reaches the blocked site, it will propagate along the circuit if the site has recovered from its refractoriness. This impulse may collide with the subsequent paced impulse, and perpetuation of this situation will result in a linking by complex collision (*B*).

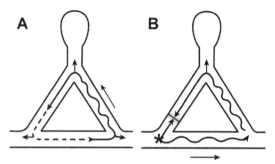

Fig. 24. Linking by complex collision during bundle branch reentry. (*A*) A bundle branch reentrant tachycardia circuit. The circuit utilizes the right bundle branch antegradely and the left bundle branch retrogradely. (*B*) During pacing from the right ventricle (*asterisk*), the paced impulse, propagating in a counterclockwise fashion, collides with the reentrant impulse propagating along the right bundle branch in the antegrade direction. The same paced impulse also traverses the septum and circulates along the circuit until it collides with the subsequent (counterclockwise) paced impulse.

will turn around and block in the AV nodal SP. This block occurs as a result of either collision (ie, linking by simple collision) of opposing antegrade and retrograde impulses or the initial block of the antegrade impulse rendering the SP refractory to the subsequent retrograde impulse (ie, linking by interference). For the atrial impulse to complete its course over the SP, the SP must regain its excitability after being penetrated in the retrograde direction (CC). This situation may be accomplished by a timely recovery of the SP and/or a distal site of retrograde block. Once the respective

atrial impulse completes its course over the SP, the AV nodal common pathway, the HPS, and the ventricle must be excitable to allow a DVR to occur. The occurrence of this phenomenon may be spontaneous or triggered by premature impulses.

3. Exclusive conduction of a supraventricular impulse over an AP may generate a BBR complex (**Fig. 38**).[43] An A2 impulse blocks in the NP and, by conducting exclusively over the AP, gives rise to a V2 impulse. Depending on the RP of the BBs, the V2 impulse, by blocking retrogradely in one BB and conducting over the contralateral BB, may set the stage for the genesis of a BBR beat (V3).

Impact of CC on Different Forms of Tachycardia

Reentrant tachycardias

For any anatomic reentrant process to occur, a reentrant circuit[130] is required in which: (1) A unidirectional block must occur to allow the impulses to circulate in only one direction; (2) in a spatial or temporal sense, the circuit must be long or slow enough to permit the reentrant wavefront to circulate without encountering any refractory tissue along the way. It becomes apparent that the initial (unidirectional) block is pivotal for the initiation of the reentrant tachycardia. In addition, the site of the initial block is equally important for both the initiation of reentry and the direction in which the reentrant impulses circulate. For instance, in the presence of an AP, the antegrade block of an A2 impulse in the AP and its conduction over the NP would initiate ORT and conversely, the A2 block in the NP and its conduction over the AP would

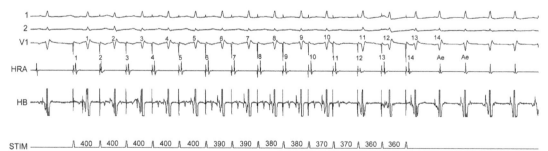

Fig. 25. Initiation of atrioventricular (AV) nodal reentry on cessation of atrial pacing. Tracings are from a patient with typical AV nodal reentrant tachycardia (AVNRT). Incremental atrial pacing from high right atrium (HRA) at cycle lengths of 400 to 360 ms is shown. The first 10 atrial impulses are conducted via the fast pathway (FP) with progressive prolongation of the AH interval, after which the 11th impulse suddenly shifts from the FP to the slow pathway (SP). Conduction over the SP persists for the subsequent atrial (#12–14) impulses. On cessation of pacing, the 14th atrial impulse initiates AVNRT. See **Fig. 26** for further explanation. HB, His bundle; STIM, stimulation marker.

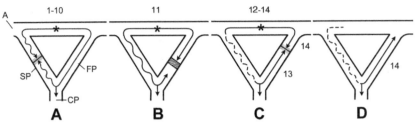

Fig. 26. Linking phenomenon in atrioventricular (AV) nodal reentrant circuit. Schematic diagrams illustrate the sequence of events occurring during atrial pacing and initiation of AV nodal reentrant tachycardia (AVNRT) shown in **Fig. 25**. Each diagram shows the AV nodal fast pathway (FP), slow pathway (SP), common pathway (CP), and the atrium (A). (*A*) The first atrial impulse completes its course over the FP and after propagating retrogradely over the SP collides with the same impulse that had penetrated the SP earlier. This linking by simple collision persists for atrial impulses 1 to 10. A less likely alternative possibility is the occurrence of linking by interference, if each successive impulse encounters the SP refractoriness owing to its earlier concealment caused by the opposing impulse. (*B*) The 11th atrial impulse blocks in the FP and continues to propagate along the SP. After completing its course over the SP and propagating retrogradely over the FP (if the latter has already recovered from its earlier refractoriness), this impulse will collide with the 12th impulse propagating over the FP antegradely. This process initiates linking by complex collision, which persists for the next several cycles (*C*). On cessation of atrial pacing, the last paced impulse (#14) does not encounter any forthcoming paced impulse to collide with, and thus by completing its retrograde course over the FP initiates AVNRT (*D*). *Asterisk* indicates pacing source.

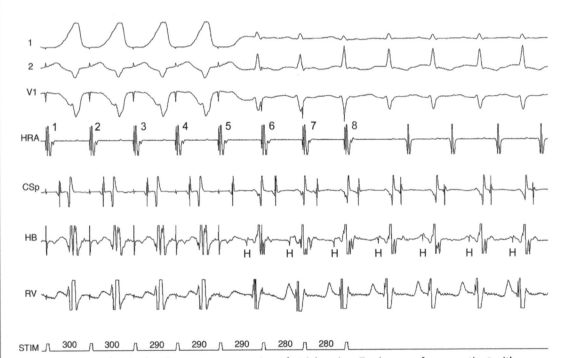

Fig. 27. Initiation of orthodromic reentry on cessation of atrial pacing. Tracings are from a patient with a manifest posteroseptal accessory pathway (AP). Incremental atrial pacing with cycle lengths (CLs) of 300 to 280 ms is shown. Antegrade AP block occurs at CL of 290 ms (atrial impulses 5–8). On cessation of atrial pacing, orthodromic reentrant tachycardia (ORT) is initiated. The reentrant circuit uses the AP retrogradely and the normal pathway (NP) antegradely. See **Fig. 28** for further explanation. CSp, proximal coronary sinus; HB, His bundle electrogram; HRA, high right atrial electrogram; RV, right ventricular electrogram; STIM, stimulation marker.

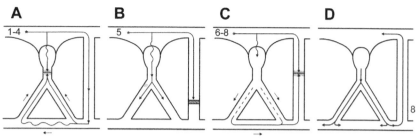

Fig. 28. Linking phenomenon in orthodromic reentrant circuit. Diagrams illustrate the sequence of events occurring during atrial pacing and initiation of orthodromic reentrant tachycardia (ORT) shown in **Fig. 27.** (*A*) Atrial impulses 1 to 4 approaching both the accessory pathway (AP) and the normal pathway (NP). Antegrade conduction over the AP occurs rapidly and each impulse, by turning around and propagating retrogradely over the NP, collides with the same impulse propagating along the NP. Therefore, linking by simple collision perpetuates along the NP, and the site of collision depends on the conduction properties of the AP versus the NP. (*B*) The fifth atrial impulse blocks in the AP and continues to propagate along the NP. After completing its course over the NP and propagating retrogradely over the AP (if the latter has already recovered from its earlier refractoriness), this impulse will collide with the subsequent (sixth) impulse propagating over the AP antegradely. This process initiates linking by complex collision, which perpetuates for the next several cycles (*C*). On cessation of atrial pacing, the last paced impulse (#8) does not encounter any forthcoming paced impulse to collide with, and thus by completing its retrograde course over the AP initiates ORT (*D*).

initiate true ART. Similarly, the retrograde block of a V2 in the NP and its conduction over the AP would set the stage for the initiation of ORT (**Fig. 39**), whereas the opposite situation may fulfill the prerequisite(s) of the initiation of ART. More specifically, in both ORT and ART, the weakest link for the initiation and maintenance of reentry is usually the AV node.[43,131] Thus during ORT initiation by V2 impulse, the site of retrograde block in the HPS is more likely to permit ORT to occur than if the AV node was the site of penetration (see **Fig. 39**).[132,133] On the other hand, induction of ART by A2 usually requires a proximal AV nodal block. Therefore, by the time the impulse has completed its course over the AP, ventricular muscle, the HPS, and the distal AV node, the

proximal AV node would have enough time to regain its excitability. Termination of a reentrant process by CC is also a common occurrence. This process is primarily accomplished when a part of the reentrant circuit becomes refractory, either spontaneously[134] or by premature impulses (**Fig. 40**).[135–137] Subthreshold stimulation may also terminate reentrant tachycardias (**Fig. 41**).[138,139] Although the underlying mechanism(s) of tachycardia termination by subthreshold stimulation may be entirely different to those of the captured beats, the former should technically be categorized as CC because, though remaining inconspicuous on the surface ECG, it still makes a critical portion of the reentrant circuit refractory to the circulating wavefront.

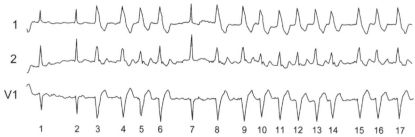

Fig. 29. Ashman phenomenon during atrial fibrillation. ECG leads show a segment of atrial fibrillation with narrow (#1, 2, and 7) and wide (#3–6, 8–17) QRS complexes. The wide QRS complexes are due to functional (left) bundle branch block (FBBB). The occurrence of FBBB is preceded by long-to-short cycle-length variations, a process also known as the Ashman phenomenon. The maintenance of FBBB is due to linking by interference (see text for further details).

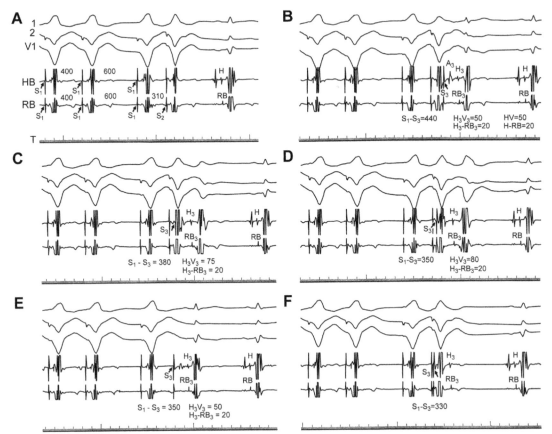

Fig. 30. Functional bundle branch block resulting from retrograde concealment in the His-Purkinje system. Tracings from top to bottom are ECG leads (1, 2, V_1), His bundle (HB), and right bundle (RB) electrograms followed by timelines (T). For all panels, programmed stimulation is performed at short-to-long (400/600) basic drive cycle lengths (simultaneous atrial and ventricular pacing), and a premature ventricular impulse with a coupling interval of 310 ms is introduced. (A) The V_2 impulse is blocked retrogradely in the His-Purkinje system as indicated by the absence of an H_2 deflection. A premature atrial impulse (A_3) is introduced after the V_2 complex, and its coupling interval (ie, S_1-S_3) is gradually shortened. A_3 conducted with morphology similar to the sinus complex at S_1-S_3 interval = 440 ms (B), functional left anterior fascicular block at S_1-S_3 = 380 ms (C), and functional left bundle branch block at S_1-S_3 = 350 ms (D). (E) Omission of the V_2 impulse at the S_1-S_3 interval, similar to that in D, results in normal conduction of the A_3 impulse, which verifies that the functional bundle branch block shown in D is due to the retrograde concealment in the His-Purkinje system. (F) Further shortening of the S_1-S_3 interval to 330 ms results in functional bilateral block, most likely in the distal bundle branches, as suggested by the presence of RB_3 potential. (*From* Jazayeri MR, Sra JJ, Akhtar M. Wide QRS complexes. Electrophysiologic basis of a common electrocardiographic diagnosis. J Cardiovasc Electrophysiol 1992;3:365–93; with permission.)

Tachycardias with V greater than A

The main characteristic of these tachycardias is the presence of AV discordance. Technically, the term AV dissociation may not be suitable nor descriptive enough for the situation. Such tachycardias have also been termed pseudo-tachycardia,[140] abrupt doubling of the ventricular rate,[141] or 1:2 tachycardia.[142] Occasionally the A/V ratio is variable and not necessarily in a constant 1:2 relationship. Two prototypes have been identified:

- *Nonreentrant supraventricular (AV nodal or junctional) tachycardia.* This tachycardia is a persistent form of a DVR phenomenon whereby successive dual AV nodal responses produce a run of tachycardia (**Fig. 42**).[141,143–148] The occurrence of this

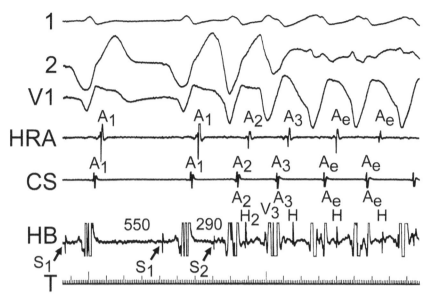

Fig. 31. Functional bundle branch block during orthodromic tachycardia induced by premature ventricular stimulation. Tracings from top to bottom are surface ECG leads (1, 2, V₁), high right atrial (HRA), coronary sinus (CS), and His bundle (HB) electrograms followed by timelines (T). This tracing was obtained from a patient with a posteroseptal accessory pathway. Programmed ventricular stimulation at a basic drive cycle length of 550 ms and a premature coupling interval of 290 ms induced a bundle branch reentrant complex (V₃), which in turn, by blocking retrogradely in the left bundle, initiated orthodromic reentrant tachycardia with functional left bundle branch block. (*From* Jazayeri MR, Sra JJ, Akhtar M. Wide QRS complexes. Electrophysiologic basis of a common electrocardiographic diagnosis. J Cardiovasc Electrophysiol 1992;3:365–93; with permission.)

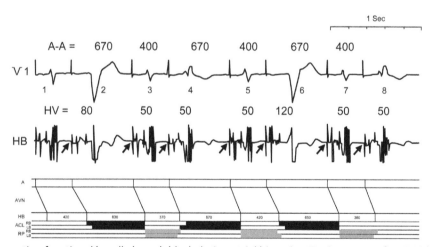

Fig. 32. Alternating functional bundle branch block during atrial bigeminy. Tracings are surface ECG leads V₁ and His-bundle electrogram (HB). A ladder diagram placed at the bottom depicts the relative activation timing of the atrium (A), atrioventricular node (AVN), and HB, in addition to the activation cycle lengths (ACL) and refractory periods (RP) of the right bundle (RB) and left bundle (LB). This segment of paced bigeminal atrial rhythm shows a series of alternating long and short cycles. For all practical purposes, the atrial impulses ending the short cycles behave as premature (A2) beats. The A2 impulses conduct with alternating functional LB and RB block. The retrograde concealed conduction of each blocked bundle via the contralateral bundle sets the stage for the occurrence of functional block in the latter during antegrade conduction of the subsequent A2. Note also that the HV interval is markedly prolonged with functional LB block (80 and 120 ms) in comparison with the other complexes (50 ms), which indicates significant conduction delay along the HB-RB axis. *Arrows* depict pacing spikes. (*Adapted from* Jazayeri MR, Sra JJ, Akhtar M. Wide QRS complexes. Electrophysiologic basis of a common electrocardiographic diagnosis. J Cardiovasc Electrophysiol 1992;3:365–93; with permission.)

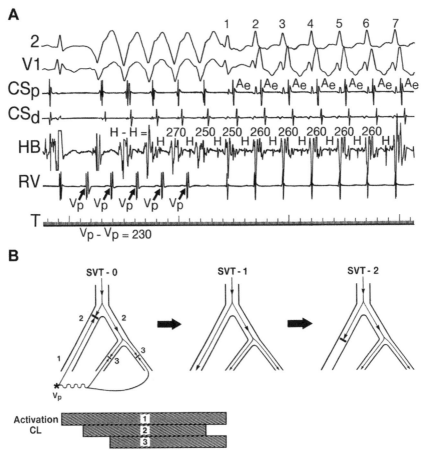

Fig. 33. Functional right bundle branch block in the second beat of supraventricular tachycardia induced by burst ventricular pacing. Tracings are from a patient with a posteroseptal accessory pathway (AP). (*A*) A 5-beat train of burst ventricular pacing (Vp-Vp) at a cycle length of 230 ms is introduced during sinus rhythm, which then induces orthodromic reentrant tachycardia (ORT). Despite constant preceding His-bundle (HB) inputs (H-H interval = 250 ms), the second beat of supraventricular tachycardia (SVT) complex exhibits functional right bundle branch block that persists in the subsequent complexes. The first marked HB potential following the third paced ventricular complex is most likely activated retrogradely, whereas subsequent H potentials are probably anterograde His potentials. Therefore, the last 2 paced complexes, while circulating around the ORT circuit, collide with the antegrade impulses propagating across the His-Purkinje system (HPS) (linking by complex collision). Of note, the SVT-1 complex is conducted with a narrow QRS complex. (*B*) The most likely mechanism of functional bundle branch block occurring in the SVT-2 complex. The last Vp, while propagating retrogradely over the AP (not shown here), also collides with the orthodromic reentrant impulse (SVT-0) generated by its prior Vp. The numbers (1–3) denote the relative activation timing of the distal and proximal segments of the bundle branches. The last Vp penetrates the bundle branches in a sequential manner, with the distal right bundle (1) activation being the earliest. Subsequently, the proximal right bundle branch (2) is activated retrogradely. Transseptal activation of the distal left bundle (3) occurs at a later time than anterograde activation of the proximal left bundle (2). The SVT-1 complex is conducted normally along the normal pathway. Horizontal bars represent the activation cycle lengths (CL) of segments 1 to 3 from the time the last Vp penetrates the HPS to the time that SVT-1 is conducted. Therefore, the activation CL of the distal right bundle (1) is much longer than the other segments, which would set the stage for the occurrence of functional right bundle branch block during propagation of the subsequent tachycardia complex (SVT-2). CSp and CSd, proximal and distal coronary sinus electrograms; RV, right ventricular electrogram; T, timelines. (*Adapted from* Gonzalez-Zuelgaray J, Sheikh S, Akhtar M. Functional bundle branch block as a delayed manifestation of retrograde concealment in the His-Purkinje system. J Cardiovasc Electrophysiol 1996;7:248–58; with permission.)

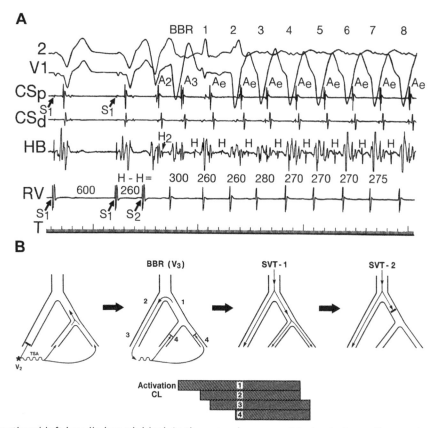

Fig. 34. Functional left bundle branch block in the second supraventricular tachycardia complex induced by bundle branch reentry. Tracings are also obtained from the same patient shown in **Fig. 33.** (*A*) Premature ventricular stimulation is performed in the right ventricle (RV). Simultaneous atrial and ventricular pacing is carried out during basic drive (S_1-S_1) with a cycle length (CL) of 600 ms. At a premature coupling interval (S_1-S_2) of 260 ms, a bundle branch reentrant (BBR) beat is generated, which in turn triggers orthodromic reentrant tachycardia (ORT). The first supraventricular tachycardia (SVT-1) complex is conducted with a narrow QRS morphology. The SVT-2 complex exhibits functional left bundle branch block that is perpetuated through the subsequent complexes. The SVT-2 complex has a normal axis as opposed to the subsequent beats, which exhibit a leftward axis. This change of axis may represent a distal shift in the site of functional block. (*B*) The most likely mechanism of functional bundle branch block in the SVT-2 complex, initiated by a BBR beat. During premature right ventricular stimulation at critical coupling intervals, the premature impulse (V_2) blocks retrogradely in the distal right bundle branch and by trans-septal activation (TSA) reaches the left bundle system. The anterograde transmission of the impulse to the ventricle via the right bundle, which has recovered from the blocked V_2, produces a BBR or V_3 complex. This process is usually a single-beat phenomenon that spontaneously terminates by blocking retrogradely in the distal left bundle. In the presence of an accessory pathway capable of retrograde conduction, the BBR may initiate ORT. The numbers (1–4) denote the relative activation timing of the distal and proximal segments of the bundle branches. The hashed bars represent the activation CL of segments 1 to 4 from the time that BBR is produced to the time that the first tachycardia complex (SVT-1) is conducted. Among different segments of the bundle branches including proximal left bundle (1), proximal right bundle (2), distal right bundle (3), and distal left bundle (4); segment 1 has the longest CL of activation. This situation would render the latter segment refractory to the next supraventricular impulse (SVT-2). CSp and CSd, proximal and distal coronary sinus electrograms; T, timelines. (*Adapted from Gonzalez-Zuelgaray J, Sheikh S, Akhtar M. Functional bundle branch block as a delayed manifestation of retrograde concealment in the His-Purkinje system. J Cardiovasc Electrophysiol 1996;7:248–58; with permission.*)

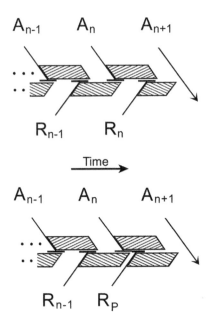

Fig. 35. Resolution of functional block. These diagrams show maintenance of functional block attributable to linking by interference (see **Fig. 21**). Both panels depict a set of antegrade (A) and retrograde (R) impulses penetrating a conductive pathway in a sequential and alternating fashion. (*Top*) Shortening of the refractory period (*hashed bars*), which allows the subsequent impulse to propagate. (*Bottom*) How a premature impulse (Rp), by "peeling back" refractoriness, allows propagation of the subsequent impulse.

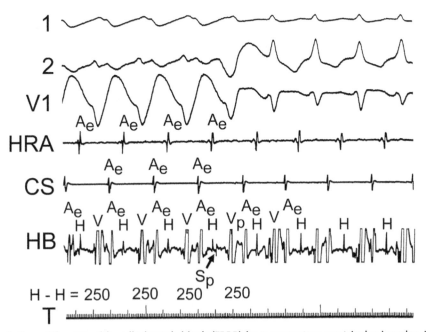

Fig. 36. Resolution of functional bundle branch block (FBBB) by a premature ventricular impulse. Tracings are from the same patient shown in **Fig. 31**. During orthodromic reentrant tachycardia with functional left bundle branch block, a premature ventricular impulse (S_p) is introduced at the time that the His bundle is refractory. Note that FBBB is resolved and the QRS complex is normalized, despite no change in the H-H interval. CS, coronary sinus electrogram; HB, His bundle electrogram; HRA, high right atrial electrogram; T, timelines. (*From Jazayeri MR, Sra JJ, Akhtar M. Wide QRS complexes. Electrophysiologic basis of a common electrocardiographic diagnosis. J Cardiovasc Electrophysiol 1992;3:365–93; with permission.*)

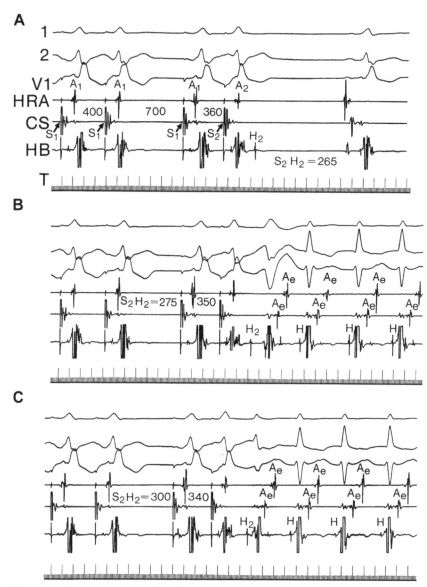

Fig. 37. Double ventricular response resulting from concomitant conduction over normal and accessory pathways. Tracings are from a patient with a posteroseptal accessory pathway (AP). Programmed atrial stimulation at the coronary sinus (CS) with short-to-long (400–700 ms) cycle lengths is shown. (*A*) At a coupling interval of 360 ms, the A_2 impulse is conducted over both the AP and normal pathway (NP) with exclusive ventricular activation (V_2) via the former. However, as a result of the retrograde concealment generated by the V_2 complex exclusively via the AP, the impulse transmitted over the NP is blocked below the His-bundle recording site. (*B*) At the S_1-S_2 interval of 350 ms, however, the A_2 impulse results in a double ventricular response (DVR), the first complex with conduction over the AP and the second with propagation via the NP. Note that the first complex is conducted with functional left bundle branch block (FBBB), which is secondary to the retrograde concealment of the second complex in the left bundle. (*C*) At the S_1-S_2 interval of 340 ms, owing to further AV nodal conduction delay (S_2H_2 = 300 ms compared with 265 ms and 275 ms shown in *A* and *B*, respectively), propagation of the A_2 impulse over NP occurs without FBBB. In both *B* and *C*, conduction of the A_2 impulse via the NP initiated orthodromic reentrant tachycardia. HB, His bundle electrogram; HRA, high right atrial electrogram; T, timelines. (*Adapted from* Jazayeri MR, Sra JJ, Akhtar M. Wide QRS complexes. Electrophysiologic basis of a common electrocardiographic diagnosis. J Cardiovasc Electrophysiol 1992;3:365–93; with permission.)

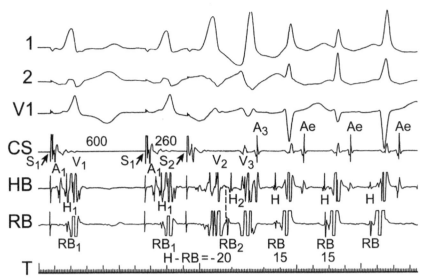

Fig. 38. Double ventricular response attributable to bundle branch reentry. Tracings are from a patient with a posteroseptal accessory pathway (AP). Programmed atrial stimulation (S1-S2) at the coronary sinus (CS) with an S1-S1 cycle length of 600 ms and an S1-S2 coupling interval of 260 ms is shown. The V_2 impulse is a preexcited complex, which is conducted exclusively over the AP. A wide QRS complex (V_3), with right bundle branch block morphology, follows the V_2 impulse, which in turn initiates orthodromic reentrant tachycardia. The right bundle (RB_2) potential precedes the His bundle (H_2) potential by 20 ms, compared with the H-RB interval of 15 ms during normally conducted supraventricular impulses. This situation indicates that the V_3 complex is indeed a bundle branch reentrant beat using the RB retrogradely and the left bundle antegradely. (*From* Jazayeri MR, Sra JJ, Akhtar M. Wide QRS complexes. Electrophysiologic basis of a common electrocardiographic diagnosis. J Cardiovasc Electrophysiol 1992;3:365–93; with permission.)

tachycardia depends on a very delicate balance between the conduction properties and recovery of excitability of the AV nodal pathways. The underlying atrial drive can be sinus rhythm, ectopic atrial rhythm, or atrial tachycardia. This phenomenon has been observed as a nonsustained form in the midst of typical AVNRT (see Fig. 22-12 of Jazayeri and colleagues[149]). It is conceivable, therefore, that in the presence of multiple AV nodal pathways a unique form of tachycardia would develop, in which the retrograde conduction is over 1 retrograde pathway and the resultant atrial impulse, in turn, conducts sequentially over 2 distinct antegrade pathways (**Fig. 43**).

- *Sinus beats alternating with interpolated premature impulses.*[139,150] An interpolated impulse (VEI or JEI) is sandwiched between 2 conducted sinus beats (**Fig. 44**). For this to occur, the extrasystole must lack retrograde VA conduction to the atrium. This scenario is usually provided by a retrograde block (CC) of the interpolated impulse in the AV node, which in turn might also lengthen

the PR interval of the subsequent sinus beat.

Pacemaker-mediated tachycardia

Patients with implanted dual-chamber pacemakers are prone to this iatrogenic arrhythmia when they have intact VA conduction.[151,152] This so-called endless loop tachycardia could last indefinitely unless the retrograde conduction is, at least temporarily, interrupted or the pacemaker ceases to pace the ventricle, at least for 1 cycle. These general principles could take place in several potential scenarios as either naturally occurring events or programmed features of the pacemakers. Approximately one-third of patients with intact VA conduction during incremental ventricular pacing demonstrate a ventricular echo beat resulting from atypical AV nodal reentry (concealed reciprocation), which is almost always a single-beat phenomenon. The resultant ventricular echo beat could terminate pacemaker-mediated tachycardia if the pacemaker senses it (**Fig. 45**). On the other hand, persistent antegrade block of the

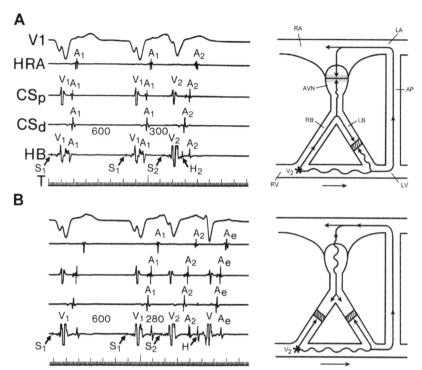

Fig. 39. Initiation of orthodromic reentry by premature ventricular impulse. Tracings are from a patient with a left-sided accessory pathway (AP). Premature ventricular stimulation (S1-S2) is done at an S1-S1 cycle length of 600 ms from the right ventricle (RV). At S1-S2 coupling interval of 280 ms, S2 conducts over the AP, as indicated by the sequence of atrial activation. The His bundle (HB) potential (H2) has emerged from the local ventricular electrogram (V2). (*A, right*) the S2 impulse propagates over the AP, then turns around in the AV node (AVN). However, the impulse approaching the AVN cannot initiate orthodromic reentrant tachycardia (ORT) because of its refractoriness caused by concealment of H2, or by collision of the 2 wavefronts in the AVN. (*B*) The S2 blocks in both bundle branches, and by conducting over the AP it initiates ORT because the bundle branches have recovered from their earlier refractoriness. CSp and CSd, proximal and distal coronary sinus electrograms; HRA, high right atrial electrogram; LA, left atrium; LB, left bundle; LV, left ventricle; RA, right atrium; RB, right bundle; T, timelines.

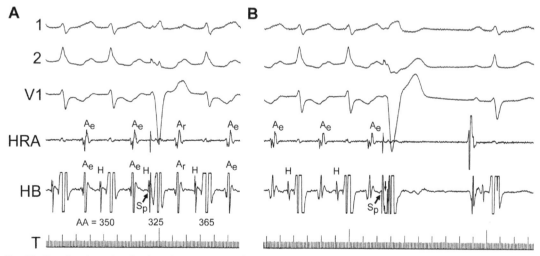

Fig. 40. Termination of orthodromic reentrant tachycardia by a premature ventricular impulse. Tracings are from a patient with a concealed accessory pathway (AP) with a long ventriculoatrial conduction time. A premature ventricular impulse (Sp) is introduced during an episode of orthodromic reentrant tachycardia (ORT). (*A*) Resetting of ORT by Sp while the latter is introduced at the time that the His bundle (HB) is refractory. This phenomenon confirms that the reentrant process uses an AP as the retrograde limb. (*B*) An Sp impulse is introduced slightly earlier than that in *A*. A small arrow indicates the timing of the HB activation, which occurs almost simultaneously with the Sp. This premature impulse terminates ORT without reaching the atrium because of retrograde concealed conduction in the AP. HRA, high right atrial electrogram; T, timelines.

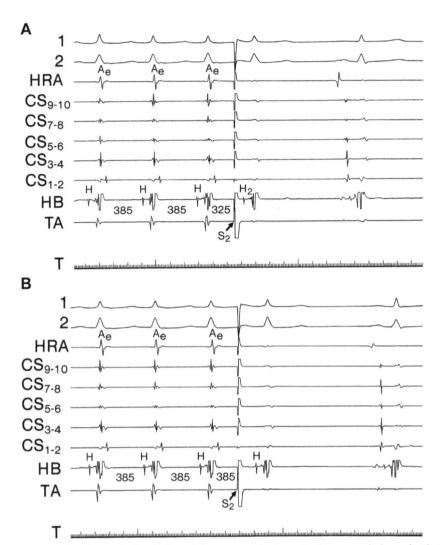

Fig. 41. Termination of atrioventricular (AV) nodal reentrant tachycardia by concealed conduction of a subthreshold impulse. Tracings are from a patient with typical AV nodal reentrant tachycardia (AVNRT). A catheter is positioned at the anterior aspect of the tricuspid septal annulus (TA) for pacing. (*A*) A premature impulse (S2) is introduced. This impulse does not invoke any atrial electrogram in the intracardiac recordings. However, it advances the His bundle (HB) potential (H$_2$), probably by pacing the HB stem. The H$_2$ impulse blocks retrogradely in the fast pathway and thereby terminates AVNRT. (*B*) The S2 may be considered a subthreshold impulse because it not only fails to capture any structure surrounding the TA but also fails to advance the HB potential. Nonetheless, it terminates AVNRT, probably the same way as the S2 does in *A*. CS, coronary sinus electrogram; HRA, high right atrial electrogram; T, timelines.

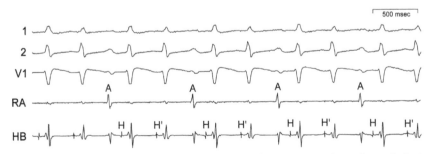

Fig. 42. Nonreentrant supraventricular tachycardia. A segment of supraventricular tachycardia is shown in a patient with dual AV nodal pathways. The QRS complexes outnumber the sinus P waves 2 to 1. Each atrial impulse (A) is conducted to the His bundle (HB) sequentially via a fast pathway (H) and a slow pathway (H'). RA, right atrial electrogram.

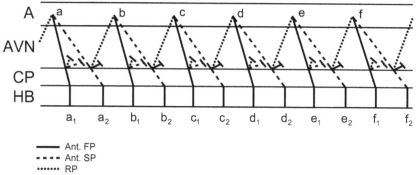

Ant. FP
---- Ant. SP
······· RP

Fig. 43. A proposed supraventricular tachycardia in the presence of multiple atrioventricular nodal (AVN) pathways. Ladder diagram shows a unique form of AVN reentrant tachycardia (AVNRT), in which 2 antegrade (Ant.) fast and slow pathways (FP and SP) and a single retrograde pathway (RP) are present. Each atrial impulse produced by conduction over the RP in turn propagates sequentially over the FP then the SP. Therefore, this would technically mimic AVNRT, except for there being twice as many ventricular impulses as atrial impulses. Propagation of atrial impulses over the FP would be incidental and not required for the maintenance of the reentrant process. As shown in the diagram, a series of intermittent retrograde concealment would be crucial and, therefore, the occurrence of such tachycardia would require a delicate balance in conduction properties and recovery of the excitability of these pathways. Furthermore, the conduction properties and recovery of the excitability of the AVN common pathway (CP), the His bundle (HB), and the ventricles must allow the maintenance of a 1:2 A-to-V relationship during this phenomenon.

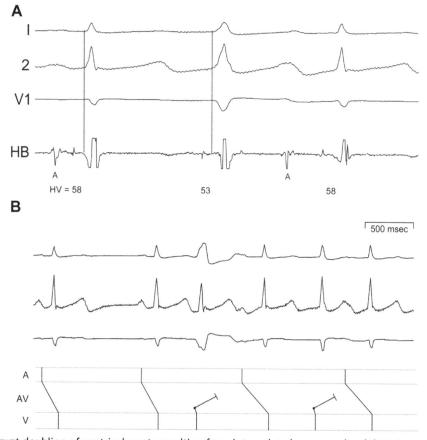

Fig. 44. Abrupt doubling of ventricular rate resulting from interpolated extrasystoles. (*A*) An interpolated junctional extrasystolic impulse (JEI) sandwiched between 2 sinus beats (SBs). The HV interval of 53 ms (vs 58 ms during SB) is in favor of the middle complex being JEI rather than a supraventricular impulse of a different origin, such as the second component of a double ventricular response. (*B*) A segment of tachycardia produced by the JEIs alternating with the SB. The JEIs block retrogradely in the AV node (ie, concealed conduction), which is crucial for the genesis of this rather unusual form of tachycardia. It should be pointed out that in the presence of retrograde ventriculoatrial conduction, the JEI would not have been interpolated, sandwiched between 2 successive SBs, and therefore this tachycardia would not have occurred.

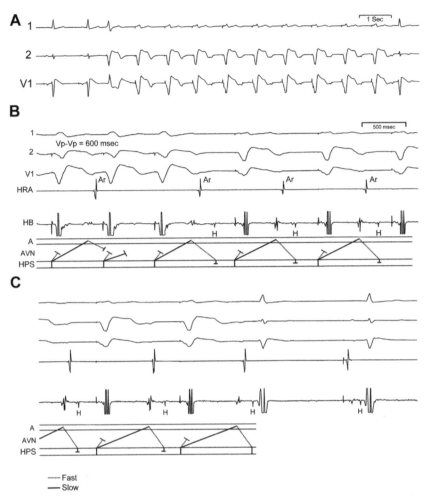

Fig. 45. Pacemaker-mediated tachycardia (PMT) and concealed reentry. Tracings are from a patient with noni-schemic cardiomyopathy and a low left ventricular ejection fraction who is status postimplantation of an implant-able cardioverter-defibrillator (ICD) device. Because of recurrent ventricular tachycardia (VT) and frequent ICD discharges, he was brought to the electrophysiology laboratory for VT ablation. As an incidental finding, he was noted to have PMT. (*A*) An episode of nonsustained PMT spontaneously initiated by a premature ventricular impulse (third complex from the left). Panels *B* and *C* are continuous. (*B, C*) The terminal portion of incremental ventricular pacing (Vp-Vp) with a cycle length of 600 ms. The first and third Vp impulses conduct retrogradely to the atrium (Ar) with a rather long ventriculoatrial (VA) conduction time. On cessation of incremental pacing, PMT ensues. All the Ar impulses after the last Vp in addition to those during PMT, in turn, produce AV nodal reentrant echo beats which, by conducting to the His bundle (HB), elicit HB potentials (H). However, the His-Purkinje system (HPS) refractoriness below the HB recording site does not allow the Ar to complete its course and reach the ven-tricles. This block below the HB (BBH) permits PMT to persist for several cycles until sudden resolution of BBH, followed by propagation to the ventricle and termination of PMT. PMT in *A* is also terminated by a conducted echo beat. AVN, atrioventricular node; HRA, high right atrial electrogram.

reciprocal beat along the NP would maintain pacemaker-mediated tachycardia.

SUMMARY

CC is a common ECG phenomenon, and its recog-nition is critical for an in-depth analysis of cardiac arrhythmias. Many simple and complex arrhyth-mias are triggered, maintained, or terminated by this interesting phenomenon. Any unexpected

rhythm-related issue detected on the surface ECG should be interpreted with adequate consid-eration for CC.

ACKNOWLEDGMENTS

The author would like to express his gratitude to Linda Jarmuskiewicz for her excellent secre-tarial assistance, and the staff of Bellin Health

Electrophysiology Laboratory for their superb technical support.

REFERENCES

1. Moukabary T. Willem Einthoven (1860–1927): father of electrocardiography. Cardiol J 2007;14:316–7.
2. Rosen M. The electrocardiogram 100 years later: electrical insights into molecular messages. Circulation 2002;106:2173–9.
3. Langendorf R. Concealed A-V conduction; the effect of blocked impulses on the formation and conduction of subsequent impulses. Am Heart J 1948; 35:542–52.
4. Englemann TW. Beobachtungen and Versuche am suspendieren Herzen. Pflugers Arch 1894;56: 149–202.
5. Ashman R. Conductivity in compressed cardiac muscle. Am J Physiol 1925;74:121–39.
6. Drury AN. Further observations upon intraauricular block produced by pressure or cooling. Heart 1925;12:143–69.
7. Lewis T, Master AM. Observations upon conduction in the mammalian heart. A-V conduction. Heart 1925;12:209–69.
8. Langendorf R, Pick A. Concealed conduction further evaluation of a fundamental aspect of propagation of the cardiac impulse. Circulation 1956;13:381–99.
9. Moe GK, Abildskov JA, Mendez C. An experimental study of concealed conduction. Am Heart J 1964;67:338–56.
10. Langendorf R, Pick A, Edelist A, et al. Experimental demonstration of concealed AV conduction in the human heart. Circulation 1965;32:386–93.
11. Moore EN. Microelectrode studies on concealment of multiple premature atrial responses. Circ Res 1966;18:660–72.
12. Moore EN. Microelectrode studies on retrograde concealment of multiple premature ventricular responses. Circ Res 1967;20:88–98.
13. Moore EN, Knoebel SB, Spear JF. Concealed conduction. Am J Cardiol 1971;28:406–13.
14. Damato AN, Lau SH. Concealed and supernormal atrioventricular conduction. Circulation 1971;43: 967–70.
15. Wu D, Denes P, Dhingra RC, et al. Quantification of human atrioventricular nodal concealed conduction utilizing S1S2S3 stimulation. Circ Res 1976; 39:659–65.
16. Wit AL, Weiss MB, Berkowitz WD, et al. Patterns of atrioventricular conduction in the human heart. Circ Res 1970;27:345–59.
17. Akhtar M, Mahmud R, Tchou P, et al. Normal electrophysiologic responses of the human heart. Cardiol Clin 1986;4:365–86.
18. Page RL, Wharton JM, Prystowsky EN. Effect of continuous vagal enhancement on concealed conduction and refractoriness within the atrioventricular node. Am J Cardiol 1996;77:260–5.
19. Fujiki A, Tani M, Mizumaki K, et al. Quantification of human concealed atrioventricular nodal conduction: relation to ventricular response during atrial fibrillation. Am Heart J 1990;120:598–603.
20. Fujiki A, Mizumaki K, Tani M. Effects of diltiazem on concealed atrioventricular nodal conduction in relation to ventricular response during atrial fibrillation in anesthetized dogs. Am Heart J 1993;125: 1284–9.
21. Lehmann MH, Mahmud R, Denker ST, et al. Effect of concealed anterograde impulse penetration on retrograde atrioventricular nodal conduction in man. Am Heart J 1987;114:1374–83.
22. Jazayeri MR, Rovang K, Van Wyhe G, et al. Recovery of excitability of retrograde atrioventricular nodal pathway following an antegrade concealment in patients with and without reentrant substrate [abstract]. Pacing Clin Electrophysiol 1990;13:556.
23. Jazayeri MR, Dhala AA, Koch K, et al. Atrioventricular nodal reentry in patients with accessory pathway. A suitable substrate for preexcited tachycardia [abstract]. Pacing Clin Electrophysiol 1991; 14:278.
24. Schuger CD, Steinman RT, Lehmann MH. Recovery of retrograde fast pathway excitability in the atrioventricular node reentrant circuit after concealed anterograde impulse penetration. J Am Coll Cardiol 1991;17:1129–37.
25. Lehmann MH, Denker S, Mahmud R, et al. Patterns of human atrioventricular nodal accommodation to a sudden acceleration of atrial rate. Am J Cardiol 1984;53:71–6.
26. Denes P, Levy L, Pick A, et al. The incidence of typical and atypical A-V Wenckebach periodicity. Am Heart J 1975;89:26–31.
27. Martin P. The influence of the parasympathetic nervous system on atrioventricular conduction. Circ Res 1977;41:593–9.
28. Prystowsky EN, Jackman WM, Rinkenberger RL, et al. Effect of autonomic blockade on ventricular refractoriness and atrioventricular nodal conduction in humans. Evidence supporting a direct cholinergic action on ventricular muscle refractoriness. Circ Res 1981;49:511–8.
29. Sadr-Ameli MA, Shenasa M, Lacombe P, et al. Effect of autonomic nervous system modulation on retrograde atrioventricular nodal conduction in human heart. Cardiovasc Res 1987;21:45–54.
30. McKinnie J, Avitall B, Caceres J, et al. Electrophysiologic spectrum of concealed intranodal conduction during atrial rate acceleration in a model of 2:1 atrioventricular block. Circulation 1989;80:43–50.
31. Shrier A, Dubarsky H, Rosengarten M, et al. Prediction of complex atrioventricular conduction rhythms

in humans with use of the atrioventricular nodal recovery curve. Circulation 1987;76:1196–205.

32. Halpern MS, Nau GJ, Levi RJ, et al. Wenckebach periods of alternate beats. Clinical and experimental observations. Circulation 1973;48:41–9.

33. Amat-y-Leon F, Chuquimia R, Wu D, et al. Alternating Wenckebach periodicity. A common electrophysiologic response. Am J Cardiol 1975;36:757–64.

34. Castellanos A, Fernandez P, Interian A Jr, et al. Dynamics of atrioventricular nodal conduction ratios during conversion of 2:1 into 3:1, 4:1 and 5:1 atrioventricular block. Am J Cardiol 1991;68:979–81.

35. Castellanos A, Cox MM, Fernandez PR, et al. Mechanisms and dynamics of episodes of progression of 2:1 atrioventricular block in patients with documented two-level conduction disturbances. Am J Cardiol 1992;70:193–9.

36. Castellanos A, Interian A Jr, Cox MM, et al. Alternating Wenckebach periods and allied arrhythmias. Pacing Clin Electrophysiol 1993;16:2285–300.

37. Young M, Gelband H, Castellanos A, et al. Reverse alternating Wenckebach periodicity. Am J Cardiol 1987;80:90–4.

38. Castellanos A, Fuenmayor AJ, Huikuri H, et al. Dynamics of atrioventricular nodal conduction ratios of reverse alternating Wenckebach periods. Am J Cardiol 1989;1(64):1047–9.

39. Steinman RT, Lehmann MH. Beat-to-beat changes in atrioventricular nodal excitability and its modulation by concealed conduction during functional 2:1 block in man. Circulation 1987;76:759–67.

40. Vereckei A, Vera Z, Pride HP, et al. Atrioventricular nodal conduction rather than automaticity determines the ventricular rate during atrial fibrillation and atrial flutter. J Cardiovasc Electrophysiol 1992;3:534–43.

41. Lehmann MH, Steinman RT. Atrioventricular and intraventricular block. In: Zipes DP, Rowland DJ, editors. Progress in Cardiology. Philadelphia: Lea and Febiger; 1988. p. 281–312.

42. Damato AN, Varghese J, Caracta AR, et al. Functional 2:1 A-V block within the His-Purkinje system. Simulation of type II second-degree A-V block. Circulation 1973;47:534–42.

43. Jazayeri MR, Sra JJ, Akhtar M. Wide QRS complexes. Electrophysiologic basis of a common electrocardiographic diagnosis. J Cardiovasc Electrophysiol 1992;3:365–93.

44. Denker S, Shenasa M, Gilbert CJ, et al. Effects of abrupt changes in cycle length on refractoriness of the His-Purkinje system in man. Circulation 1983;67:60–8.

45. Chiale PA, Sanchez RA, Franco DA, et al. Overdrive prolongation of refractoriness and fatigue in the early stages of human bundle branch disease. J Am Coll Cardiol 1994;23:724–32.

46. Dhingra RC, Rosen KM, Rahimtoola SH. Wenckebach periods with repetitive block. Evaluation with His bundle recording. Am Heart J 1973;86:444–8.

47. Moe GK, Abildskov JA. Observations on the ventricular dysrhythmia associated with atrial fibrillation in the dog. Circ Res 1964;14:447–60.

48. Moore EN. Observations on concealed conduction in atrial fibrillation. Circ Res 1967;21:201–8.

49. Moore EN, Spear JF. Electrophysiological studies on atrial fibrillation. Heart Vessels Suppl 1987;2:32–9.

50. Cohen SI, Lau SH, Berkowitz WD, et al. Concealed conduction during atrial fibrillation. Am J Cardiol 1970;25:416–9.

51. van den Berg MP, Haaksma J, Brouwer J, et al. Heart rate variability in patients with atrial fibrillation is related to vagal tone. Circulation 1997;96:1209–16.

52. Toivonen L, Kadish A, Kou W, et al. Determinants of the ventricular rate during atrial fibrillation. J Am Coll Cardiol 1990;16:1194–200.

53. Bootsma BK, Hoelsen AJ, Strackee J, et al. Analysis of R-R Intervals in patients with atrial fibrillation at rest and during exercise. Circulation 1970;41:783–94.

54. Blanck Z, Dhala AA, Sra J, et al. Characterization of atrioventricular nodal behavior and ventricular response during atrial fibrillation before and after a selective slow-pathway ablation. Circulation 1995;91:1086–94.

55. Markowitz SM, Stein KM, Lerman BB. Mechanism of ventricular rate control after radiofrequency modification of atrioventricular conduction in patients with atrial fibrillation. Circulation 1996;94:2856–64.

56. Stein KM, Walden J, Lippman N, et al. Ventricular response in atrial fibrillation: random or deterministic? Am J Physiol 1999;277:H452–8.

57. Akhtar M, Gilbert CJ, Wolf FG, et al. Retrograde conduction in the His-Purkinje system. An analysis of routes of impulse propagation using His and right bundle branch recordings. Circulation 1979;59:1252–65.

58. Akhtar M. Retrograde conduction in man. Pacing Clin Electrophysiol 1981;4:548–62.

59. Josephson M, Kastor JA. His-Purkinje conduction during retrograde stress. J Clin Invest 1978;61:171–7.

60. Denker S, Lehmann MH, Mahmud R, et al. Divergence between refractoriness of His-Purkinje system and ventricular muscle with abrupt changes in cycle length. Circulation 1983;68:1212–21.

61. Akhtar M, Damato AN, Batsford WP, et al. A comparative analysis of antegrade and retrograde conduction patterns in man. Circulation 1975;52:766–78.

62. Akhtar M, Damato AN, Ruskin JN, et al. Antegrade and retrograde conduction characteristics in three patterns of paroxysmal atrioventricular junctional reentrant tachycardia. Am Heart J 1978;95:22–42.

63. Lehmann MH, Denker S, Mahmud R, et al. Functional His-Purkinje system behavior during sudden ventricular rate acceleration in man. Circulation 1983;68:767–75.

64. Schamroth L, Marriott HJ. Concealed ventricular extrasystoles. Circulation 1963;27:1043–9.

65. Schamroth L. Genesis and evolution of ectopic ventricular rhythm. Br Heart J 1966;28:244–57.

66. Schamroth L. Interpolated extrasystoles. S Afr Med J 1967;41:919–22.

67. Schamroth L, Surawicz B. Concealed interpolated A-V junctional extrasystoles and A-V junctional parasystole. Am J Cardiol 1971;27:703–7.

68. Rosen KM, Ehsani AA, Sinno MZ, et al. Simultaneous block proximal and distal to His bundle. An example of concealed "concealed conduction". Arch Intern Med 1973;131:588–90.

69. Katz LN, Langendorff R, Cole SL. An unusual effect of interpolated ventricular premature systoles. Am Heart J 1944;28:167–76.

70. Langendorf R, Mehlman JS. Blocked (nonconducted) A-V nodal premature systoles imitating first and second degree A-V block. Am Heart J 1947;34:500–6.

71. Marriott HJ, Bradely SM. Main-stem extrasystoles. Circulation 1957;16:544–7.

72. Rosen KM, Rahimtoola SH, Gunnar RM. Pseudo A-V block secondary to premature nonpropagated His bundle depolarizations: documentation by His bundle electrocardiography. Circulation 1970;42:367–73.

73. Chung EK. A reappraisal of concealed atrioventricular conduction. Am Heart J 1971;82:408–16.

74. Massumi RA, Ertem GE, Vera Z. Aberrancy of junctional escape beats. Evidence for origin in the fascicles of the left bundle branch. Am J Cardiol 1972;29:351–9.

75. Massumi RA, Hilliard G, DeMaria A, et al. Paradoxic phenomenon of premature beats with narrow QRS in the presence of bundle-branch block. Circulation 1973;47:543–53.

76. Cannom DS, Gallagher JJ, Goldreyer BN, et al. Concealed bundle of His extrasystoles simulating nonconducted atrial premature beats. Am Heart J 1972;83:777–9.

77. Lindsay AE, Schamroth L. Atrioventricular junctional parasystole with concealed conduction simulating second degree atrioventricular block. Am J Cardiol 1973;31:397–9.

78. Castellanos A, Befeler B, Myerburg RJ. Pseudo AV block produced by concealed extrasystoles arising below the bifurcation of the His bundle. Br Heart J 1974;36:457–61.

79. Fisch C, Zipes DP, McHenry PL. Electrocardiographic manifestations of concealed junctional ectopic impulses. Circulation 1976;53:217–23.

80. Pick A, Langendorf R. Specific mechanisms of various disorders of impulse formation, conduction, and their combinations. In: Pick A, Langendorf R, editors. Interpretations of complex arrhythmias. Philadelphia: Lea and Febiger; 1979. p. 367–578.

81. Camous JP, Baudouy M, Guarino L, et al. Effects of an interpolated premature ventricular contraction on the AV conduction of the subsequent premature atrial depolarization. An apparent facilitation. J Electrocardiol 1980;13:353–7.

82. Fisch C. Concealed conduction. Cardiol Clin 1983;1:63–74.

83. Fisch C. Concealed conduction at the AV nodal level. In: Mazgalev T, Dreifus LS, Michelson EL, editors. Electrophysiology of sinoatrial and atrioventricular nodes. New York: Alan R Liss, Inc; 1988. p. 287–300.

84. Fisch C. Concealed conduction. In: Jalife J, Zipes DP, editors. Cardiac electrophysiology: from cell to bedside. Philadelphia: WB Saunders; 1995. p. 961–9.

85. Damato AN, Varghese PJ, Lau SH, et al. Manifest and concealed reentry. A mechanism of AV nodal Wenckebach phenomenon. Circ Res 1972;30:283–92.

86. Gallagher JJ, Damato AN, Varghese PJ, et al. Manifest and concealed reentry: a mechanism of A-V nodal Wenckebach in man. Circulation 1973;47:752–7.

87. Langendorf R, Pick A. Manifestations of concealed reentry in the atrioventricular junction. Eur J Cardiol 1973;1:11–21.

88. Shenasa M, Denker S, Mahmud R, et al. Atrioventricular nodal conduction and refractoriness after intranodal collision from antegrade and retrograde impulses. Circulation 1983;67:651–60.

89. Lehmann MH, Mahmud R, Denker S, et al. Retrograde concealed conduction in the atrioventricular node: differential manifestations related to level of intranodal penetration. Circulation 1984;70:392–401.

90. Mahmud R, Lehmann M, Denker S, et al. Atrioventricular sequential pacing: differential effect on retrograde conduction related to level of impulse collision. Circulation 1983;68:23–32.

91. Mahmud R, Denker S, Lehmann MH, et al. Effect of atrioventricular sequential pacing in patients with no ventriculoatrial conduction. J Am Coll Cardiol 1984;4:273–7.

92. Li H, Yee R, Thakur RK, et al. The effect of variable retrograde penetration on dual AV nodal pathways: observations before and after slow pathway ablation LDD. Pacing Clin Electrophysiol 1997;20:2146–53.

93. Moe GK, Childers RW, Merideth J. Appraisal of "supernormal" A-V conduction. Circulation 1968; 38:5–28.

94. Cranefield PF, Hoffman BF. Conduction of the cardiac impulse. II. Summation and inhibition. Circ Res 1971;28:220–33.

95. Zipes DP, Mendez C, Moe GK. Evidence for summation and voltage dependency in rabbit atrioventricular nodal fibers. Circ Res 1973;32:170–7.

96. Antzelevitch C, Moe GK. Electrotonic inhibition and summation of impulse conduction in mammalian Purkinje fibers. Am J Physiol 1983;245:H42–53.

97. Fisch C, Greenspan K. Wedensky's observations. Circulation 1967;35:819–20.

98. Akhtar M, Gilbert CJ, Al-Nouri M, et al. Electrophysiologic mechanisms for modification and abolition of atrioventricular junctional tachycardia with simultaneous and sequential atrial and ventricular pacing. Circulation 1979;60:1443–54.

99. Mahmud R, Denker ST, Tchou PJ, et al. Modulation of conduction and refractoriness in atrioventricular junctional reentrant circuit. Effect on reentry initiated by atrial extrastimulus. J Clin Invest 1988;81:39–46.

100. Moe GK, Mendez C, Han J. Aberrant A-V impulse propagation in the dog heart. A study of functional bundle branch block. Circ Res 1965;16:261–86.

101. Moe GK, Mendez C. Functional block in the intraventricular conduction system. Circulation 1971; 43:949–54.

102. Wellens HJJ, Durrer D. Supraventricular tachycardia with left aberrant conduction due to retrograde invasion into the left bundle branch. Circulation 1968;38:474–9.

103. Jazayeri MR, Deshpande SS, Sra JS, et al. Retrograde (transseptal) activation of right bundle branch during sinus rhythm. J Cardiovasc Electrophysiol 1993;4:280–7.

104. Rosenbaum MB, Elizari MV, Lazzari JO, et al. The differential electrocardiographic manifestations of hemiblocks, bilateral bundle branch block, and trifascicular blocks. In: Schlant RC, Hurst WJ, editors. Advances in electrocardiography. New York: Grune & Stratton; 1972. p. 145–82.

105. Lehmann MH, Denker S, Mahmud R, et al. Linking: a dynamic electrophysiologic phenomenon in macroreentry circuits. Circulation 1985;71:254–65.

106. Castellanos A, Portillo B, Zaman L, et al. Linking phenomenon during atrial stimulation with accessory pathways. Am J Cardiol 1986;58:964–9.

107. Lehmann MH, Steinman RT. Linking by collision initiated in the absence of preexisting reentrant tachycardia. Am J Cardiol 1988;61:354–60.

108. Okumura K, Henthorn RW, Epstein AE, et al. Further observations on transient entrainment: importance of pacing site and properties of the components of the reentry circuit. Circulation 1985;72:1293–307.

109. El-Sherif N, Gough WB, Restivo M. Reentrant ventricular arrhythmias in the late myocardial infarction period: 14. Mechanisms of resetting, entrainment, acceleration, or termination of reentrant tachycardia by programmed electrical stimulation. Pacing Clin Electrophysiol 1987;10:341–71.

110. Stevenson WG, Sager PT, Friedman PL. Entrainment techniques for mapping atrial and ventricular tachycardias. J Cardiovasc Electrophysiol 1995;6: 201–16.

111. Cohen SI, Lau SH, Haft JI, et al. Experimental production of aberrant ventricular conduction in man. Circulation 1967;36:673–85.

112. Cohen SI, Lau SH, Stein E, et al. Variations of aberrant ventricular conduction in man: evidence of isolated and combined block within the specialized conduction system. An electrocardiographic and vectorcardiographic study. Circulation 1968;38: 899–916.

113. Denker ST, Gilbert CJ, Shenasa M, et al. An electrocardiographic–electrophysiologic correlation of aberrant ventricular conduction in man. J Electrocardiol 1983;16:269–77.

114. Chilson DA, Zipes DP, Heger JJ, et al. Functional bundle branch block: discordant response of right and left bundle branches to changes in heart rate. Am J Cardiol 1984;54:313–6.

115. Fisch C. Aberration: seventy five years after Sir Thomas Lewis. Br Heart J 1983;50:297–302.

116. Lehmann MH, Denker S, Mahmud R, et al. Electrophysiologic mechanisms of functional bundle branch block at onset of induced orthodromic tachycardia in the Wolff-Parkinson-White syndrome. Role of stimulation method. J Clin Invest 1985;76:1566–74.

117. Miles WM, Prystowsky EN. Alteration of human right bundle branch refractoriness by changes in duration of the atrial drive train. Circulation 1986; 73:244–8.

118. Gouaux JL, Ashman R. Auricular fibrillation with aberration simulating ventricular paroxysmal tachycardia. Am Heart J 1947;34:366–73.

119. Cohen SI, Lau SH, Scherlag BJ, et al. Alternate patterns of premature ventricular excitation during induced atrial bigeminy. Circulation 1969;39: 819–29.

120. Denker S, Lehmann M, Mahmud R, et al. Effects of alternating cycle lengths on refractoriness of the His-Purkinje system. J Clin Invest 1984;74: 559–70.

121. Stark S, Farshidi A. Mechanism of alternating bundle branch aberrancy with atrial bigeminy. Electrocardiographic-electrophysiologic correlate. J Am Coll Cardiol 1985;5:1491–5.

122. Gozalez-Zuelgaray J, Sheikh S, Akhtar M, et al. Functional bundle branch block as a delayed manifestation of retrograde concealment in the

His-Purkinje system. J Cardiovasc Electrophysiol 1996;7:248–58.

123. Jazayeri MR, Caceres J, Tchou P, et al. Electrophysiologic characteristics of sudden QRS axis deviation during orthodromic tachycardia. Role of functional fascicular block in localization of accessory pathway. J Clin Invest 1989;83:952–9.

124. Myerburg RJ. The gating mechanism in the distal atrioventricular conducting system. Circulation 1971;43:955–60.

125. Akhtar M, Gilbert C, Al-Nouri M, et al. Site of conduction delay during functional block in the His-Purkinje system in man. Circulation 1980;61:1239–48.

126. Lehmann MH, Denker S, Mahmud R, et al. Postextrasystolic alterations in refractoriness of the His-Purkinje system and ventricular myocardium in man. Circulation 1984;69:1096–102.

127. Akhtar M, Damato AN, Lau SH, et al. Clinical uses of His bundle electrocardiography. Part III. Am Heart J 1976;91:805–9.

128. Josephson ME, Seides SF, Damato AN. Wolff-Parkinson-White syndrome with 1:2 atrioventricular conduction. Am J Cardiol 1976;37:1094–6.

129. Wu D, Denes P, Dhingra R, et al. New manifestations of dual A-V nodal pathways. Eur J Cardiol 1975;2:459–66.

130. Mines GR. On circulating excitations in heart muscles and their possible relation to tachycardia and fibrillation. Trans R Soc Can 1914;8:43–52.

131. Lehmann MH, Tchou P, Mahmud R, et al. Electrophysiological determinants of antidromic reentry induced during atrial extrastimulation. Insights from a pacing model of Wolff-Parkinson-White syndrome. Circ Res 1989;65:295–306.

132. Akhtar M, Shenasa M, Schmidt DH. Role of retrograde His Purkinje block in the initiation of supraventricular tachycardia by ventricular premature stimulation in the Wolff Parkinson-White syndrome. J Clin Invest 1981;67:1047–55.

133. Akhtar M, Lehmann MH, Denker ST, et al. Electrophysiologic mechanisms of orthodromic tachycardia initiation during ventricular pacing in the Wolff-Parkinson-White syndrome. J Am Coll Cardiol 1987;9:89–100.

134. Ross DL, Farre J, Bar FW, et al. Spontaneous termination of circus movement tachycardia using an accessory pathway. Incidence, site of block and mechanisms. Circulation 1981;63:1129–39.

135. Moe GK, Cohen W, Vick RL. Experimentally induced paroxysmal A-V nodal tachycardia in the dog. Am Heart J 1963;65:87–92.

136. Massumi RA, Kistin AD, Tawakkol AA. Termination of reciprocating tachycardia by atrial stimulation. Circulation 1967;36:637–43.

137. Barold SS, Linhart JW, Samet P, et al. Supraventricular tachycardia initiated and terminated by a single electrical stimulus. Am J Cardiol 1969;24:37–41.

138. Shenasa M, Cardinal R, Kus T, et al. Termination of sustained ventricular tachycardia by ultrarapid subthreshold stimulation in humans. Circulation 1988;78(5 Pt 1):1135–43.

139. Shenasa M, Fromer M, Borggrefe M, et al. Subthreshold electrical stimulation for termination and prevention of reentrant tachycardias. J Electrocardiol 1992;24(Suppl):25–31.

140. Massumi RA. Atrioventricular junctional rhythms. In: Mandel WJ, editor. Cardiac arrhythmias. Their mechanisms, diagnosis, and management. Philadelphia: JB Lippincott; 1987. p. 235–60.

141. Massumi R, Shehata M. Doubling of the ventricular rate by interpolated junctional extrasystoles resembling supraventricular tachycardia. Pacing Clin Electrophysiol 2010;33:945–9.

142. Germano JJ, Essebag V, Papageorgiou P, et al. Concealed and manifest 1:2 tachycardia and atrioventricular nodal reentrant tachycardia: manifestations of dual atrioventricular nodal physiology. Heart Rhythm 2005;2:536–9.

143. Csapo G. Paroxysmal nonreentrant tachycardias due to simultaneous conduction in dual atrioventricular nodal pathways. Am J Cardiol 1979;43:1033–45.

144. Buss J, Kraatz J, Stegaru B, et al. Unusual mechanism of PR interval variation and nonreentrant supraventricular tachycardia as manifestation of simultaneous anterograde fast and slow conduction through dual atrioventricular nodal pathways. Pacing Clin Electrophysiol 1985;8:235–41.

145. Kim SS, Lal R, Ruffy R, et al. Paroxysmal nonreentrant supraventricular tachycardia due to simultaneous fast and slow pathway conduction in dual atrioventricular node pathways. J Am Coll Cardiol 1987;10:456–61.

146. Li HG, Klein GJ, Natale A, et al. Nonreentrant supraventricular tachycardia due to simultaneous conduction over fast and slow AV node pathways: successful treatment with radiofrequency ablation. Pacing Clin Electrophysiol 1994;17:1186–93.

147. Arena G, Bongiorni MG, Soldati E, et al. Incessant nonreentrant atrioventricular nodal tachycardia due to multiple nodal pathways treated by radiofrequency ablation of the slow pathways. J Cardiovasc Electrophysiol 1999;10:1636–42.

148. Yokoshiki H, Sasaki K, Shimokawa J, et al. Nonreentrant atrioventricular nodal tachycardia due to triple nodal pathways manifested by radiofrequency ablation at coronary sinus ostium. J Electrocardiol 2006;39:395–9.

149. Jazayeri MR, Keelan ET, Jazayeri MA. Atrioventricular nodal reentrant tachycardia: current

understanding and controversies. In: Shenasa M, Hindricks G, Borggrefe M, et al, editors. Cardiac mapping. 4th edition. Oxford(UK): Wiley-Blackwell Publishing Ltd; 2013. p. 224–48.

150. Massumi RA. Interpolated His Bundle extrasystoles. An unusual cause of tachycardia. Am J Med 1970;49:265–70.

151. Furman S, Fisher JD. Endless loop tachycardia in an AV universal [DDD] pacemaker. Pacing Clin Electrophysiol 1982;5:486–9.

152. Mahmud R, Denker S, Lehmann M, et al. Functional characteristics of retrograde conduction in a pacing model of endless loop tachycardia. J Am Coll Cardiol 1984;3:1488–99.

Electrocardiographic Characteristics of Ventricular Arrhythmia in Inherited Channelopathies

Nilubon Methachittiphan, MD[a],
Peerawut Deeprasertkul, MD[a], Mark S. Link, MD[b],*

KEYWORDS

- Long-QT syndrome • Short-QT syndrome • Brugada syndrome
- Catecholaminergic polymorphic ventricular tachycardia • Ventricular fibrillation

KEY POINTS

- Ventricular arrhythmias in idiopathic VT often present as monomorphic VT, and the overall prognosis is usually benign. Ventricular arrhythmias in channelopathies usually are polymorphic VT and ventricular fibrillation, and the prognosis is more variable.
- Since ventricular arrhythmias in some type of channelopathies can often be fatal, recognizing their ECG patterns is important.
- Some types of channelopathies require further testing such as exercise stress test, EP study, and genetic testing, which will help with risk stratification and prevention of sudden cardiac death by defibrillators in high risk patients.

INTRODUCTION

Ventricular arrhythmias occurring in a structurally normal heart generally account for between 5% and 15% of all patients presenting with ventricular arrhythmias.[1] These arrhythmias can be divided into idiopathic ventricular arrhythmia, in which there is no known ion mutation or genetic component, and inherited ion channelopathies, in which gene mutations causing ion-channel dysfunction play an important role in the mechanism of ventricular tachycardia (VT).[2,3] Arrhythmias may also be characterized as monomorphic or polymorphic (**Fig. 1**). Ventricular arrhythmias in idiopathic VT often present as monomorphic VT, and the overall prognosis is usually benign. However, ventricular arrhythmias in channelopathies usually are polymorphic VT and ventricular fibrillation (VF), and the prognosis is more variable.

Sudden cardiac arrests (SCA) in patients with structurally normal hearts are usually confined to those with channelopathies, although rarely SCA may be secondary to idiopathic VT or Wolff-Parkinson-White (WPW) syndrome. In the last 15 years, the results of mutation screening (molecular autopsy) in sudden unexplained death syndrome or sudden infant death syndrome have been reported in several studies. Although the yield of molecular autopsy reported by different studies is highly variable, ranging from 4% to 30%, a positive genetic test may allow the extension of genotyping to family members of those affected to reduce additional deaths in the family.[1]

The authors have nothing to disclose.

[a] Department of Medicine, University of Texas Medical Branch, 301 University Boulevard 5.106 John Sealy Annex, Galveston, Texas 77555-0553, USA; [b] Department of Medicine, Tufts Medical Center, 800 Washington Street, Box # 197, Boston, MA 02111, USA

* Corresponding author.

E-mail address: mlink@tuftsmedicalcenter.org

Card Electrophysiol Clin 6 (2014) 419–432
http://dx.doi.org/10.1016/j.ccep.2014.05.013
1877-9182/14/$ – see front matter © 2014 Elsevier Inc. All rights reserved.

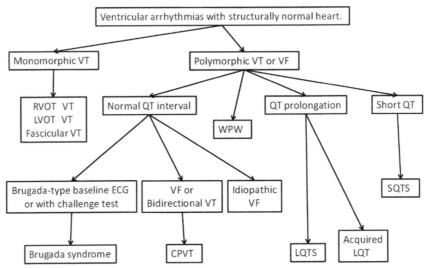

Fig. 1. Proposed clinical approach to ventricular tachycardia with a structurally normal heart. CPVT, catecholaminergic polymorphic ventricular tachycardia; LQT, long QT; LQTS, long-QT syndrome; LVOT, left ventricular outflow tract; RVOT, right ventricular outflow tract; SQTS, short-QT syndrome; VF, ventricular fibrillation; VT, ventricular tachycardia; WPW, Wolff-Parkinson-White syndrome.

LONG-QT SYNDROME

Background

Long-QT syndrome (LQTS) is caused by cardiac ion-channel abnormalities involved in repolarization. Patients with this syndrome have an increased risk for SCA. LQTS was first described in 1957 by Jervell and Lange-Nielsen.[4] This syndrome was found in children with deafness, recurrent syncope, SCA, and QT prolongation. Homozygous mutation in recessive manifestation in the KCNQ1 gene was found to be responsible for this disorder. Subsequently, Romano and colleagues[5] and Ward and colleagues reported another congenital long QT (LQT), which had an autosomal dominance pattern of inheritance. To date 13 types of LQT have been described, and more will certainly be discovered with time.

Genetics and Pathogenesis

More than 300 gene mutations have been found to be related to LQT in 13 different genes.[6] However, most patients (75%) are those with LQT1, LQT2, and LQT3.[7,8] Repolarization abnormalities in LQT can be due to a decrease in repolarizing potassium currents or inappropriate late entry of sodium currents into cardiac myocytes.[9] In LQT1, a KCNQ1 defect is responsible for slowly acting repolarizing potassium currents (I_{Ks}), whereas in LQT2 rapidly repolarizing potassium channel (I_{Kr}) defective genes (KCNH2) are found. Mutations in these potassium channels account for delayed repolarization.[10] In LQT3, a prolonged QT interval is caused by mutations of sodium channel protein (SCN5A), leading to persistent inward sodium currents. Mutations in this gene cause failure of the sodium channel to close after ventricular depolarization.[10]

Electrocardiographic Characteristics

An LQT diagnosis is traditionally described as greater than 460 milliseconds in women and greater than 450 milliseconds in men.[11] However, there is an overlap in QTc for those with LQTS and those without the syndrome. The 95th-percentile values of normal distribution of QT intervals are the same as the QTc, so 2.5% of individuals without LQTS will have a prolonged QTc. In addition, approximately 10% to 30% of LQT cases may have normal QTc at rest.[12] The QT interval can be altered by heart rate, age, gender, electrolyte disturbances, and medications. Thus, electrocardiograms (ECGs) with prolonged QT interval do not necessarily indicate that affected individuals have LQTS. The positive predictive value for diagnosis of LQTS with this cutoff (>460 milliseconds in women and >450 milliseconds in men) is less than 1%. However, the longer the QTc, the more likely an individual has the diagnosis of LQTS. At a QTc of 500 milliseconds, nearly all will have LQTS.[13]

Accurate measurement of QT interval is essential for the diagnosis of LQTS; errors in measurements by physicians and the dynamic nature of QT intervals account for the misdiagnosis of LQTS, and are often observed.[14] The QT interval should be obtained manually from 3 to 5 cardiac cycles, and should be made in leads II, V5, and

V6.[15] Because heart rate can affect QT intervals, a correction formula for QT interval is proposed.[16] The Bazzett correction formula (QTc = QT/√RR, expressed in seconds) is most commonly used. However, this correction is not as accurate at heart rates greater than 100 beats/min or less than 60 beats/min.[17] At present, the guideline recommends a linear regression formula for QT correction.[11]

The morphologies of T wave differ among LQT subtypes. In LQT1, the T wave appears broad and is not shortened with exercise (**Fig. 2**). A bifid or notched T wave is observed in LQT2 (**Fig. 3**), and the T wave in LQT3 is narrow and tall with a long isoelectric segment (**Fig. 4**).[18] In addition, macroscopic T-wave alternans, defined as a beat-by-beat variation in amplitude in T wave, is a marker of electrical instability.[19]

QT interval is the most powerful predictor of cardiac events.[20–23] Priori and colleagues[20] demonstrated that patients with LQT mutations, who had QTc of less than 440 milliseconds, had a less than 20% risk of cardiac events, whereas for those with QTc greater than 498 milliseconds the risk for cardiac events was greater than 70%. This study concluded that the features predicting high risk (>50%) for sudden death include QTc of more than 500 milliseconds in carriers of LQT1 or

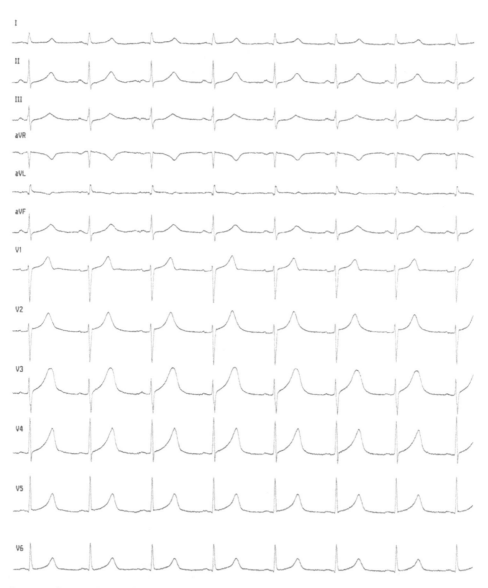

Fig. 2. Electrocardiogram (ECG) of a patient with LQT1. Note the long and broad T wave. (*Courtesy of* S. Priori, MD, Pavia, Italy and A. Mazantti, MD, Pavia, Italy.)

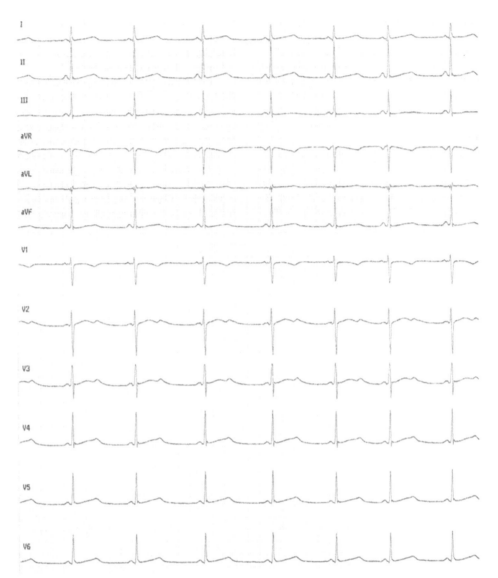

Fig. 3. ECG of patient with LQT2. Note the notched and bifid T wave. (*Courtesy of* S. Priori, MD, Pavia, Italy and A. Mazantti, MD, Pavia, Italy.)

LQT2, and in male carriers of LQT3. On the other hand, patients carrying LQT1, and male carriers of LQT2 with QTc of less than 500 milliseconds, are considered low risk. Current expert consensus suggests that high risk presents when QTc is greater than 500 milliseconds, and becomes extremely high when QTc is greater than 600 milliseconds. Overt T-wave alternans represents electrical instabilities and needs protective measures. Patients with syncope or SCA in the first year of life, and patients suffering from cardiac events despite medical therapies, are considered as high risk. Patients with low risk include those with concealed mutations and asymptomatic LQT1 males.[24]

Syncope in patients with LQTs usually is a result of polymorphic VT, also described as torsades de pointes (TdP) (**Fig. 5**). It is commonly preceded by a pause followed by an extrasystole (short-long-short RR interval).[25] Bradycardia can be responsible for syncope in patients with LQT3.[26,27]

Clinical Manifestation and Diagnosis

Patients with LQTS commonly present with palpitations, presyncope, syncope, or SCA. Most patients develop ventricular arrhythmia by physical stress or emotional stress, triggered especially by loud noises or occurring while sleeping.[28–30] Triggers in LQTS are gene-specific.[31] I_{Ks} channels in LQT1 are adrenergic-sensitive.[32] The

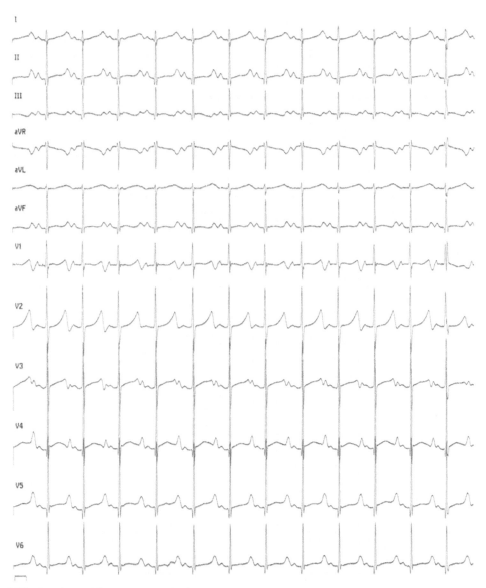

Fig. 4. ECG of patient with LQT3. Note the long isoelectric ST segment and then the late T wave. (*Courtesy of* S. Priori, MD, Pavia, Italy and A. Mazantti, MD, Pavia, Italy.)

prolongation of QT interval and cardiac events in LQT1 occur with exercise or epinephrine challenge test.[33] Patients with LQT2 often have cardiac events while asleep or triggered by an alarm clock.[34] LQT3 arises when the inactivation process of sodium channels is interfered with, and usually occurs during sleep.

A thorough history is critical to establishing a diagnosis of this syndrome in suspected cases. Imaging modalities are helpful in excluding structural abnormalities. Secondary causes of prolonged QT need to be considered before diagnosing LQTS. The Schwartz scoring system has been widely accepted for identifying LQTS,

although it does not include genetic testing.[35] A detailed family history can possibly give clues not only of cardiac history in the family but also of other unexpected deaths without apparent causes, such as dying while swimming or driving. The genetic data of affected family members can be helpful.

An exercise stress test may be helpful to demonstrate the change of QT interval with exertion.[33,36] Abnormal QTc interval (>470 milliseconds), 2 to 3 minutes after the recovery phase in exercise test, is considered abnormal.[37,38] Epinephrine challenge testing has also been used to identify patients with LQT1 gene mutations.

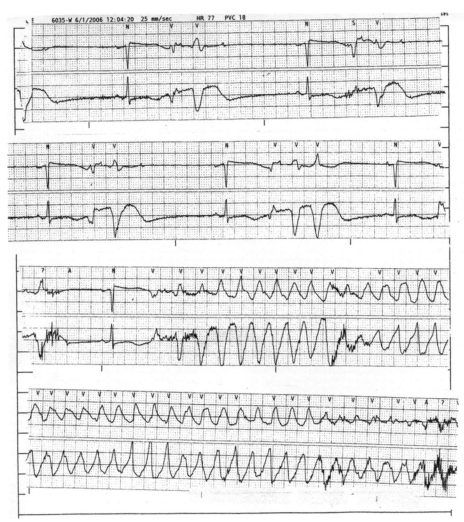

6035-W 6/1/2006 12:04:20   25 mm/sec   HR 77   PVC 18

Fig. 5. An ECG tracing of a 63-year-old man not known to have long QT. He developed a marked QTc prolongation and torsades de pointes after a single dose of dofetilide.

Genetic testing may help in suspected cases. In patients with clinical diagnosis, a genetic test can yield positivity up to 90%.[39,40] However, a negative test does not exclude the possibility of LQTS. Further analysis would help confirm the significance of positive genetic mutations related to functionality. Genetic testing may help identify concealed LQTS, because 20% to 50% of carriers have normal QTc.

Management

Because of the rarity of disease, randomized controlled trials have not been conducted. In addition, the heterogeneity in subtypes and severity further complicates the analysis of treatment strategies. The main approaches include; avoiding QT-prolonging agents; β-blockade therapy; and implantable cardioverter-defibrillators (ICDs) for those at risk of SCA.

β-Blockade therapy has been used in patients with LQTS since the 1970s, especially long-acting agents.[30] Goals of therapy aim at decreasing the exercise heart rate by 20%. Several reports have shown survival benefit in symptomatic patients with gene mutations. This effect is more apparent in LQT1 than in LQT2 and LQT3. Propranolol and nadolol have been shown to reduce the recurrence of symptoms. The mechanism of efficacy involves the blockade of late sodium currents.[41]

Left cardiac sympathetic denervation (LCSD) requires removal of ganglia T1 to T4, which results in decreased norepinephrine release at the ventricular level.[42] LCSD also helps reduce multiple shocks in patients with LQTS who have ICDs.

ICDs are widely considered in patients at high risk of sudden death, including those with symptoms before puberty, those with QTc greater than 500 milliseconds, and those with syncope while on β-blockers.

SHORT-QT SYNDROME
Background

Short-QT syndrome (SQTS) is an inherited disorder associated with a markedly short QT interval on ECGs with ventricular arrhythmia (**Fig. 6**), and was first reported relatively recently.[43] Data concerning this disease are lacking primarily because of its rarity. SQTS was first described when 4 patients with atrial arrhythmia and SCA were found to have an extremely short QT interval.[43] Since then more than 100 cases have been reported, and several studies have supported the pathophysiology of shortened QT intervals in SCA.

Genetics and Pathogenesis

Six different genes have been found to be related to SQTS. These genes encode different cardiac ion channels, and classify SQTS into 6 subtypes. Many of these gene mutations were also involved in LQTs. For example, most patients with SQT1, the most common form, were linked to *KCNH2* gene, which is found in LQT2.[44] *KCNH2* mutation is also found in Brugada-type ECGs.[45] Another example, L-type calcium channel gene mutations, were also found in some patients with SQTS, which manifests with a normal QT interval but has the features of Brugada syndrome (BS) and SQTS.[46]

The shortening of repolarization occurs with reduction in inward calcium currents or increased outward potassium currents. The curtailments of the action potential are heterogeneous in epicardium, myocardium, and endocardium. This dispersion promotes the initiation of arrhythmia in SQTS.[47,48] Premature beats that generate arrhythmia may involve a phase-2 reentry or late phase-3 reentry.[48,49] (T_{peak}-T_{end})/QT ratio was proposed as an index of dispersion of repolarization, and was found to be elevated in most cases of SQTS.[50,51]

ECG Characteristics

The shortening of QT interval is essential in establishing the diagnosis; however, the lower limit of QT interval remains unclear.[52] From reported SQT cases, the range of QT interval has frequent overlap with those QT intervals in healthy individuals. Rautaharju and colleagues[53] proposed the formula predicted QT (QTp) = 656/(1 + heart rate/100). This study demonstrated that a QT interval that was less than 88% of QTp is equivalent to 2 standard deviations below the mean of QT interval, and therefore considered abnormal. In SQTS, typical ECG findings include: QT less than 360 milliseconds; absence of ST segment; tall and peaked T waves in precordial leads; poor rate adaptation of QT interval; and prolonged T_{peak}-T_{end} and (T_{peak}-T_{end})/QT ratio.[50,51] SQTS may also have different ECG features including Brugada types or J-point elevation.[54] Measuring QT should be obtained when heart rate is less than 80 beats/min. Bazett's formula may overestimate the QT interval when the heart rate is fast;

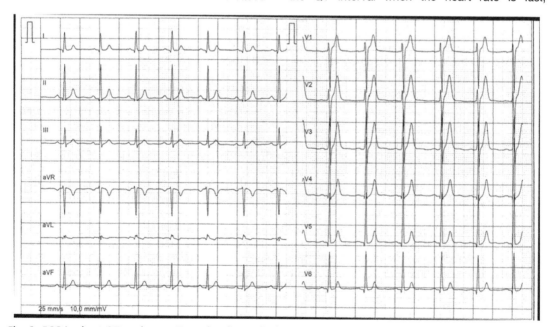

Fig. 6. ECG in short-QT syndrome. Note also the peaked T waves. (*Courtesy of* M. Borggreffee.)

therefore, Holter monitoring or long-term ECG recording is helpful for QT analysis when there is a slower heart rate. SQT subtypes have a distinctive T wave.[55] SQT1 and SQT2 generally show a symmetric tall peak T wave, whereas SQT3 has an asymmetric T wave.

Clinical Manifestation and Diagnosis

Clinical presentations of SQTS vary. Symptoms include syncope, palpitation, atrial fibrillation (AF), and SCA. Most affected patients are in the first year of life or between 20 and 40 years of age, predominantly male.[56] No apparent triggers have been identified, but from recent studies most patients experienced events while sleeping. Detailed history and physical examination are essential to establishing a diagnosis. AF is common in patients with SQTS. Therefore, SQTS should be suspected in young patients with lone AF and short QT interval. The applicability of the SQT score remains unclear. In a recent study, 5 from 8 (62%) patients with diagnosed SQT who suffered from cardiac arrest had a low score.[56]

Electrophysiologic study (EPS) may help in the diagnosis of SQTS. Most SQT patients show extremely short atrial and ventricular effective refractory periods.[55,57–59] Programmed stimulation with 3 stimuli induced both AF and VF in many patients (60%). Genetic testing may help in suspected cases based on ECG and clinical history. Because of the rarity of the disease, Gollob and colleagues[60] have proposed the diagnostic criteria for SQTS. However, these criteria still require further validation, even though the modified version has already been proposed.[60] Other possible causes should also be considered, such as normal variant SQT interval (most of the cases of SQT), drug intoxication, electrolyte imbalances, and deceleration-dependent shortening of QT interval.[43]

Treatment

If the diagnosis is definitive, the only treatment for SQTS is ICDs, because patients with SQTS are at very high risk for SCA.[61] Only 60% of cases have inducibility for ventricular arrhythmia from EPS, so a negative test should not hinder the recommendation that those with clear SQT should receive ICDs. Antiarrhythmic drugs are used as an adjunctive therapy to ICDs, unless patients refuse or are not candidates for ICDs. Data regarding pharmacotherapy for SQTS are limited, and there have been reports on medication in only SQT1.[62] Hydroquinidine, disopyramide, and amiodarone were found to prolong the QT interval.[63–65]

BRUGADA SYNDROME
Background

BS is characterized by ventricular arrhythmias mostly occurring at rest or during sleep, in the presence of fever, or after a large meal.[66,67] The prevalence varies among different populations with many of the cases involving Asians, especially in males, despite the autosomal dominant inheritance. Because the ECG patterns can be dynamic and are often concealed, it is difficult to estimate the true prevalence of BS in the general population. In reports from Japan, the prevalence of type 1 Brugada pattern ECGs were present in 0.7% to 1.0% of the population.[68,69] In 2 studies from the United States, the prevalence were found to be 0.4% and 0.012%.[70,71] Depending on the diagnostic criteria, the prevalence of BS was observed to range from 3% to 24% in patients with idiopathic VF.

Genetics and Pathogenesis

BS has autosomal dominant inheritance with variable expression. The first and most well-known mutation related to BS is the SCN5A gene mutation. This mutation leads to a defect in the α subunit of the cardiac sodium channel. However, only 18% to 30% of affected families have an identified abnormality of SCN5A genes.[72] Hence, It is possible that additional genetic abnormalities may also produce the phenotypic characteristics of BS. The defective myocardial sodium channels result in localized conduction blocks and shortened refractory periods, thereby providing arrhythmogenic substrates for localized reentry. The short coupled ventricular premature beats (VPBs) that result from phase-2 reentry may precipitate sustained ventricular arrhythmias.[73]

ECG Characteristics

The ECG findings during sinus rhythm have distinctive patterns, which can be dynamic or concealed. The classic type 1 BS includes ST elevation (>2 mm), descending with upward convexity, and inverted T wave in the right precordial leads (Fig. 7). This pattern is also called pseudo–right bundle branch block (RBBB). However, unlike RBBB, the widened and slurred S wave is absent in the Brugada pattern. Moving right precordial leads up to the second intercostal space or using bipolar chest leads may increase the sensitivity of detecting these abnormalities.[72] Type 2 and type 3 patterns have a "saddle-back" ST-T wave configuration. The ST segment descends toward the baseline, then rises again to an upright or biphasic T wave. The ST segment is elevated greater than

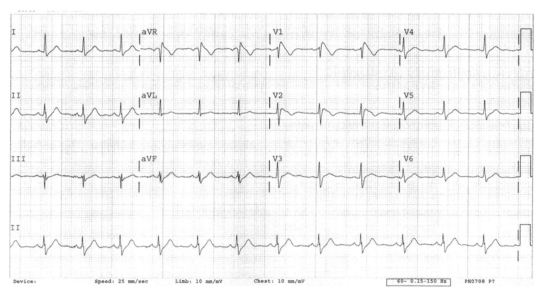

Fig. 7. A 12-lead ECG of a 41-year-old man who presented with syncope secondary to a ventricular arrhythmia. Baseline ECG is as shown. Note the ST elevation, descending with upward convexity, and inverted T wave in the right precordial leads, consistent with type 1 Brugada pattern. The patient eventually received an implantable cardioverter-defibrillator for secondary prevention.

1 mm in type 2 and <1 mm in type 3. ECG abnormalities can be accentuated by increased parasympathetic tone, fever, cocaine abuse, or psychotropic drugs, including cyclic antidepressant and neuroleptic drug overdose. Fragmented QRS (fQRS), defined as additional spikes within the QRS complex, can be found in 43% of BS patients. It is also more often seen in BS patients with VF than in those without VF, and more so in BS patients with *SCN5A* mutation than in those without *SCN5A* mutation. As a result, fQRS has been proposed to be a predictor of prognosis of BS.[74,75]

Clinical Manifestation and Diagnosis

SCA can be the first clinical event in one-third of patients. Arrhythmic events usually occur between the ages of 22 and 65 years, and are more common at night during sleep, when patients have higher parasympathetic tone. SCA is usually not related to exercise. Frequent spontaneous VPBs are often present before the onset of arrhythmia.[76] Patients with BS may also be at increased risk of atrial arrhythmia, most notably AF.[77]

BS is definitively diagnosed when a type 1 ST-segment elevation is observed in more than 1 right precordial lead (V1–V3) in the presence or absence of a sodium channel–blocking agent, and in conjunction with one of the following: documented VF, polymorphic VT, a family history of SCA at younger than 45 years, coved-type ECGs in family members, inducibility of VT with programmed electrical stimulation, syncope, or nocturnal

agonal respiration.[72] For type 2 or 3 BS pattern, the diagnosis should be considered if type 1 BS appears on challenge test with a sodium-channel blocker, in conjunction with one of the aforementioned conditions. Sodium-channel blockers can transiently induce type 1 BS changes and can also induce VPBs or VTs in patients with BS, particularly in symptomatic patients.[78] There is no consensus on the value of the EPS in predicting outcomes. EPS can be considered for assessment of supraventricular arrhythmia.

Management

For prevention of ventricular arrhythmia, patients should be advised to avoid medications that can induce arrhythmia in BS (www.BrugadaDrug.org), and fever should be treated aggressively. Unfortunately, the only therapy that has proven efficacy is ICD. ICD therapy should be considered in patients with prior SCA, history of syncope (without other explanation), or history of VT. In patients who continue to have frequent ICD discharges, antiarrhythmics can be considered. Amiodarone is the drug of choice, but quinidine is a possible alternative.[79,80] Isoproterenol is reasonable for the treatment of electrical storms. Catheter ablation over the right ventricular outflow tract epicardium[81] and endocardium[82] were found to normalize the Brugada ECG patterns and decrease episodes of ventricular arrhythmia/VF storms in recent small studies. Genetic testing, which involves sequencing of *SCN5A* mutations, should be performed in conjunction with clinical and ECG correlation, under the supervision of specialists who have expertise in this area.

CATECHOLAMINERGIC POLYMORPHIC VENTRICULAR TACHYCARDIA
Background

Catecholaminergic polymorphic ventricular tachycardia (CPVT) is a rare inherited arrhythmia syndrome, characterized by adrenergic mediated polymorphic ventricular tachyarrhythmia. The mortality rate of CPVT is extremely high, up to 50% by the age of 20 years if untreated. Estimated rates of cardiac events at 4 and 8 years were 33% and 58% in CPVT patients without β-blockade therapies. The earlier onset of the disease correlates with poorer prognosis.[83]

Genetics and Pathogenesis

Thus far there are 3 identified mutations found to be related to CPVT. The first identified, and most common, mutation is in genes encoding human cardiac ryanodine receptors (*RYR2*). This mutation is an autosomal dominant form. Recent studies have shown that other forms of mutations are associated with CPVT, namely *CASQ2* and *TRDN*. Both forms have autosomal recessive inheritance. These mutations result in spontaneous calcium release from sarcoplasmic reticulum, and eventually produce delayed afterdepolarization that may trigger arrhythmias. This pathologic spontaneous calcium release is enhanced by β-adrenergic stimulation.

ECG Characteristics

In CPVT, baseline 12-lead ECGs do not show any abnormality and cardiac imaging is typically unremarkable. Ventricular ectopies emerge with increased frequency as heart rate increases. Initially monomorphic VPBs may appear, then deteriorate to polymorphic VPBs, and eventually bidirectional or polymorphic VT, or VF (**Fig. 8**).

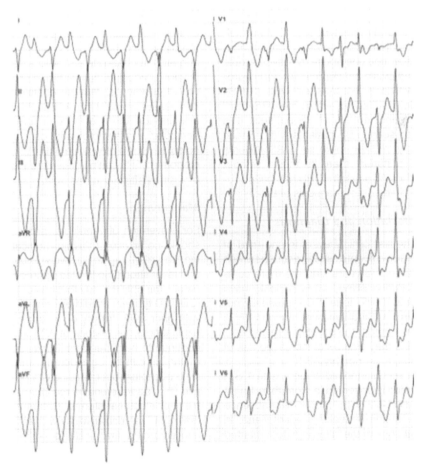

Fig. 8. Bidirectional ventricular tachycardia in a patient with catecholaminergic polymorphic ventricular tachycardia. (*Courtesy of* S. Priori, MD, Pavia, Italy and A. Mazantti, MD, Pavia, Italy.)

Although bidirectional VT is a hallmark of CPVT, its sensitivity and specificity is low. Of note, other conditions that can cause bidirectional VT include digoxin toxicity myocarditis, myocardial infarction, and Andersen-Tawil syndrome (ventricular arrhythmias, periodic paralysis, and dysmorphic features.)

Clinical Presentation and Diagnosis

Classic CPVT usually presents at the age of 3 to16 years with syncope, aborted SCA, or SCA. Patients with CPVT tend to experience an event during emotional or physical stress, including swimming. RYR2 mutations have also been identified in sudden infant death syndrome. The gold standard for diagnosis is exercise testing with a treadmill or a bicycle ergometer. During the exercise testing, typical arrhythmia usually starts with VPBs, with left bundle branch block (LBBB) superior-axis and RBBB inferior-axis morphologies. VPBs can progress to bidirectional VTs, characterized by an RBBB pattern with 180° alternating QRS axis from beat to beat. Eventually, ventricular arrhythmia can deteriorate to VF. Supraventricular tachycardia has also been reported during exercise testing. Epinephrine infusion has lower sensitivity than exercise testing, and programmed ventricular pacing in EPS unreliably triggers ventricular arrhythmia.

Management

Because of the high mortality rate, all clinically or genetically diagnosed CPVT patients should be aggressively treated. Patients are advised to avoid competitive sports. β-Blockers are the mainstay of medical treatment, and the highest tolerable dose is recommended. Flecanide has been proposed to have some efficacy in CPVT. LCSD has been reported to have excellent results in patients who are not well controlled by medical treatment. ICD therapy is recommended in patients with previous aborted cardiac arrest and those with sustained or intolerant VT despite β-blocker treatment. However, several case reports have reported that ICD may be proarrhythmic because of appropriate and inappropriate shocks causing increased catecholamine release and triggered ventricular storms. A recent retrospective review of 24 patients reported that the efficacy of ICD in CPVT depends on the mechanism of arrhythmia. VFs are uniformly treated with shock therapies, but polymorphic bidirectional VTs are not.[84] Family screening is mandatory because most common mutations in CPVTs, RYR2 gene mutations, are autosomal dominant. Asymptomatic carriers of RYR2 mutations are often detected. A small number of the mutation carriers have apparently normal phenotype, even with provocative tests; however, they do experience syncope and SCA. This finding implies that asymptomatic patients are not guaranteed protection from the occurrence of polymorphic VT.[85]

REFERENCES

1. Napolitano C, Bloise R, Monteforte N, et al. Sudden cardiac death and genetic ion channelopathies: long QT, Brugada, short QT, catecholaminergic polymorphic ventricular tachycardia, and idiopathic ventricular fibrillation. Circulation 2012;125: 2027–34.
2. Nathani P, Shetty S, Lokhandwala Y. Ventricular tachycardia in structurally normal hearts: recognition and management. J Assoc Physicians India 2007;55(Suppl):33–8.
3. Srivathsan K, Lester SJ, Appleton CP, et al. Ventricular tachycardia in the absence of structural heart disease. Indian Pacing Electrophysiol J 2005;5: 106–21.
4. Jervell A, Lange-Nielsen F. Congenital deafmutism, functional heart disease with prolongation of the Q-T interval and sudden death. Am Heart J 1957;51:59–68.
5. Romano C, Gemme G, Pongiglione R. Rare cardiac arrhythmia of the pediatric age. II. Syncopal attacks due to paroxysmal ventricular fibrillation. (presentation of the first case in Italian pediatric literature). Clin Pediatr (Bologna) 1963;45:656–83 [in Italian].
6. Splawski I, Shen J, Timothy KW, et al. Spectrum of mutations in long-QT syndrome genes. KVLQT1, HERG, SCN5A, KCNE1, and KCNE2. Circulation 2000;102:1178–85.
7. Schwartz PJ, Crotti L, Insolia R. Long-QT syndrome: from genetics to management. Circ Arrhythm Electrophysiol 2012;5:868–77.
8. Ackerman MJ, Priori SG, Willems S, Berul C, et al. HRS/EHRA expert consensus statement on the state of genetic testing for the channelopathies and cardiomyopathies: this document was developed as a partnership between the Heart Rhythm Society (HRS) and the European Heart Rhythm Association (EHRA). Europace 2011;13:1077–109.
9. Moss AJ, Kass RS. Long QT syndrome: from channels to cardiac arrhythmias. J Clin Invest 2005;115: 2018–24.
10. Goldenberg I, Moss AJ. Long QT syndrome. J Am Coll Cardiol 2008;51:2291–300.
11. Rautaharju PM, Surawicz B, Gettes LS, et al, American Heart Association Electrocardiography and Arrhythmias Committee, Council on Clinical Cardiology, American College of Cardiology Foundation, Heart Rhythm Society. AHA/ACCF/HRS

recommendations for the standardization and interpretation of the electrocardiogram: part IV: the ST segment, T and U waves, and the QT interval: a scientific statement from the American Heart Association Electrocardiography and Arrhythmias Committee, Council on Clinical Cardiology; the American College of Cardiology Foundation; and the Heart Rhythm Society. Endorsed by the International Society for Computerized Electrocardiology. J Am Coll Cardiol 2009;53:982–91.

12. Ackerman MJ, Khositseth A, Tester DJ. Congenital long QT syndrome in electrical diseases of the heart; genetic mechanism, treatment, prevention. New York: Springer Publishing; 2008. p. 462–82.

13. Schwartz PJ, Ackerman MJ. The long QT syndrome: a transatlantic clinical approach to diagnosis and therapy. Eur Heart J 2013;34:3109–16.

14. Perkiomaki JS, Zareba W, Nomura A, et al. Repolarization dynamics in patients with long QT syndrome. J Cardiovasc Electrophysiol 2002;13: 651–6.

15. Cowan JC, Yusoff K, Moore M, et al. Importance of lead selection in QT interval measurement. Am J Cardiol 1988;61:83–7.

16. Bazzett H. An analysis of the time-relations of electrocardiograms. Ann Noninvasive Electrocardiol 1997;2:177–94.

17. Luo S, Michler K, Johnston P, et al. A comparison of commonly used QT correction formulae: the effect of heart rate on the QTc of normal ECGs. J Electrocardiol 2004;37(Suppl):81–90.

18. Moss AJ, Zareba W, Benhorin J, et al. ECG T-wave patterns in genetically distinct forms of the hereditary long QT syndrome. Circulation 1995;92:2929–34.

19. Zareba W, Moss AJ, le Cessie S, et al. T wave alternans in idiopathic long QT syndrome. J Am Coll Cardiol 1994;23:1541–6.

20. Priori SG, Schwartz PJ, Napolitano C, et al. Risk stratification in the long-QT syndrome. N Engl J Med 2003;348:1866–74.

21. Kimbrough J, Moss AJ, Zareba W, et al. Clinical implications for affected parents and siblings of probands with long-QT syndrome. Circulation 2001; 104:557–62.

22. Hobbs JB, Peterson DR, Moss AJ, et al. Risk of aborted cardiac arrest or sudden cardiac death during adolescence in the long-QT syndrome. JAMA 2006;296:1249–54.

23. Sauer AJ, Moss AJ, McNitt S, et al. Long QT syndrome in adults. J Am Coll Cardiol 2007;49:329–37.

24. Priori SG, Wilde AA, Horie M, et al, Document Reviewers. Executive summary: HRS/EHRA/APHRS expert consensus statement on the diagnosis and management of patients with inherited primary arrhythmia syndromes. Europace 2013;15: 1389–406.

25. Viskin S, Fish R, Zeltser D, et al. Arrhythmias in the congenital long QT syndrome: how often is torsade de pointes pause dependent? Heart 2000;83:661–6.

26. Viskin S, Alla SR, Barron HV, et al. Mode of onset of torsade de pointes in congenital long QT syndrome. J Am Coll Cardiol 1996;28:1262–8.

27. Lupoglazoff JM, Denjoy I, Villain E, et al. Long QT syndrome in neonates: conduction disorders associated with HERG mutations and sinus bradycardia with KCNQ1 mutations. J Am Coll Cardiol 2004;43: 826–30.

28. Moss AJ, McDonald J. Unilateral cervicothoracic sympathetic ganglionectomy for the treatment of long QT interval syndrome. N Engl J Med 1971; 285:903–4.

29. Moss AJ, Schwartz PJ, Crampton RS, et al. The long QT syndrome: a prospective international study. Circulation 1985;71:17–21.

30. Schwartz PJ, Periti M, Malliani A. The long Q-T syndrome. Am Heart J 1975;89:378–90.

31. Kapplinger JD, Landstrom AP, Salisbury BA, et al. Distinguishing arrhythmogenic right ventricular cardiomyopathy/dysplasia-associated mutations from background genetic noise. J Am Coll Cardiol 2011;57:2317–27.

32. Wang Q, Curran ME, Splawski I, et al. Positional cloning of a novel potassium channel gene: KVLQT1 mutations cause cardiac arrhythmias. Nat Genet 1996;12:17–23.

33. Vyas H, Hejlik J, Ackerman MJ. Epinephrine QT stress testing in the evaluation of congenital long-QT syndrome: diagnostic accuracy of the paradoxical QT response. Circulation 2006;113:1385–92.

34. Schwartz PJ, Priori SG, Spazzolini C, et al. Genotype-phenotype correlation in the long-QT syndrome: gene-specific triggers for life-threatening arrhythmias. Circulation 2001;103:89–95.

35. Schwartz PJ, Moss AJ, Vincent GM, et al. Diagnostic criteria for the long QT syndrome. An update. Circulation 1993;88:782–4.

36. Swan H, Viitasalo M, Piippo K, et al. Sinus node function and ventricular repolarization during exercise stress test in long QT syndrome patients with KvLQT1 and HERG potassium channel defects. J Am Coll Cardiol 1999;34:823–9.

37. Schwartz PJ, Crotti L. QTc behavior during exercise and genetic testing for the long-QT syndrome. Circulation 2011;124:2181–4.

38. Horner JM, Horner MM, Ackerman MJ. The diagnostic utility of recovery phase QTc during treadmill exercise stress testing in the evaluation of long QT syndrome. Heart Rhythm 2011;8:1698–704.

39. Tester DJ, Will ML, Haglund CM, et al. Effect of clinical phenotype on yield of long QT syndrome genetic testing. J Am Coll Cardiol 2006;47:764–8.

40. Van Langen IM, Birnie E, Alders M, et al. The use of genotype-phenotype correlations in mutation

analysis for the long QT syndrome. J Med Genet 2003;40:141–5.

41. Besana A, Wang DW, George AL Jr, et al. Nadolol block of Nav1.5 does not explain its efficacy in the long QT syndrome. J Cardiovasc Pharmacol 2012; 59:249–53.

42. Schwartz PJ, Stone HL. Left stellectomy and denervation supersensitivity in conscious dogs. Am J Cardiol 1982;49:1185–90.

43. Gussak I, Brugada P, Brugada J, et al. Idiopathic short QT interval: a new clinical syndrome? Cardiology 2000;94:99–102.

44. Tester DJ, Ackerman MJ. Genetics of cardiac arrhythmia. In: Libby P, BR, Mann DL, et al, editors. Braunwald's heart disease. 9th edition. Philadelphia: Saunders; 2012. p. 81–90.

45. Sun Y, Quan XQ, Fromme S, et al. A novel mutation in the KCNH2 gene associated with short QT syndrome. J Mol Cell Cardiol 2011;50:433–41.

46. Templin C, Ghadri JR, Rougier JS, et al. Identification of a novel loss-of-function calcium channel gene mutation in short QT syndrome (SQTS6). Eur Heart J 2011;32:1077–88.

47. Patel C, Antzelevitch C. Cellular basis for arrhythmogenesis in an experimental model of the SQT1 form of the short QT syndrome. Heart Rhythm 2008;5:585–90.

48. Extramiana F, Antzelevitch C. Amplified transmural dispersion of repolarization as the basis for arrhythmogenesis in a canine ventricular-wedge model of short-QT syndrome. Circulation 2004;110:3661–6.

49. Burashnikov A, Antzelevitch C. Late-phase 3 EAD. A unique mechanism contributing to initiation of atrial fibrillation. Pacing Clin Electrophysiol 2006; 29:290–5.

50. Anttonen O, Vaananen H, Junttila J, et al. Electrocardiographic transmural dispersion of repolarization in patients with inherited short QT syndrome. Ann Noninvasive Electrocardiol 2008;13:295–300.

51. Gupta P, Patel C, Patel H, et al. T(p-e)/QT ratio as an index of arrhythmogenesis. J Electrocardiol 2008;41:567–74.

52. Cross B, Homoud M, Link M, et al. The short QT syndrome. J Interv Card Electrophysiol 2011;31: 25–31.

53. Rautaharju PM, Zhou SH, Wong S, et al. Sex differences in the evolution of the electrocardiographic QT interval with age. Can J Cardiol 1992;8:690–5.

54. Antzelevitch C, Pollevick GD, Cordeiro JM, et al. Loss-of-function mutations in the cardiac calcium channel underlie a new clinical entity characterized by ST-segment elevation, short QT intervals, and sudden cardiac death. Circulation 2007;115: 442–9.

55. Priori SG, Pandit SV, Rivolta I, et al. A novel form of short QT syndrome (SQT3) is caused by a mutation in the KCNJ2 gene. Circ Res 2005;96:800–7.

56. Mazzanti A, Kanthan A, Monteforte N, et al. Novel insights in the natural history of Short QT Syndrome. J Am Coll Cardiol 2013;63:1300–8.

57. Gaita F, Giustetto C, Bianchi F, et al. Short QT syndrome: a familial cause of sudden death. Circulation 2003;108:965–70.

58. Giustetto C, Di Monte F, Wolpert C, et al. Short QT syndrome: clinical findings and diagnostic-therapeutic implications. Eur Heart J 2006;27:2440–7.

59. Bellocq C, van Ginneken AC, Bezzina CR, et al. Mutation in the KCNQ1 gene leading to the short QT-interval syndrome. Circulation 2004;109: 2394–7.

60. Gollob MH, Redpath CJ, Roberts JD. The short QT syndrome: proposed diagnostic criteria. J Am Coll Cardiol 2011;57:802–12.

61. Bjerregaard P, Gussak I. Short QT syndrome: mechanisms, diagnosis and treatment. Nat Clin Pract Cardiovasc Med 2005;2:84–7.

62. Gaita F, Giustetto C, Bianchi F, et al. Short QT syndrome: pharmacological treatment. J Am Coll Cardiol 2004;43:1494–9.

63. Mizobuchi M, Enjoji Y, Yamamoto R, et al. Nifekalant and disopyramide in a patient with short QT syndrome: evaluation of pharmacological effects and electrophysiological properties. Pacing Clin Electrophysiol 2008;31:1229–32.

64. Lu LX, Zhou W, Zhang X, et al. Short QT syndrome: a case report and review of literature. Resuscitation 2006;71:115–21.

65. Giustetto C, Schimpf R, Mazzanti A, et al. Long-term follow-up of patients with short QT syndrome. J Am Coll Cardiol 2011;58:587–95.

66. Amin AS, Meregalli PG, Bardai A, et al. Fever increases the risk for cardiac arrest in the Brugada syndrome. Ann Intern Med 2008;149:216–8.

67. Ikeda T, Abe A, Yusu S, et al. The full stomach test as a novel diagnostic technique for identifying patients at risk of Brugada syndrome. J Cardiovasc Electrophysiol 2006;17:602–7.

68. Matsuo K, Akahoshi M, Nakashima E, et al. The prevalence, incidence and prognostic value of the Brugada-type electrocardiogram: a population-based study of four decades. J Am Coll Cardiol 2001;38:765–70.

69. Miyasaka Y, Tsuji H, Yamada K, et al. Prevalence and mortality of the Brugada-type electrocardiogram in one city in Japan. J Am Coll Cardiol 2001;38:771–4.

70. Monroe MH, Littmann L. Two-year case collection of the Brugada syndrome electrocardiogram pattern at a large teaching hospital. Clin Cardiol 2000;23:849–51.

71. Patel SS, Anees S, Ferrick KJ. Prevalence of a Brugada pattern electrocardiogram in an urban population in the United States. Pacing Clin Electrophysiol 2009;32:704–8.

72. Antzelevitch CBP, Borggrefe M, Brugada J, et al. Brugada syndrome: report of the second consensus conference. Heart Rhythm 2005;2: 429–40.

73. Aiba T, Shimizu W, Hidaka I, et al. Cellular basis for trigger and maintenance of ventricular fibrillation in the Brugada syndrome model: high-resolution optical mapping study. J Am Coll Cardiol 2006;47: 2074–85.

74. Priori SG, Gasparini M, Napolitano C, et al. Risk stratification in Brugada syndrome: results of the PRELUDE (PRogrammed ELectrical stimUlation preDictive valuE) registry. J Am Coll Cardiol 2012; 59:37–45.

75. Morita H, Kusano KF, Miura D, et al. Fragmented QRS as a marker of conduction abnormality and a predictor of prognosis of Brugada syndrome. Circulation 2008;118:1697–704.

76. Kakishita M, Kurita T, Matsuo K, et al. Mode of onset of ventricular fibrillation in patients with Brugada syndrome detected by implantable cardioverter defibrillator therapy. J Am Coll Cardiol 2000;36:1646–53.

77. Kusano KF, Taniyama M, Nakamura K, et al. Atrial fibrillation in patients with Brugada syndrome relationships of gene mutation, electrophysiology, and clinical backgrounds. J Am Coll Cardiol 2008;51: 1169–75.

78. Morita H, Morita ST, Nagase S, et al. Ventricular arrhythmia induced by sodium channel blocker in patients with Brugada syndrome. J Am Coll Cardiol 2003;42:1624–31.

79. Belhassen B, Glick A, Viskin S. Efficacy of quinidine in high-risk patients with Brugada syndrome. Circulation 2004;110:1731–7.

80. Marquez MF, Salica G, Hermosillo AG, et al. Ionic basis of pharmacological therapy in Brugada syndrome. J Cardiovasc Electrophysiol 2007;18:234–40.

81. Nademanee K, Veerakul G, Chandanamattha P, et al. Prevention of ventricular fibrillation episodes in Brugada syndrome by catheter ablation over the anterior right ventricular outflow tract epicardium. Circulation 2011;123:1270–9.

82. Sunsaneewitayakul B, Yao Y, Thamaree S, et al. Endocardial mapping and catheter ablation for ventricular fibrillation prevention in Brugada syndrome. J Cardiovasc Electrophysiol 2012;23(Suppl 1): S10–6.

83. Leenhardt A, Denjoy I, Guicheney P. Catecholaminergic polymorphic ventricular tachycardia. Circ Arrhythm Electrophysiol 2012;5:1044–52.

84. Miyake CY, Webster G, Czosek RJ, et al. Efficacy of implantable cardioverter defibrillators in young patients with catecholaminergic polymorphic ventricular tachycardia: success depends on substrate. Circ Arrhythm Electrophysiol 2013;6:579–87.

85. Hayashi M, Denjoy I, Extramiana F, et al. Incidence and risk factors of arrhythmic events in catecholaminergic polymorphic ventricular tachycardia. Circulation 2009;119:2426–34.

Electrophysiological Basis of ECG Characteristics of Torsades de Pointes in Long QT Syndrome

Nabil El-Sherif, MD[a,b,*], Gioia Turitto, MD[c],
Mohamed Boutjdir, PhD[a], Sajin Pilai, MD[d], Bryan Otte, MA[e],
Roland Pedalino, MD[f]

KEYWORDS

- Long QT syndrome • Torsades de pointes • Dispersion of repolarization • Bigeminal rhythm
- T-wave alternans • Mapping

KEY POINTS

- In the long QT syndrome, prolonged repolarization is associated with increased spatial dispersion of repolarization.
- Prolongation of repolarization also acts as a primary step for the generation of early afterdepolarizations (EADs).
- The focal EAD-induced triggered beats can infringe on the underlying substrate of inhomogeneous repolarization to initiate polymorphic reentrant ventricular tachycardia.

INTRODUCTION

Both congenital and acquired long QT syndromes (LQTS) are caused by abnormalities (intrinsic and/or acquired) of the ionic currents underlying repolarization. Prolongation of the repolarization phase acts as a primary step for the generation of early afterdepolarizations (EADs). EAD-induced triggered beats arise predominantly from the Purkinje network.[1] In LQTS, prolonged repolarization is associated with increased spatial dispersion of repolarization.[2,3] The focal EAD-induced triggered beats can infringe on the underlying substrate of inhomogeneous repolarization to initiate polymorphic reentrant ventricular tachycardia (VT).[3] Torsades de pointes (TdP) is an ear-pleasing term that describes an eye-catching form of polymorphic VT. The term was first coined by Dessertenne[4] who described its electrocardiographic (ECG) pattern of continuously changing morphology of the QRS complexes that seem to twist around an imaginary baseline. The quasi-musical term and the intriguing ECG pattern have caught the attention of electrophysiologists for years and have been, to some extent, a driving force behind the focused interest into the role of genetics and cardiac ion channel pathophysiology in cardiac arrhythmias in general.[5] More importantly, it is useful to focus attention on the role of dispersion of ventricular repolarization in the genesis of malignant VTs.

There is more than one electrophysiologic mechanism for polymorphic VT, and an understanding of these mechanisms can be of valuable help in the proper management of individual

Supported in part by Veterans Administration and the Narrows Institute for Biomedical Research.
[a] State University of New York, Downstate Medical Center, Brooklyn, New York; [b] Cardiology Division, New York Harbor VA Healthcare System, Brooklyn, New York; [c] Electrophysiology Service, New York Methodist Hospital, Brooklyn, New York; [d] Cardiac Telemetry Service, New York Harbor VA Healthcare System, Brooklyn, New York; [e] Cardiology Research Program, New York Harbor VA Healthcare System, Brooklyn, New York; [f] Cardiology Section, Kings County Hospital, Brooklyn, New York
* Corresponding author.
E-mail address: nelsherif@aol.com

Card Electrophysiol Clin 6 (2014) 433–444
http://dx.doi.org/10.1016/j.ccep.2014.05.011
1877-9182/14/$ – see front matter Published by Elsevier Inc.

patients. The most appropriate way to classify polymorphic VT is whether it is associated with normal or prolonged QT interval. The electrophysiologic mechanisms of these 2 types of polymorphic VT may be different. The term *TdP* should be reserved for use with the LQTS. However, not all patients with LQTS have polymorphic VT with a characteristic TdP configuration[6]; this classic configuration can be seen in some cases without a prolonged QT interval.[7]

ECG CHARACTERISTICS OF TDP

In an analysis of more than 250 different episodes of nonsustained VT obtained from 54 patients with congenital or acquired LQTS, the arrhythmia

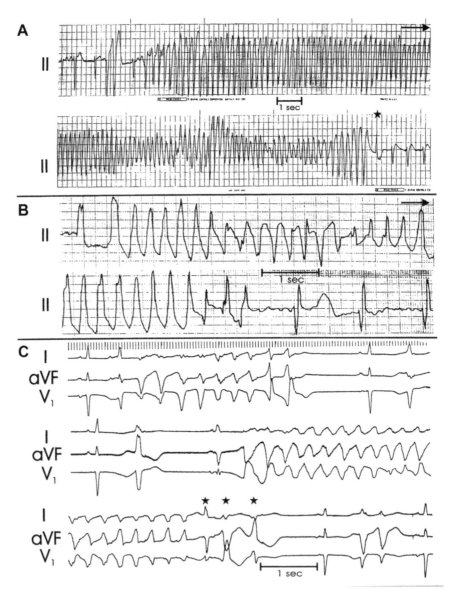

Fig. 1. Three ECG examples of acquired LQTS and TdP. (*A*) ECG of a 23-year-old woman who was positive for human immunodeficiency virus and receiving pentamidine. The patient was admitted with severe diarrhea and hypokalemia. (*B*) ECG of a 62-year-old man with hypertension and chronic atrial fibrillation who was receiving digoxin and hydrochlorothiazide and had a potassium level of 3.2 mEq/L. The TdP tachycardia developed 12 hours after the patient received a total of 4 tablets of quinidine gluconate in an attempt to restore normal sinus rhythm. (*C*) ECG of a 64-year-old man receiving procainamide for suppression of very frequent ventricular premature complexes. Stars mark ectopic beats. The horizontal *arrow* in panels *A* and *B* represent continuous recordings. (*From* El-Sherif N, Turitto G. The long QT syndrome and torsade de pointes. Pacing Clin Electrophysiol 1999;22:91–110; with permission.)

ranged in length from 3 beats (the definition of non-sustained VT) up to 156 beats (**Fig. 1A**), with an average length of 18 ± 8 beats. The cycle length (CL) of these episodes ranged from 186 to 399 milliseconds, with an average of 276 ± 42 milliseconds. The VT was frequently preceded by a variable period of bigeminal rhythm caused by one or 2 premature ventricular beats coupled to the prolonged QT segment of the preceding basic beat (see **Fig. 1A, C**). Following the termination of an episode of fast VT, it is not uncommon to see one or more ectopic beats of variable configuration occurring at a much longer CL compared with that of the VT (see beats marked by stars in **Fig. 1**). The change in the QRS configuration

during VT can take several forms. During a very fast VT, periodic decrease in the amplitude of the entire QRS-T complex is seen with less distinct shifts in the QRS axis (see **Fig. 1A**). In VTs with relatively slower rates, the classic twisting of the QRS axis from a predominantly positive to a predominantly negative configuration with a variable number of transitional complexes and vice versa is commonly seen (see **Fig. 1B**). Sometimes, a polymorphic QRS configuration is seen without any of the 2 previously characteristic patterns (as verified in multiple simultaneous leads, see **Fig. 1C**, middle recording). Different patterns can be seen in different VT episodes from the same patient (see **Fig. 1C**).

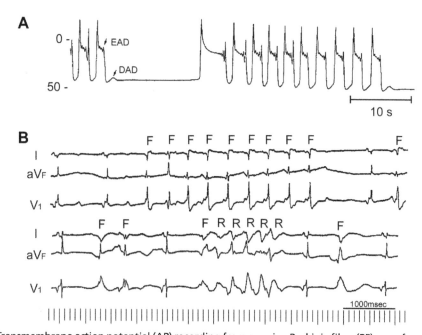

Fig. 2. (A) Transmembrane action potential (AP) recording from a canine Purkinje fiber (PF) superfused with 20 mM cesium chloride (a surrogate experimental model for LQT2). The recording illustrates the bradycardia-dependent prolongation of AP duration associated with membrane oscillation characteristic of EADs. It also shows that complete repolarization of the AP is followed by a subthreshold delayed afterdepolarization (DAD). The latter is explained by increased intracellular Ca^{2+} associated with the prolonged AP duration triggering a transient inward current. This almost-forgotten observation strongly suggests that some VT and ectopic beats in LQTS could be secondary to DADs. (B) Corroboration of the observation in (A) from the canine AP-A surrogate model of LQT3. The top ECG tracing was obtained 10 minutes after infusion of AP-A and shows moderate prolongation of the QT interval and a run of nonsustained monomorphic VT at a rate of 150 beats per minute. The VT starts with a late couple beat that is well beyond the end of the QT interval of the preceding sinus beat. Tridimensional mapping of activation showed that the VT arose as a focal discharge (F) from the same subendocardial site. For all practical purposes, the F could be attributed to DAD-triggered activity. The bottom ECG tracing was obtained from the same experiment 10 minutes later and shows further prolongation of the QT interval. The ectopic beats labeled F now seem to be coupled to the end of the prolonged QT interval of the preceding sinus beats. The middle of the tracing illustrates a 6-beat run of polymorphic VT. Tridimensional mapping shows that the first beat arose from a subendocardial focal site attributed to EAD-triggered activity, whereas subsequent beats were caused by reentrant excitation (R) in the form of continuously varying scroll waves. (*From* [A] Hoffman BF, Rosen MR. Cellular mechanisms for cardiac arrhythmias. Circ Res 1981;49:1–15, with permission; and [B] El-Sherif N. Mechanism of ventricular arrhythmias in the long QT syndrome: on hermeneutics. J Cardiovasc Electrophysiol 2001;12:973–6, with permission.)

436

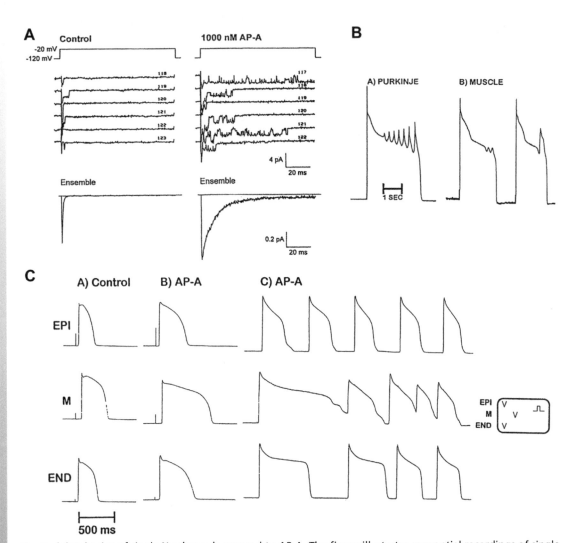

Fig. 3. (*A*) Behavior of single Na channels exposed to AP-A. The figure illustrates sequential recordings of single Na channel current responses during depolarizing steps from −120 to −20 mV from rabbit cardiac myocytes. (*Left panel*) Recordings under control conditions. (*Right panel*) Recordings from a patch exposed to 1000 nM of AP-A. At −20 mV, control Na channels opened briefly, on average only once, very soon after the potential step. In contrast, Na channels exposed to AP-A showed long-lasting bursts consisting of repetitive long openings interrupted by brief closures. Some of the bursts lasted for the entire duration of the potential step. The ensemble currents from both patches are shown on the bottom. The control ensemble current shows fast relaxation. Conversely, the ensemble current of the Na channel exposed to AP-A shows markedly slowed relaxation, with the current failing to relax completely by the end of the 95-m step. Kinetic analysis suggested that AP-A results in modal gating behavior of the Na channel. (*B*) AP recordings from a Purkinje fiber (PF) in an endocardial preparation and from a midmyocardial (M) cell, from a transmural strip, both isolated from the left ventricle of a 10-week-old puppy and placed in the same chamber and superfused with 50 µg/L AP-A. The 2 preparations were stimulated at a CL of 3000 milliseconds. The PF shows a series of EADs that increased gradually in amplitude before final repolarization. However, the first AP of the M cell showed marked prolongation of APD and low amplitude EADs at the end of phase 2. The subsequent AP showed the occurrence of a potential at the end of phase 2 that is more representative of an electrotonic interaction rather than an EAD. This observation is emphasized in (*C*), which shows simultaneous recordings from a subepicardial (EPI) cell, M cell, and a subendocardial (END) cell from a transmural strip isolated from the left ventricle of a 12-week-old puppy and transfused with 50 µg/L AP-A. The preparation was stimulated at a CL of 4000 milliseconds. Control recordings show the characteristic prolongation of APD of the M cell compared with EPI and END cells. AP-A resulted in prolongation of all 3 cell types, but the effect was more marked in the M cell. (*C*) Spontaneous regular activity arose in the preparation at a CL of 1200 milliseconds. There was a 1:1 response in the EPI cell but irregular responses in the M and END cells. In particular, the M cell, which had a markedly prolonged APD, showed an inflection on phase 3, suggestive of electrotonic interaction. There was also evidence of asynchronous activation in the preparation (possible substrate for reentrant excitation). (*From* El-Sherif N, Turitto G. The long QT syndrome and torsade de pointes. Pacing Clin Electrophysiol 1999;22:91–110; with permission.)

Monomorphic nonsustained VT is infrequently seen in patients with LQTS.[6] The rate of the monomorphic VT is relatively slow compared with the more common polymorphic VT in the same patient. The same phenomenon was also seen in the AP-A surrogate model of LQT3 (**Fig. 2**). The monomorphic VT was caused by repetitive unifocal activity, which is most probably caused by delayed afterdepolarization (DAD)–triggered activity.[8] This could be understood considering that the prolonged action potential (AP), the hallmark of LQTS, is associated with elevated intracellular calcium and the tendency to develop DADs following the spontaneous termination of the fast polymorphic VT. This mechanism is also the probable explanation of the beats marked by stars in **Fig. 1**.

A PARADIGM OF TDP FROM ION CHANNELS TO ECG

An in vivo canine model of LQTS and TdP was developed using the neurotoxins Anthopleurin-A (AP-A)[9] or ATX-II.[10] These agents act by slowing sodium (Na) channel inactivation resulting in a sustained inward current during the plateau and prolongation of the AP duration (APD).[11,12] The experimental model anticipated by 7 years the discovery of a genetic mutation of the Na channel subunit (SCN5A) in patients with LQT3.[13] The mutant channels were shown to generate a sustained inward current during depolarization quite similar to the Na channel exposed to AP-A or ATX-II.[14] Although the model is a surrogate of LQT3, the basic electrophysiologic mechanism of TdP in this model seems to apply, with some necessary modifications to all forms of congenital and acquired LQTS. In a series of reports, a paradigm of the mechanisms of TdP that extends from an ion channel abnormality to an arrhythmia with a characteristic ECG morphology was elucidated.[3,8–12,15]

Fig. 3A illustrates the behavior of single Na channels exposed to AP-A. **Fig. 3**B demonstrates the effects of AP-A on the AP of a canine Purkinje fiber (PF) from an endocardial preparation and a midmyocardial (M) cell from a transmural strip that were placed in the same chamber and superfused with the same concentration of AP-A. The drug resulted in prolongation of the APD of the PF and the development of a series of EADs. However, the drug resulted in marked prolongation of APD of the M cell and low-amplitude EADs at the end of phase 2. The subsequent AP showed the occurrence of a potential at the end of phase 2 that is more representative of an electrotonic interaction rather than an EAD. This observation is emphasized in **Fig. 3**C, which shows simultaneous recordings from a subepicardial (Epi) cell, M cell,

and a subendocardial (End) cell from a transmural strip isolated from the left ventricular (LV) free wall of a 12-week-old puppy and superfused with AP-A. The recording illustrates the differential marked lengthening of the AP of the M cell compared with both Epi and End cells; the development of conduction block between the Epi and M cells and the occurrence of asynchronous activation in the slice is suggestive of reentrant excitation.

THE MECHANISM OF TWISTING QRS MORPHOLOGY OF TDP

Since the initial description of TdP tachyarrhythmia by Dessertenne,[4] many electrophysiologists have been intrigued by the QRS morphologic characteristic of the arrhythmia, sometimes at the expense of proposing a cohesive electrophysiologic mechanism. The original hypothesis proposed by Dessertenne[4] was that the change of the QRS axis was caused by 2 competing foci. Several investigators proposed explanations based on shifting circus movement reentry. In a study of reentrant activity in isolated cardiac muscle, Pertsov and colleagues[16] suggested that a spiral wave of reentrant excitation migrating along the epicardial surface could explain the twisting QRS morphology of TdP. Abildskov and Lux[17] used a computer model consisting of a pathway with short refractory periods bisecting regions with longer refractory periods. Premature stimulation from the region with shorter refractoriness initiated figure-8 circus movement reentry with progressive migration of the site of the reentrant circuit. A contrasting hypothetical model by Antzelevitch and Sicouri[2] proposed an M column of functional barrier created by the population of M cells with longer refractory periods. A premature activation wave front arising outside the barrier would propagate along the edge of the column, enter the M region after expiration of its refractoriness, and then reenter at the border to initiate circus movement. Repetition of this type of circus movement with progressively shifting sites of reentry could yield the electrical migration characteristic of TdP.

The authors have described a novel mechanism for the classic twisting configuration of the QRS of TdP arrhythmia in the AP-A surrogate model of LQT3. The transition of the QRS axis was attributed to bifurcation of a single circulating wave front into 2 simultaneous independent wave fronts, followed by termination (extinction) of one of the wave fronts.[15] A period of transitional complexes covering more than one cycle is associated with a gradual dominance of one of the 2 wave fronts before termination of the other wave front (**Fig. 4**).

SHORT-LONG CARDIAC SEQUENCE AND THE ONSET OF TDP

One or more short-long cardiac cycles, usually the result of a ventricular bigeminal rhythm, frequently precede the onset of malignant ventricular tachyarrhythmias. This is seen in patients with organic heart disease and apparently normal QT intervals[18] as well as in patients with either the congenital[19] or acquired[20,21] LQTS (see **Fig 1A**). The electrophysiological mechanisms that underlie this relationship was investigated in the canine AP-A model.[22] The bigeminal beats consistently arose from an End focal activity from the same or different sites, whereas TdP was caused by encroachment of the focal activity on a substrate of dispersion of repolarization to induce reentrant

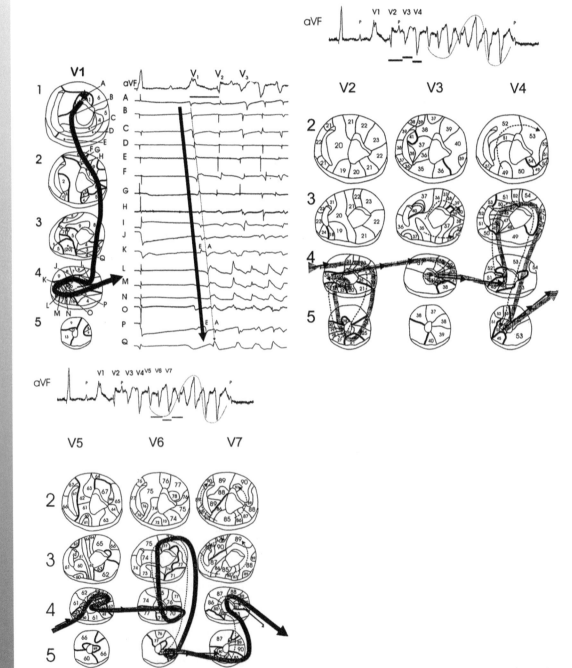

Fig. 4. Tridimensional ventricular activation patterns of a 12-beat nonsustained TdP VT. See Figure legend on opposite page.

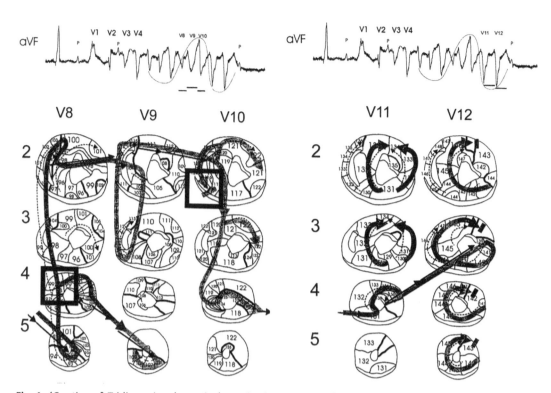

Fig. 4. (*Continued*) Tridimensional ventricular activation patterns of a 12-beat nonsustained TdP VT. The maps are presented as if the heart was cut transversely into 5 sections, oriented with the basal section on top and the apical section on bottom, and labeled 1 to 5. The activation isochrones were drawn as closed contour at 20-millisecond intervals and labeled as 1, 2, 3 and so on to make it easier to follow the activation patterns of successive beats of the VT. Functional conduction block is represented in the maps by heavy solid lines. The thick bars under the surface ECG lead mark the time intervals covered by each of the tridimensional maps. The V1 beat arose as a focal subendocardial activity (*star in section 1*). The selected local electrograms recorded along the reentrant pathway during the V1 illustrate complete diastolic bridging during the first reentrant cycle of 400-millisecond duration. Bipolar electrograms recorded from the very slow conducting component of the circuit in section 4 had a wide multicomponent configuration. Electrograms recorded in close proximity to arcs of functional conduction block had double potentials representing an electrotonic potential (E) and an activation potential (A), respectively. Note that the electrotonic potentials were synchronous with activation at the opposite side of arcs of functional block (electrograms J, K, and Q). All subsequent beats of TdP were caused by reentrant excitation with varying configuration of the reentrant circuit. The twisting QRS pattern was more evident in lead aVF during the second half of the VT episode. The transition in QRS axis (between V7 and V1O) correlated with the bifurcation of a predominantly single rotating wavefront (scroll) into 2 separate simultaneous wave fronts rotating around the LV and right ventricle (RV) cavities. The final transition in QRS axis (between V10 and V11) correlated with the termination of the RV circuit and the reestablishment of a single LV circulating wave front. P, P waves.(*From* El-Sherif N, Turitto G. The long QT syndrome and torsade de pointes. Pacing Clin Electrophysiol 1999;22:91–110; with permission.)

arrhythmias. In the presence of a multifocal bigeminal rhythm, TdP followed the focal activity that had a critical site of origin and local coupling interval in relation to the underlying pattern of dispersion of repolarization that promoted reentry. In the presence of a unifocal bigeminal rhythm, the following mechanisms for the onset of TdP were observed: (1) A second focal activity from a different site infringed on the dispersion of repolarization of the first focal activity to initiate reentry. (2) A slight lengthening of the preceding CLs resulted in increased dispersion of repolarization at key sites caused by the differential increase of local repolarization at M zones compared with epicardial zones. The increased dispersion of repolarization resulted in de novo arcs of functional conduction block and slowed conduction to initiate reentry. Thus, the transition of a bigeminal rhythm to TdP was caused by well-defined electrophysiologic changes with predictable consequences that promoted reentrant excitation.

QT/T-WAVE ALTERNANS AND TDP

It has long been known that tachycardia-dependent T-wave alternans (TWA) occurs in patients with the congenital or idiopathic form of the LQTS and may presage the onset TdP.[23,24] Manifest TWA is more frequent in congenital LQTS compared with the acquired form (**Fig. 5**). The frequency of occurrence of TWA is usually proportional to the length of the corrected QT (QT_C) interval in the ECG. TWA occurred in one or more occasions during an average 4-year follow-up in 21% of the patients with a QT_C greater than 0.60 seconds but in less than 0.2% of the patients with QT_C less than 0.50 seconds.[25] Patients

with advanced forms of TWA (those with bidirectional beat-to-beat changes in T-wave polarity) were younger, had longer QT_C values, had a higher incidence of complex ventricular tachyarrhythmias, and were more likely to experience a cardiac event (syncope or cardiac arrest) than those with less advanced forms of TWA (those without bidirectional beat-to-beat changes in T-wave polarity).

Interest in repolarization alternans is attributed to the hypothesis that it may reflect an underlying increased dispersion of repolarization. Although overt TWA in the ECG is not common, in recent years, digital signal processing techniques have made it possible to detect subtle degrees of TWA. This suggests that the phenomenon may

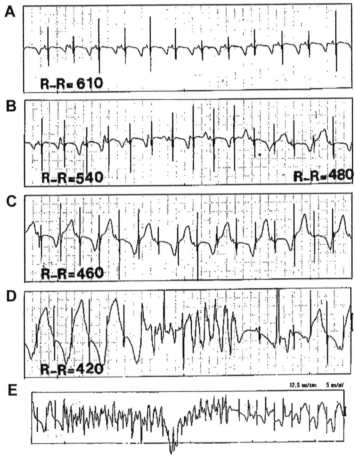

Fig. 5. Tachycardia-dependent QT alternans (TWA) from a newborn baby with Romano-Ward LQTS. The figure illustrates the development of TWA with gradual acceleration of the heart rate. At a cardiac CL (R-R) of 610 milliseconds (*A*), the QTU interval was 440 to 480 milliseconds, and TWA was not discernable. Gradual shortening of the CL to 540 milliseconds resulted in TWA that became more prominent at shorter CLs (*B, C*). In (*D*), on further shortening of the CL to 420 milliseconds, TWA was markedly exaggerated and was associated with the onset of nonsustained polymorphic VT with a twisting QRS morphology characteristic of TdP. (*E*) Recorded at reduced paper speed to illustrate the onset and termination of a longer run of TdP that was also associated with marked TWA at a sinus CL of 420 to 440 milliseconds. (*From* Habbab MA, El-Sherif N. TU alternans, long QTU, and torsade de pointes: clinical and experimental observations. Pacing Clin Electrophysiol 1992;15:916–31; with permission.)

be more prevalent than previously recognized and may represent an important marker of vulnerability to ventricular tachyarrhythmias in general.[26]

The electrophysiologic basis of arrhythmogenicity of TWA in LQTS has been investigated in the AP-A-model of LQT3.[27] TWA could be concordant or discordant. The arrhythmogenicity of discordant TWA is primarily caused by the greater degree of spatial dispersion of repolarization during alternans (**Fig. 6**). The dispersion of repolarization was most marked between M and epicardial zones in the LV free wall. In the presence of a critical degree of dispersion of repolarization, the activation wave front of focal premature beat could be blocked between these zones to initiate reentrant excitation and polymorphic VT. Two factors contributed to the modulation of repolarization during TWA, resulting in greater magnitude of dispersion of repolarization between M and epicardial zones at critical short CL: (1) differences in restitution kinetics at M sites, characterized by larger activation-recovery intervals (ΔARI) and a slower time constant compared with epicardial sites, and (2) differences in the diastolic interval that would result in different input to the restitution curve at the same constant CL. The longer ARI of M sites resulted in shorter diastolic interval during the first short cycle, and thus a greater degree of ARI shortening.

An important observation was that marked repolarization alternans could be present in local electrograms without manifest alternation of the QT/T segment in the surface ECG. Manifest alteration in the ECG was seen at critically short CLs associated with reversal of the gradient of repolarization between epicardial and M sites, with a consequent reversal of polarity of the intramyocardial QT wave in alternate cycles. This observation provides the rationale for the digital signal processing techniques that attempt to detect subtle degrees of TWA.[26]

THE MECHANISM OF PERPETUATION OF TDP: REPETITIVE FOCAL ACTIVITY VERSUS REENTRANT EXCITATION

An important question regarding the electrophysiologic mechanism of VT in the LQTS is the role that EADs play in the generation of TdP. There is a wide consensus that TdP is initiated by EADs. However, there is some controversy as to whether the tachyarrhythmia is sustained by repetitive rapid firing of EADs from several foci[28–30] or EADs account only for the initiation of the arrhythmia.[3] In the latter case, the tachyarrhythmia will be caused by the interaction of the EAD-triggered premature activation with an underlying substrate of dispersion of repolarization. The later mechanism was shown in simulation studies[31] and was documented in the canine LQT3 model using tridimensional mapping of activation[3] The original experimental study of the canine surrogate model of LQT3 has addressed this issue.[1] Using a Purkinje-muscle preparation it was shown that EADs arose from PF and conducted to overlying myocardium with varying degrees of conduction delay through Purkinje-muscle junctions. In 2 more studies, the role of the Purkinje network in TdP was investigated in experimental models of LQT2[29] and LQT3[32] by chemically ablating the endocardium. The 2 studies came to different conclusions. In one study, ablating the endocardium did not abolish the spontaneous development of TdP.[29] In the other study, ablating the endocardium abolished the spontaneous development of TdP, but the arrhythmia could still be induced by premature stimulation acting on a substrate of dispersion of repolarization to initiate reentrant excitation.[32] The 2 studies used epicardial mapping of optical APs. Optical mapping techniques, although providing more direct and possibly more accurate evaluation of the spatial changes in cardiac

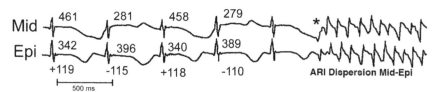

Fig. 6. Mechanism of arrhythmogenicity of discordant TWA: Extracellular electrogram recordings from an epicardial (Epi) and midmyocardial (Mid) sites from the canine AP-A model of TdP. Numbers above the tracings are calculated activation-recovery intervals (ARI). Numbers below the tracings are dispersion of ARI between Epi and Mid sites. The tracing illustrates marked discordant TWA between the 2 sites. The first 5 beats represent regular ventricular pacing at 500-millisecond cycle length. The sixth beat is a spontaneous premature focal discharge (*asterisk*) that resulted in a functional conduction block between Epi and Mid sites and initiated TdP arrhythmia. (*From* Verrier L, Kligenheben T, Malik M, et al. Microvolt T-wave alternans: physiologic basis, methods of measurement, and clinical utility–consensus guidelines by International Society for Holter and Noninvasive Electrocardiology. J Am Coll Cardiol 2011;58:1309–24; with permission.)

repolarization compared with extracellular electrograms, are currently incapable of analyzing the tridimensional properties of cardiac repolarization.[33] Although the different results could be attributed to the difference between experimental models of LQTS (ie, LQT2 vs LQT3 and so forth), this is unlikely considering the largely similar basic electrophysiologic substrate of VT in LQTS. A more plausible explanation is the adequacy of complete endocardial ablation.

This question was readdressed in a subsequent report in the AP-A surrogate model of LQT3 using endocardial ablation and tridimensional mapping (**Fig. 7**).[34] The study clearly established that in the LQTS, the focal activity generated in Purkinje tissue is the only trigger for TdP by acting on an underlying substrate of dispersion of myocardial repolarization to induce reentrant excitation. This mechanism is further documented by the ability to induce reentrant excitation by an appropriately coupled premature stimulus following complete ablation of endocardium. The premature activation acted on the underlying intramural substrate of dispersion of repolarization to induce reentrant excitation. Although the study would not exclude the possibility that successive EADs from multiple Purkinje foci may be both the initiators as well as the perpetuators of TdP, this is very unlikely for

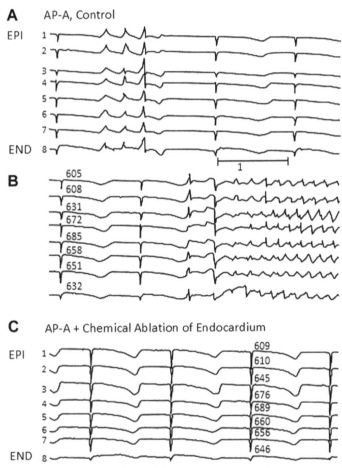

Fig. 7. Endocardial ablation and TdP: Recordings of 8 unipolar transmural electrograms from the free LV wall from the canine AP-A model of LQT3. Ventricular pacing was maintained at 1000 milliseconds. (*A, B*) Images obtained following AP-A infusion and illustrate a short run (*A*) and a long run (*B*) of ventricular tachyarrhythmia (VAs). The numbers in (*B*) represent ARIs across the LV wall. Note the markedly prolonged ARIs, with the longest ARIs in midventricular sites. (*C*) Recordings from the same sites following endocardial ablation of the endocardium and demonstrates the absence of any significant changes in ARI following ablation. Spontaneous VAs were no longer observed. However, a critically timed premature stimulation can induce VAs by acting on the underlying dispersion of repolarization to initiate reentrant activation (not shown). EPI, epicardial; END, endocardial. (*From* Caref EB, Boutjdir M, Himel HD, et al. role of subendocardial Purkinje network in triggering torsade de pointes arrhythmia in experimental long QT syndrome. Europace 2008;10:1218–23; with permission.)

the following argument: EADs induced in PF in the LQTS are bradycardia dependent. The initiation of TdP tachyarrhythmia is implicitly associated with shortening of successive cardiac CL, which should mitigate against the induction of further EADs unless some Purkinje foci have entrance block but no exit block. This situation is probably conceivable only for one or 2 subsequent beats as has been demonstrated in mapping studies. These studies have shown that, in most TdP, only the first one or 2 beats are of End focal origin, whereas successive beats are the result of reentrant excitation.[3]

SUMMARY

The electrophysiologic mechanisms of LQTS and TdP are a prime example of how genetics, molecular biology, ion channels, and cellular and organ physiology coupled with clinical observations are the optimal paradigm for the advancement of medical knowledge in general.[35]

REFERENCES

1. El-Sherif N, Craelius W, Boutjdir M, et al. Early afterdepolarizations and arrhythmogenesis. J Cardiovasc Electrophysiol 1990;1:145–60.
2. Antzelevich C, Sicouri S. Clinical relevance of cardiac arrhythmias generated by afterdepolarizations: role of M cells in the generation of U waves. Triggered activity and torsade de pointes. J Am Coll Cardiol 1994;23:259–77.
3. El-Sherif N, Caref EB, Yin H, et al. The electrophysiological mechanism of ventricular tachyarrhythmias in the long QT syndrome: tridimensional mapping of activation and recovery patterns. Circ Res 1996;79: 474–92.
4. Dessertenne F. La tachycardie ventriculaire a deux foyers opposes variables. Arch Mal Coeur Vaiss 1996;59:263–72.
5. Roden DM, Lazzara R, Rosen M, et al. Multiple mechanisms in the long QT syndrome. Current knowledge, gaps, and future directions. Circulation 1996;94:1996–2012.
6. Jackman WM, Clark M, Friday KJ, et al. Ventricular tachyarrhythmias in the long QT syndrome. Med Clin North Am 1984;68:1079–104.
7. Leenhardt A, Glaser E, Burguera M, et al. Short-coupled variant of torsade de pointes. A new electrocardiographic entity in the spectrum of idiopathic ventricular tachyarrhythmias. Circulation 1994;89: 206–15.
8. E-Sherif N. Mechanism of ventricular arrhythmias in the long QT syndrome: on hermeneutics. J Cardiovasc Electrophysiol 2001;12:973–6.
9. El-Sherif N, Zeiler RH, Craelius W, et al. QTU prolongation and polymorphic ventricular tachyarrhythmias due to bradycardia-dependent early afterdepolarizations. Circ Res 1988;63:286–305.
10. Boutjdir M, El-Sherif N. Pharmacological evaluation of early afterdepolarizations induced by sea anemone toxin (ATXII) in dog heart. Cardiovasc Res 1991;25:815–9.
11. El-Sherif N, Fozzard HA, Hanck DA. Dose-dependent modulation of the cardiac sodium channel by the sea anemone toxin ATXII. Circ Res 1992;70: 285–301.
12. Boutjdir M, Restivo M, Wei Y, et al. Early afterdepolarization formation in cardiac myocytes: analysis of phase plane patterns, action potential, and membrane currents. J Cardiovasc Electrophysiol 1994;5: 609–20.
13. Wang Q, Shen J, Splawski I, et al. SCN5A mutations associated with an inherited cardiac arrhythmia, long QT syndrome. Cell 1995;80:805–11.
14. Bennett PB, Yazawa K, Makita N, et al. Molecular mechanism for an inherited cardiac arrhythmia. Nature 1995;376:683–5.
15. El-Sherif N, Chinushi M, Caref EB, et al. Electrophysiological mechanism of the characteristic electrocardiographic morphology of torsade de pointes tachyarrhythmias in the long QT syndrome. Detailed analysis of ventricular tridimensional activation patterns. Circulation 1997;96:4392–9.
16. Pertsov AM, Davidenko JM, Salomonz B, et al. Spiral waves of activation underlie reentrant activity in isolated cardiac muscle. Circ Res 1993;72:631–50.
17. Abildskov J, Lux RL. The mechanism of simulated torsades de pointes in computer model of propagated excitation. J Cardiovasc Electrophysiol 1993; 4(5):547–60.
18. Leclercq F, Maison-Blanche P, Cauchemez B, et al. Respective role of sympathetic tone and cardiac pauses in the genesis of 62 cases of ventricular fibrillation recorded during Holter monitoring. Eur Heart J 1988;9:1276–83.
19. Viskin S, Alla SR, Barron HV, et al. Mode of onset of torsades de pointes in congenital long QT syndrome. J Am Coll Cardiol 1996;28:1262–8.
20. Roden DM, Woosley RL, Primm RK. Incidence and clinical features of the quinidine associated long QT syndrome: implications for patient care. Am Heart J 1986;111:1088–93.
21. Kay GN, Plumb VJ, Arciniegas JG, et al. Torsades de pointes: the long-short initiating sequence and other clinical features: observations in 32 patients. J Am Coll Cardiol 1990;2:806–17.
22. El-Sherif N, Chinushi M, Restivo M, et al. Electrophysiologic basis of the arrhythmogenicity of short-long cardiac sequences that precede ventricular tachyarrhythmias in the long QT syndrome [abstract]. Pacing Clin Electrophysiol 1998;21:852.
23. Schwartz PJ, Malliani A. Electrical alternation of the T-wave: clinical and experimental evidence of its

relationship with the sympathetic nervous system and with the long Q-T syndrome. Am Heart J 1975; 89:45–50.

24. Habbab MA, El-Sherif N. TU alternans, long QTU, and torsade de pointes: clinical and experimental observations. Pacing Clin Electrophysiol 1992;15:916–31.

25. Moss AJ. Long QT syndrome. In: Podrid PJ, Kowey PR, editors. Cardiac arrhythmias. Mechanisms, diagnosis, and management. Baltimore (MD): Williams & Wilkins; 1995. p. 1110–20.

26. Verrier L, Kligenheben T, Malik M, et al. Microvolt T-wave alternans: physiological basis, methods of measurement, and clinical utility- consensus guidelines by International Society for Holter and Noninvasive Electrocardiology. J Am Coll Cardiol 2011;58: 1309–24.

27. Chinushi M, Restivo M, Caref EB, et al. Electro-physiological basis of the arrhythmogenicity of QT/T alternans in the long QT syndrome: tridimensional analysis of the kinetics of cardiac repolarization. Circ Res 1998;83:614–28.

28. Asano Y, Davidenko JM, Baxter WT, et al. Optical mapping of drug-induced polymorphic arrhythmias and torsade de pointes in the isolated rabbit heart. J Am Coll Cardiol 1997;29:831–42.

29. Choi BR, Burton F, Salama G. Cytosolic Ca2+ triggers early afterdepolarization and torsade de pointes in rabbit hearts with type 2 long QT syndrome. J Physiol 2002;543:615–31.

30. Boulaksil M, Jungschleger JG, Antoons G, et al. Drug-induced torsade de pointed arrhythmias in the chronic AV block dog are perpetuated by focal activity. Circ Arrhythm Electrophysiol 2011; 4:566–76.

31. Abidskov JA, Lux RL. Simulated torsade de pointes. The role of conduction defects and mechanism of QRS rotation. J Electrocardiol 2000;33:55–64.

32. Restivo M, Caref EB, Kozhevnikov DO, et al. Spatial dispersion of repolarization is a key factor in the arrhythmogenicity of long QT syndrome. J Cardiovasc Electrophysiol 2004;15:1–9.

33. El-Sherif N. The challenge of cardiac tridimensional mapping. Heart Rhythm 2007;4:1437–40.

34. Caref EB, Boutjdir M, Himel HD, et al. Role of subendocardial Purkinje network in triggering torsade de pointes arrhythmia in experimental long QT syndrome. Europace 2008;10:1218–23.

35. El-Sherif N, Turitto G. The long QT syndrome and torsade de pointes. Pacing Clin Electrophysiol 1999;22:91–110.

Atrioventricular Conduction Disease and Block

Leila Laroussi, MD, FRCPC, Nitish Badhwar, MBBS, FACC, FHRS*

KEYWORDS

- AV block • Wenckebach • 2:1 AV block • Intra-His and infra-His block • Pacemaker indication

KEY POINTS

- A prolonged PR interval and second-degree Mobitz type 1 atrioventricular (AV) block are generally benign conditions and do not require treatment.
- Second-degree Mobitz type 2 AV block, high-degree AV block, and complete heart block are usually intra-His or infra-His processes and require pacemaker implantation.
- In 2:1 AV block, it can be difficult to determine the level of block, and further diagnostic maneuvers are needed.

INTRODUCTION

The atrioventricular (AV) conduction system contains the AV node (AVN), the penetrating bundle of His (HB), and the right and left bundle branches, which divide distally into thinner branches of the Purkinje fibers network.[1]

The AV node is located in the anterior aspect of the Koch triangle, defined by the coronary sinus ostium inferiorly, the tendon of Todaro posteriorly, and the septal leaflet of the tricuspid valve anteriorly.

Electrical impulses originate in the sinus node and are transmitted from the atrium to the ventricle through the AV node and the HB. The conduction in the AV node is decremental to allow optimal ventricular filling. This delay is influenced by autonomic tone and heart rate. Conduction through the HB is rapid and does not vary with heart rate. Conduction slowing or block can occur in the AV node, the HB, or both, and characteristic electrocardiogram (ECG) patterns occur. Prognosis depends on the location and severity of block. In general, the prognosis is better when the block is above the AV node (supra-His), whereas block below the AV node (intra-His or infra-His) portends a higher risk of progression to a complete heart block.[2] Symptoms caused by AV block can include fatigue, lightheadedness, and syncope; persistent high-grade AV block can result in heart failure caused by bradycardia and loss of AV synchrony. AV block also predisposes to ventricular arrhythmias.

ELECTROCARDIOGRAPHIC PATTERN

First-degree AV Block

First-degree AV block, or conduction delay, is defined as a PR interval exceeding 200 milliseconds (**Fig. 1**). It often reflects incipient AV nodal disease, although it can be a normal finding in patients at rest with high vagal tone, particularly highly trained athletes. It becomes more common with age (5% of men >60 years old) and with structural heart disease.[3]

The site of block is found in the compact AVN in 85% of patients, but could be located at any level of the AV conduction system. If the QRS is wide, the origin is infranodal in 45% of cases.[3]

Second-degree AV Block

Second-degree AV block is divided into Mobitz type I and type II, from the ECG pattern. It is

The authors have nothing to disclose.
Section of Electrophysiology, Division of Cardiology, University of California, San Francisco, 500 Parnassus Avenue, MUE-431, San Francisco, CA 94143-1354, USA
* Corresponding author.
E-mail address: badhwar@medicine.ucsf.edu

Card Electrophysiol Clin 6 (2014) 445–458
http://dx.doi.org/10.1016/j.ccep.2014.05.015
1877-9182/14/$ – see front matter © 2014 Elsevier Inc. All rights reserved.

cardiacEP.theclinics.com

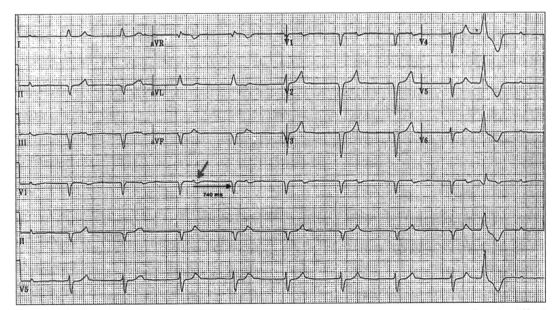

Fig. 1. First-degree AV block. In this ECG, the P wave (*red arrow*) is in the middle of the T wave and can be difficult to see. Every QRS is preceded by a P wave, the PP interval is regular, and the PR measures 740 milliseconds. The ECG shows first-degree AV block (or conduction delay) with a very long PR interval.

important to differentiate between both types, because the prognosis and management are different.

Mobitz type I, second-degree AV block

In typical Mobitz type I second-degree AV block (also called Wenckebach) the PR interval lengthens gradually until a nonconducted sinus beat occurs, and shortens on the following beat (Wenckebach conduction). The RR interval shortens progressively; the RR interval containing the blocked P wave is shorter than the sum of 2 PP intervals (**Fig. 2**). However, atypical Wenckebach in which the PR does not increase progressively is occasionally observed, although the longest PR interval always precedes the nonconducted P wave. This condition is caused by PP interval variation and inconstancy of the RP interval induced by changes in the autonomic nervous system (**Fig. 3**).[4]

In general, type I second-degree AV block suggests a supra-His level of block and is associated with a more benign prognosis.[2] It is common to observe this phenomenon in healthy patients with high vagal tone, particularly when asleep.

Wenckebach in the His-Purkinje system (HPS) is rare and only seen in pathologic conditions. Thus, type I second-degree AV block has a benign prognosis only when it is caused by supra-His block, which is usually the case when the QRS complex is narrow. When the QRS is wide, for example in the presence of bundle branch block (BBB), the level of block during Wenckebach conduction is still more likely to be in the AVN, but rarely can be seen in the HPS. In these circumstances, small PR increment preceding block is often observed.[4]

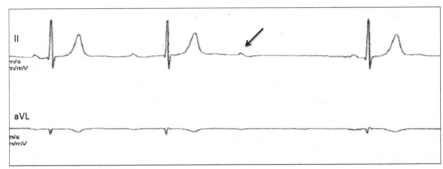

Fig. 2. Type 1 second-degree AV block. A typical Wenckebach with a 3:2 pattern; the PR increases gradually until a P wave is blocked (*arrow*). The PR interval after the pause is shorter than the last conducted PR interval.

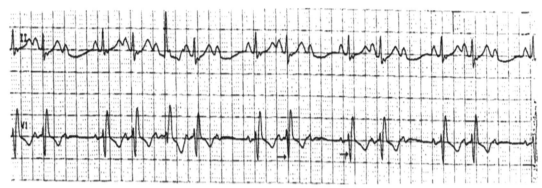

Fig. 3. Type 1 second-degree AV block. An atypical Wenckebach with a 3:2 pattern; the PR does not increase gradually, but the last PR (*black arrows*) preceding the blocked P wave is longer than the one following it.

Patients with Wenckebach conduction are typically asymptomatic, although some feel some heart rhythm irregularities. Mobitz-I second-degree AV block is also a physiologic phenomenon observed at high heart rates (especially with pacing) caused by rate-dependent refractoriness of the AV node.

Mobitz type II, second-degree AV block

In Mobitz type II AV block, the PR interval remains constant before a nonconducted sinus beat. Intermittent nonconducted P waves are observed and the pause following the nonconducted P wave is equal to the sum of the 2 preceding beats (**Fig. 4**).[4] Type II block is usually located in the infra-His conduction system (wide QRS in 80% of cases) but can also happen in the HB (narrow QRS in 20% of cases). It has a higher rate of progression to complete heart block.[2]

Some patients with Mobitz type II block are asymptomatic; others can feel irregularities of the heart rate, fatigue, and exercise intolerance. Episodes of presyncope and syncope strongly suggest disease progression.

2:1 AV Block

A 2:1 AV block occurs when 2 sinus P waves at a constant rate occur for every QRS. It is often difficult to determine whether the block is located at the level of the AV node or is infranodal. Because type 1 and type 2 AV block are based on the ECG, clinicians should not categorize 2:1 AV block as either type. However, some indices can help determine the level of the block. A long rhythm strip can show changing conduction ratio and changes of the PR interval suggesting a block at the AV nodal level. A conducted PR interval shorter than 160 milliseconds and a wide QRS complex favor a diagnosis of infra-His block. A very long PR interval (>300 milliseconds) and narrow QRS favor the presence of AV nodal block. During exercise or with atropine, when the atrial rate augments, AV nodal block tends to improve, whereas infranodal block tends to worsen (**Fig. 5**, **Table 1**).[4] During carotid sinus massage (CSM), there is an increased vagal stimulation that worsens the AV nodal block. However, in infranodal block, as the atrial rate decreases, the conduction improves (**Fig. 6**).

High-degree AV Block

High-grade AV block is defined by intermittent block of 2 or more consecutive P waves.[4] The site of block can be the AVN or the HPS. When the conducted QRS is narrow and intermittent Wenckebach is observed, it is most likely that

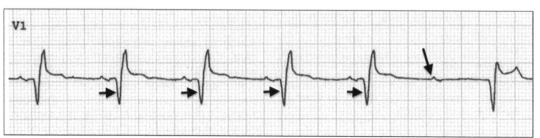

Fig. 4. Type 2 second-degree AV block. The PR (*black arrows*) is normal and stable until a nonconducted P wave occurs. Note the wide QRS with a right BBB morphology. The last beat is a junctional escape beat; it is wide and has the same morphology as the conducted QRS.

A

B

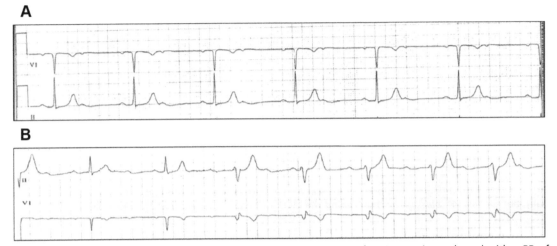

Fig. 5. A 2:1 AV block. (*A*) In this strip, 2:1 AV block is present; every other P wave is conducted with a PR of 160 milliseconds. (*B*) This strip is from the same patient. When the atrial rate increases, the patient develops complete heart block with a wide escape, which is consistent with infranodal AV block.

the block is at the AV nodal level. If the QRS is wide and the block worsens with exercise or atropine, the HPS is probably the site of the block.

One important differential diagnosis to keep in mind is pseudo–AV block, which can happen when a His extrasystole occurs soon after the preceding sinus beat. In this case, the His extrasystole is concealed, and when the next sinus impulse arrives the HB is refractory and fails to conduct. On the ECG, a blocked sinus P wave is seen. Therefore, on surface ECG, it can mimic Mobitz II, high-degree, or complete heart block (depending on the frequency of the His extrasystoles). The presence of inverted P waves, conducted and nonconducted, suggests the presence of concealed His extrasystoles. An invasive electrophysiology (EP) study can confirm the diagnosis, which is usually benign.

Third-degree AV Block and AV Dissociation

Patients with type II second-degree and high-degree AV block have a higher rate of progression

to third-degree (complete) AV block (CHB), particularly in the setting of intraventricular conduction abnormalities.

Third-degree AV block is characterized by a complete failure of P waves to conduct to the ventricle. AV dissociation is present, and the atrial rate is regular and faster than the ventricular rate. The escape rhythm can be junctional (narrow QRS and heart rate [HR] usually more than 40 beats per minute [bpm]) or ventricular (wide QRS and HR <40 bpm) (**Fig. 7**). Ventriculophasic sinus arrhythmia can be observed in 30% to 40% of patients with complete AV block and can lead to a misdiagnosis of blocked premature atrial contraction.[4] During atrial fibrillation, the presence of a slow regular ventricular rhythm is always consistent with the presence of underlying complete AV block (**Fig. 8**).

Third-degree AV block and consequent AV dissociation are almost always symptomatic, although the symptoms can vary in severity from mild dizziness and exercise intolerance to syncope or even sudden death, depending on the rate of the escape rhythm.

Paroxysmal AV Block

Advanced second-degree and third-degree AV block can be paroxysmal with long intervening periods of 1:1 AV conduction.

Paroxysmal block can follow a premature beat (atrial or ventricular) and is also called bradycardia-dependent AV block. It is thought to be a local disorder of the HPS caused by a local phase 4 block after a critical change of the H-H interval (**Fig. 9**). During a long pause, and a long diastolic interval, the HPS fibers depolarize

Table 1 Differential diagnosis of 2:1 AV block		
	Above the Node	**Below the Node**
PR interval (ms)	>200	<160
QRS width (ms)	<100	>120
Atropine/ exercise	Improves conduction to 1:1	Increases block
Carotid sinus massage	Increases block	Improves conduction to 1:1

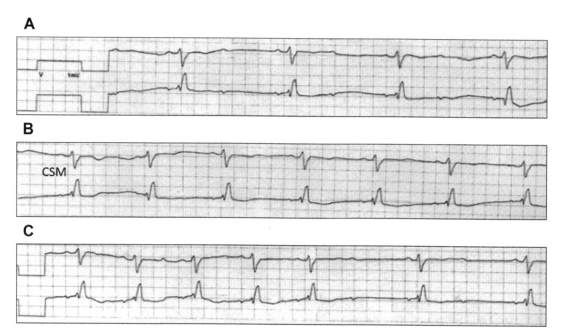

Fig. 6. A 2:1 AV block. (*A*) In this strip, only every other P wave is conducted, with a PR of 140 milliseconds and a right BBB is present. (*B*) The same patient during CSM. When the atrial rate decreases, the patient's conduction improves to 1:1. (*C*) When the CSM stops, 2:1 conduction resumes, which is consistent with an infranodal AV block.

spontaneously and become refractory to a subsequent impulse. This is thought to occur because of Na+ channel inactivation at higher resting membrane potentials.[5]

Paroxysmal AV block is highly associated with recurrent syncope bradycardia-related ventricular arrhythmias and warrants permanent pacemaker implantation.

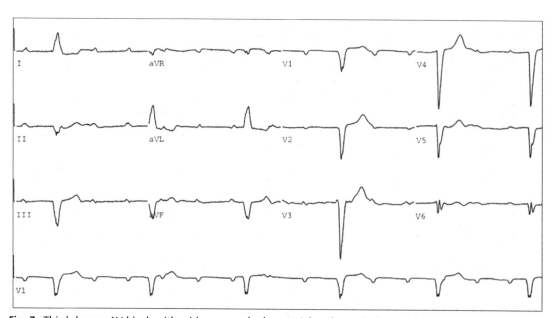

Fig. 7. Third-degree AV block with wide escape rhythm. Atrial and ventricular activities are completely dissociated. The ventricular rate is slower than the atrial rate and regular. The QRS is wide, suggesting a ventricular escape rhythm. (*Courtesy of* Dr Henry Hsia, VA Medical Center, University of California, San Francisco, San Francisco, CA.)

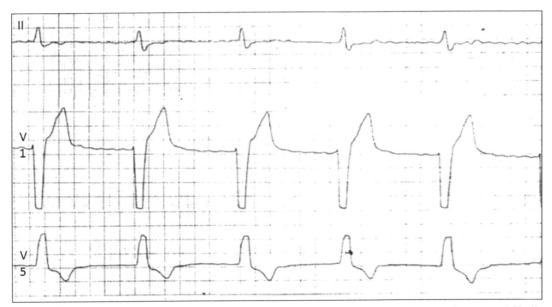

Fig. 8. Atrial fibrillation with AV dissociation. There are no P waves and the underlying rhythm is atrial fibrillation. The ventricular rate is slow and completely regular, suggesting complete AV block. The wide QRS is probably a ventricular escape rhythm.

Vagotonic AV Block

Brief periods of heart block can occur in situations of high vagal tone, in which AV block is transient or occurs exclusively during sleep and is accompanied by an adequate ventricular escape rhythm. Slowing of the sinus rhythm (prolongation of the PP interval) typically precedes the vagotonic block. This condition can also be observed during CSM and during vasovagal syncope. Vagotonic AV block is usually benign and no treatment is required. However, in some patients with prolonged periods of asystole, permanent pacing may be used to relieve symptoms.

NONINVASIVE AND INVASIVE TESTING

Because the prognosis of AV block depends on the site of the block, determining whether the level of block is nodal or infranodal is important. This can often be determined by noninvasive testing. The baseline ECG is helpful, but sometimes additional tests are needed to clarify the site of block.

Exercise testing can evaluate the response to higher adrenergic tone. In 2:1 AV block, if the block is at the level of the AV node, AV conduction improves (from to 2:1 to 3:2, for example); however, if the block is infranodal, it can worsen (from 2:1 to 3:1, for example.) Because AV block can be intermittent, prolonged ambulatory monitoring such as with Holter monitors, event monitors, or loop event recorders is a practical aid to making the correct diagnosis.

Invasive EP study may be required when symptoms are profound or result in injury, or if there is a high degree of suspicion that infranodal disease is present. With rapid atrial pacing, physiologic Wenckebach conduction can be provoked and is

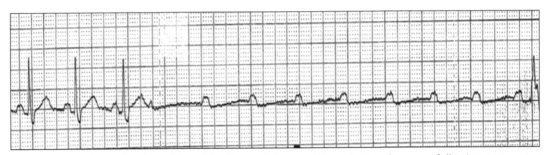

Fig. 9. Paroxysmal complete heart block. The first part shows a 1:1 conduction; however, following a premature atrial contraction, there is complete AV block (phase IV block).

a normal physiologic response. It is characterized by progressive prolongation of the AH interval until an atrial deflection is not followed by a His and ventricular deflection (**Fig. 10**). Abnormal AVN conduction produces Wenckebach at slower atrial pacing than is normally seen (cycle length longer than 500 milliseconds).

In AV nodal block, of any degree, an HB deflection does not follow the atrial depolarization. An escape rhythm (usually junctional, if present) is preceded by a His deflection with an HV within normal range (35–55 milliseconds), indicating that conduction below the level of the AV node is preserved. Sometimes, atropine or isoproterenol can be used to enhance conduction through the AV node and stress the HPS in the presence of a long Wenckebach cycle length.

In the presence of infra-His disease, a prolonged His potential duration or a split His potential can occasionally be observed (**Fig. 11**). Also, a Wenckebach block conduction pattern can be observed between the 2 His deflections; the interval between the split His gradually prolongs until the second His deflection is dropped, and the electrical impulse is not conducted to the ventricle (**Fig. 12**).

When the level of block is below the HB, there is usually an increased HV interval with the presence of a His deflection not conducted to the ventricle (type 2 second-degree pattern in the ECG). The HV interval can, rarely, increase progressively until a His deflection is not followed by a ventricular activation (infranodal type 1 second-degree pattern in the ECG). Procainamide, a class Ia antiarrhythmic drug, is known to stress the HPS conduction. Procainamide infusion during an EP study increases the HV interval from 10% to 20%. In the presence of a prolonged HV interval, infusion of procainamide leading to complete AV block or an HV interval greater than 100 milliseconds is considered pathologic and usually indicates the need for permanent pacing (**Fig. 13**).[6,7]

It is important to recognize the existence of physiologic infra-His block during pacing. Any pacing maneuver using premature extrastimuli that results in a long-short sequence to the HPS can lead to an infra-His phase 3 block (**Fig. 14**), which is normal and does not warrant treatment. Infra-His block with pacing at a constant short coupling interval (cycle length <350 milliseconds) can also be physiologic.

CAUSES OF AV BLOCK
Acquired AV Block

Drugs
Almost any medication with electrophysiologic effects on the conduction system can cause AV conduction delay or block.

β-Blockers and digoxin act indirectly on the AV node through modulation of autonomic tone. Calcium channel blockers act directly to slow conduction in the AV node. Class 1 antiarrhythmic drugs delay conduction in the HPS and can lead to nodal and infranodal block. However, it is rare for drugs to induce high-degree AV block in patients without underlying conduction disorders.

Overdose of any of the drugs mentioned earlier can lead to AV block or prolonged sinus pauses. Other medications with effects on the conduction system, such as tricyclic antidepressants,

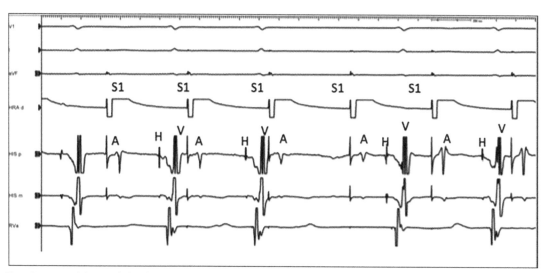

Fig. 10. AV nodal Wenckebach. In this intracardiac electrogram, during rapid atrial pacing the AH interval gradually increases until an A deflection is not followed by H or V deflection. The block is therefore at the nodal level and is physiologic.

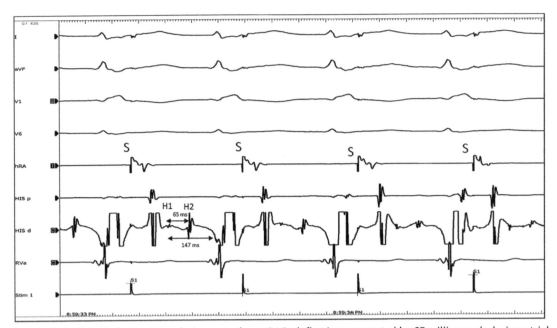

Fig. 11. Split His. This intracardiac electrogram shows 2 His deflections separated by 65 milliseconds during atrial pacing. Although the apparent HV interval is only mildly prolonged, the true HV interval (measured from the first H to the earliest ventricular activity in the electrocardiogram) is very long (147 milliseconds), which is an example of intra-His delay. (*Courtesy of* Dr Henry Hsia, VA Medical Center, University of California, San Francisco, San Francisco, CA.)

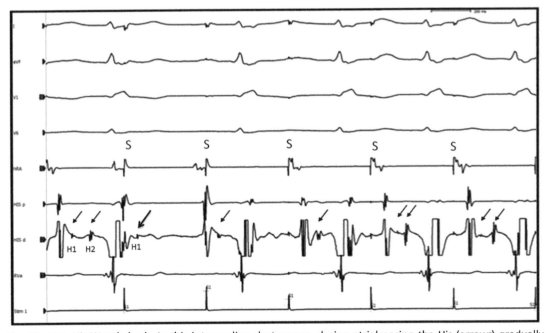

Fig. 12. Intra-His Wenckebach. In this intracardiac electrogram, during atrial pacing the His (*arrows*) gradually splits and the interval between the 2 His deflections increases. The third arrow shows only 1 His deflection, which is blocked. This deflection is an intra-His Wenckebach. (*Courtesy of* Dr Henry Hsia, VA Medical Center, University of California, San Francisco, San Francisco, CA.)

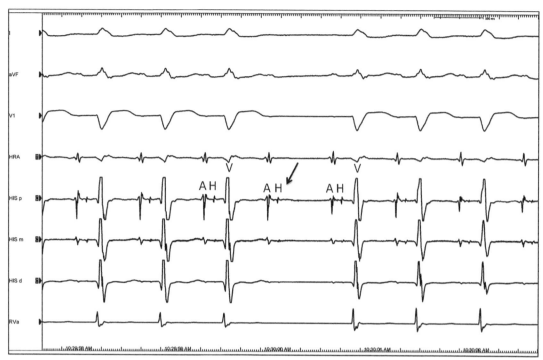

Fig. 13. Procainamide-induced infra-His block. In this intracardiac electrogram, after procainamide infusion, the atrial activity is followed intermittently by a His deflection but no ventricular activity (the arrow indicates the His block).

antipsychotics, and anticholinergic drugs, have also been reported to provoke different degrees of AV block after overdose.

Iatrogenic

AV block is a well-known complication of many cardiac surgical procedures; it is often transient, caused by local inflammation to the conduction tissue. However, if it persists for more than 2 to 5 days after surgery, patients may require a permanent pacemaker. Overall, in noncongenital cardiac surgeries, the pacemaker implant rate is reported to be 0.8% to 2.1%.[8,9]

Because of the proximity of the His bundle to the aortic valve, persistent high-degree AV block is highly prevalent after surgical aortic valve replacement (6%) or transcatheter aortic valve replacement (27%–33% with the CoreValve and 4%–12% with the Edwards Sapien valve).[10]

In patients with hypertrophic obstructive cardiomyopathy requiring a procedure to relieve the left ventricular outflow tract obstruction, 50% develop a transient third-degree AV block and 10% to 20% require a pacemaker if treated by septal alcohol ablation; 2% require a pacemaker if a surgical myomectomy is performed.[11]

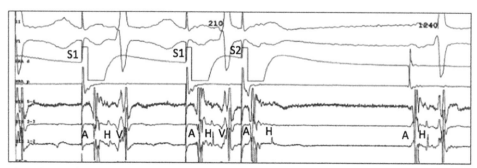

Fig. 14. Physiologic infra-His block. This intracardiac electrogram shows a premature atrial extrastimulus (S2) that results in a long-short sequence to the HPS and a blocked His signal (H).

Permanent complete AV block can complicate catheter ablation procedures of AVN reentrant tachycardia, septal accessory pathways, and para-Hisian ventricular tachycardia.

In addition, right-sided and left-sided heart catheterizations have been reported to induce transient heart block through mechanical pressure with the HB region, particularly in patients with underlying conduction disorders like left BBB or right BBB. These occurrences of heart block nearly always reverse with time.

Ischemic

AV block occurs as frequently as 25% in the setting of acute myocardial infarction (MI).[5] First-degree and Mobitz-I second-degree AV block is usually secondary to an increased vagal tone in the setting of inferior MI (Bezold-Jarisch reflex). Often transient and asymptomatic, they have not been associated with adverse outcomes after MI and acutely respond well to atropine. Temporary tranvenous pacing may be required in the acute MI setting.

Mobitz-II second-degree AV block is usually associated with HB ischemia and can progress to complete heart block. This condition is more commonly associated with anterior MI or new left BBB.

Third-degree AV block can occur in inferior or anterior MI and the prognosis varies. During inferior MI, the site of block is usually the AVN; the escape rhythm is junctional and AV conduction often recovers. AV block in this setting may respond to vagolytic or adrenergic drugs. However, atropine should be administered carefully in the setting of a wide QRS because it may exacerbate infranodal block or lead to worsened ischemia.

In anterior MI, third-degree AV block is caused by ischemia of the HB or the right or left bundle branches. It is less likely to be reversible and is associated with higher risk of ventricular fibrillation, Killip 3 and 4 heart failure, and increased mortality. The escape rhythm is usually wide and very slow (<40 bpm). Bundle branch or bifascicular block or type-II second-degree block usually precedes third-degree AV block in anterior MI, and temporary pacing may be required.

In chronic ischemic heart disease, fibrotic changes can lead to persistent AV block of any type. Also, transient AV block can occur in the setting of angina.

Degenerative

Age-related fibrotic degenerative changes of the conduction system, also known as Lev disease or Lenegre-Lev syndrome, are the most common causes of AV block, accounting for more than 50% of AV block in adults.[5] This disorder is usually progressive and can affect all parts of the conduction system. It is a primary degenerative condition hastened by hypertension and atherosclerosis.

Also, extensive calcification of the aortic annulus in aortic valve disease can extend to the adjacent His bundle and lead to progressive heart block.

Systemic diseases

Many systemic conditions have been associated with AV block.

Myotonic dystrophy is the most common inherited neuromuscular disorders in adults. Through a fatty infiltration and fibrosis mechanism, a high proportion of these patients present with variable degrees of AV block. Up to 42% have a 1st-degree AV block on ECG at initial presentation of the disease (aged 20–25 years). It is reported that 3.3% of patients evolve to complete heart block at 10 years but 11% die suddenly, likely underestimating the prevalence of the disease.[12]

Differing degrees of AV block have been reported in various neuromuscular diseases such as Emery-Dreifuss muscular dystrophy, facioscapulohumeral muscular dystrophy, Becker muscular dystrophy, Kearns-Sayre syndrome, Erb dystrophy, and peroneal muscular dystrophy.

Sarcoidosis is a multisystem disease characterized by noncaseous granulomatous infiltration of tissues. Between 20% and 30% of patients with sarcoidosis have cardiac involvement on autopsies and 30% develop third-degree AV block.[13]

Other infiltrative diseases such as amyloidosis, hemochromatosis, and primary tumors of the heart are reported to be associated with AV block.

Lyme disease is a tick-borne infection endemic in the north east of the United States. It is a multisystemic disease that involves the heart in 10% of cases. The most common cardiac manifestation is transient complete heart block and antibiotic treatment can completely reverse the disease.[14] The block typically occurs at the level of the AV node. Young patients in endemic areas who present with complete AV block should have Lyme disease excluded before implanting a permanent pacemaker.

Chagas disease is a parasitic infection widely prevalent in South America. Approximately 36% of patients have some degree of AV block, mainly first degree (24.6%). Complete heart block was observed in 8.2% and is correlated with increased mortality.[15]

Tuberculosis, measles, and mumps can also result in various degree of AV block.

Infective endocarditis with aortic valve involvement can cause AV block by infectious infiltration

Table 2
Indications for permanent pacemaker in acquired AV block

Third-degree and advanced second-degree AV block at any anatomic level associated with bradycardia with symptoms (including heart failure) or ventricular arrhythmias presumed to be caused by AV block	Class 1 LOE C
Third-degree and advanced second-degree AV block at any anatomic level associated with arrhythmias and other medical conditions that require drug therapy that results in symptomatic bradycardia	Class 1 LOE C
Third-degree and advanced second-degree AV block at any anatomic level in awake, symptom-free patients in sinus rhythm, with documented periods of asystole greater than or equal to 3.0 s or any escape rate <40 bpm, or with an escape rhythm that is below the AV node	Class 1 LOE C
Third-degree and advanced second-degree AV block at any anatomic level in awake, symptom-free patients with AF and bradycardia with 1 or more pauses of at least 5 s or longer	Class 1 LOE C
Third-degree and advanced second-degree AV block at any anatomic level after catheter ablation of the AV junction	Class 1 LOE C
Third-degree and advanced second-degree AV block at any anatomic level associated with postoperative AV block that is not expected to resolve after cardiac surgery	Class 1 LOE C
Third-degree and advanced second-degree AV block at any anatomic level associated with neuromuscular diseases with AV block, such as myotonic muscular dystrophy, Kearns-Sayre syndrome, Erb dystrophy (limb-girdle muscular dystrophy), and peroneal muscular atrophy, with or without symptoms	Class 1 LOE B
Second-degree AV block with associated symptomatic bradycardia regardless of type or site of block	Class 1 LOE B
Asymptomatic persistent third-degree AV block at any anatomic site with average awake ventricular rates of 40 bpm or faster if cardiomegaly or LV dysfunction is present or if the site of block is below the AV node	Class 1 LOE B
Second-degree or third-degree AV block during exercise in the absence of myocardial ischemia	Class 1 LOE C
Persistent third-degree AV block with an escape rate >40 bpm in asymptomatic adult patients without cardiomegaly	Class 2a LOE C
Asymptomatic second-degree AV block at intra-His or infra-His levels found at electrophysiologic study	Class 2a LOE B
First-degree or second-degree AV block with symptoms similar to those of pacemaker syndrome or hemodynamic compromise	Class 2a LOE B
Asymptomatic type II second-degree AV block with a narrow QRS When type II second-degree AV block occurs with a wide QRS, including isolated right BBB, pacing becomes a class I recommendation	Class 2a LOE B
Neuromuscular diseases such as myotonic muscular dystrophy, Erb dystrophy (limb-girdle muscular dystrophy), and peroneal muscular atrophy with any degree of AV block (including first-degree AV block), with or without symptoms, because there may be unpredictable progression of AV conduction disease	Class 2b LOE B
AV block in the setting of drug use and/or drug toxicity when the block is expected to recur even after the drug is withdrawn	Class 2b LOE B

Abbreviations: AF, atrial fibrillation; LOE, level of evidence; LV, left ventricular.

Adapted from Epstein AE, DiMarco JP, Ellenbogen KA. 2012 ACCF/AHA/HRS focused update incorporated into the ACCF/AHA/HRS 2008 guidelines for device-based therapy of cardiac rhythm abnormalities: a report of the American College of Cardiology Foundation/American Heart Association Task Force on Practice Guidelines and the Heart Rhythm Society. Circulation 2013;127(3):e283–352.

of the AV node. It is usually a sign of extensive disease and an urgent surgical intervention is warranted.

In addition, rheumatic diseases such as scleroderma, rheumatoid arthritis, systemic lupus erythematosus (SLE), ankylosing spondylitis, polymyositis, polyarteritis nodosa, and Wegener granulomatosis can also cause AV block.

Hereditary AV Block and Channelopathies

Rare cases of familial forms of AV block have been described. Mutation of the SCN5A gene (encoding for cardiac sodium channel) has been clearly associated with this progressive conduction disease. This gene mutation is also associated with Brugada syndrome and long QT syndrome (LQTS) type 3. In Brugada syndrome, prolonged PR and HV intervals are frequently seen (50%) and there are case reports of overlapping syndromes of Brugada and familial high-degree AV block.

Other genes that have been correlated with familial cardiac conduction disease include KCNJ2 (encoding for cardiac potassium channel) or PRKAG2 (encoding for a subunit of the adenosine monophosphate-activated protein kinase) described in patients with Wolff-Parkinson-White (WPW) syndrome and AV conduction disorders.[16]

In LQTS, when a very long QT interval is present, a functional block between the HB and the ventricular muscle can be seen. This block is caused by prolonged ventricular refractoriness and can lead to 2:1 AV block with severe and symptomatic bradycardia.[17,18]

Congenital AV Block

The incidence of congenital complete AV block varies from 1 in 15,000 to 1 in 22,000 live births. The site of block is usually high (AV node) and the escape rhythm is narrow at acceptable HRs (40–60 bpm).[19] The most common cause is maternal SLE, accounting for 60% to 90% of congenital AV block. The maternal antibodies cross the placenta and affect the embryonic development of the AVN and HPS with fatty replacement of the AVN. Approximately 40% of cases of congenital CHB do not present until childhood (5–6 years of age). The clinical manifestations vary from asymptomatic to reduced exercise tolerance to exercise-induced presyncope or syncope.

However, 50% of patients with congenital CHB have concurrent congenital heart malformations. These include, but are not limited to, transposition of the great arteries, congenitally corrected transposition of the great arteries, left isomerism and polysplenia syndrome, AV-canal defect, tricuspid atresia, and Ebstein anomaly of the tricuspid valve.[20]

Also, repair of any congenital disease can lead to transient or permanent AV block, which can appear early after surgery but also manifest many years later.

MANAGEMENT AND TREATMENT

Prognosis of patients with isolated first-degree AV block and Mobitz type-II second-degree AV block is excellent, and pacemaker implantation is, in general, not indicated in asymptomatic patients. However, a few indications for pacing are recognized.

Some patients with marked first-degree AV block (PR interval >0.3 seconds) have symptoms that may warrant pacemaker implantation. In these patients, ventricular activation is so delayed that the subsequent atrial activation occurs shortly after the QRS complex on the surface ECG, resulting in atrial contraction against closed AV valves, which can cause impaired ventricular filling and diastolic AV valvular regurgitation. Thus, restoration of AV synchrony with dual-chamber pacing and a normal AV delay is often required to solve the problem.

Table 3 Indications for permanent pacemaker after the acute phase of myocardial infarction	
Persistent second-degree AV block in the HPS with alternating BBB or third-degree AV block within or less than the HPS after ST-segment increase MI	Class 1 LOE B
Transient advanced second-degree or third-degree infranodal AV block and associated BBB. If the site of block is uncertain, an electrophysiologic study may be necessary	Class 1 LOE B
Persistent and symptomatic second-degree or third-degree AV block	Class 1 LOE C
Persistent second-degree or third-degree AV block at the AV node level, even in the absence of symptoms	Class 2b LOE B

Adapted from Epstein AE, DiMarco JP, Ellenbogen KA. 2012 ACCF/AHA/HRS focused update incorporated into the ACCF/AHA/HRS 2008 guidelines for device-based therapy of cardiac rhythm abnormalities: a report of the American College of Cardiology Foundation/American Heart Association Task Force on Practice Guidelines and the Heart Rhythm Society. Circulation 2013;127(3):e283–352.

Table 4
Indications for permanent pacemaker in congenital third-degree AV block

Congenital third-degree AV block with a wide QRS escape rhythm, complex ventricular ectopy, or ventricular dysfunction	Class 1 LOE B
Congenital third-degree AV block in the infant with a ventricular rate <55 bpm or with congenital heart disease and a ventricular rate <70 bpm	Class 1 LOE C
Congenital third-degree AV block beyond the first year of life with an average HR <50 bpm, abrupt pauses in ventricular rate that are 2 or 3 times the basic cycle length, or associated with symptoms caused by chronotropic incompetence	Class 1 LOE C
Congenital third-degree AV block in asymptomatic children or adolescents with an acceptable rate, a narrow QRS complex, and normal ventricular function	Class 2b LOE B

Adapted from Epstein AE, DiMarco JP, Ellenbogen KA. ACC/AHA/HRS 2008 guidelines for device-based therapy of cardiac rhythm abnormalities: executive summary. A report of the American College of Cardiology/American Heart Association Task Force on Practice Guidelines (Writing Committee to revise the ACC/AHA/NASPE 2002 guideline update for implantation of cardiac pacemakers and antiarrhythmia devices). J Am Coll Cardiol 2008;51(21):2085–105.

Patients with several neuromuscular diseases, such as myotonic dystrophy, often have rapidly progressive atrioventricular conduction system disease. Even in asymptomatic patients with these disorders, marked first-degree AV block should prompt consideration of pacemaker implantation as a prophylactic measure.

From the point of view of cardiac pacing, advanced second-degree AV block and third-degree AV block should be grouped together in a single high-risk category; pacemaker implantation is the only reasonable treatment when reversible causes cannot be identified.

When paroxysmal heart block cannot be attributed to reversible causes, pacemaker implantation is an indication in almost all clinical situations.[21,22]

The principal recommendations for a permanent pacemaker implant are summarized in **Tables 2–4**.

SUMMARY

AV conduction disorders are common in aging populations. Clinical manifestations vary from asymptomatic to syncope and even sudden cardiac death secondary to ventricular arrhythmias. The prognosis strongly depends on the site of the block, and the ECG remains the key feature to identify this. However, electrophysiologic study and maneuvers can help in specific cases.

REFERENCES

1. Ho SY, Ernst S. Electrical anatomy and accessory pathways. In: Ho SY, Ernst S, editors. Anatomy for cardiac electrophysiologists: a practical handbook. Minneapolis (MN): Cardiotext; 2012. p. 67–96.
2. Dhingra RC, Denes P, Wu D, et al. The significance of second degree atrioventricular block and bundle branch block. Observations regarding site and type of block. Circulation 1974;49(4):638–46.
3. Barrero Garcia M, Talajic M. Atrioventricular conduction disorders. In: Barrero Garcia M, Khairy P, Macle L, et al, editors. Electrophysiology for clinicians. Minneapolis (MN): Cardiotext; 2011. p. 44–62.
4. Surawicz B, Knilans T. Atrioventricular block; concealed conduction; gap phenomenon. In: Surawicz B, Knilans T, editors. Chou's electrocardiography in clinical practice. 6th edition. Philadelphia: Saunders Elsevier; 2008. p. 456–80.
5. Ziad IF, Miller JM, Zipes DP. Atrioventricular conduction abnormalities. In: Ziad IF, Miller JM, Zipes DP, editors. Clinical arrhythmology and electrophysiology; a companion to Braunwald's heart disease. 2nd edition. Philadelphia: Saunders Elsevier; 2012. p. 175–93.
6. Tonkin AM, Heddles WF, Tornos P. Intermittent atrioventricular block: procainamide administration as a provocative test. Aust N Z J Med 1978;8:594–602.
7. Twidale N, Heddle WF, Tonkin AM. Procainamide administration during electrophysiology study–utility as a provocative test for intermittent atrioventricular block. Pacing Clin Electrophysiol 1988;11(10):1388–97.
8. Emlein G, Huang SK, Pires LA, et al. Prolonged bradyarrhythmias after isolated coronary artery bypass graft surgery. Am Heart J 1993;126:1084–90.
9. Goldman BS, Hill TJ, Weisel RD, et al. Permanent cardiac pacing after open-heart surgery: acquired heart disease. Pacing Clin Electrophysiol 1984;7(3 Pt 1): 367–71.
10. Bleiziffer S, Ruge H, Hörer J, et al. Predictors for new-onset complete heart block after transcatheter aortic valve implantation. JACC Cardiovasc Interv 2010;3:524–30.
11. Gersh B, Phil D, Maron BJ. 2011 ACCF/AHA guideline for the diagnosis and treatment of hypertrophic cardiomyopathy; a report of the American College of Cardiology Foundation/American Heart Association Task Force on Practice Guidelines developed in collaboration with the American Association for Thoracic Surgery, American Society of

Echocardiography, American Society of Nuclear Cardiology, Heart Failure Society of America, Heart Rhythm Society, Society for Cardiovascular Angiography and Interventions, and Society of Thoracic Surgeons. J Am Coll Cardiol 2011;58(25):e212–60.

12. Philips MF, Harper PS. Cardiac disease in myotonic dystrophy. Cardiovasc Res 1997;33:13–22.

13. Sekhri V, Sanal S, DeLorenzo LJ, et al. Cardiac sarcoidosis: a comprehensive review. Arch Med Sci 2011;7(4):546–54.

14. Naik M, Kim D, O'Brien F, et al. Images in cardiovascular medicine. Lyme carditis. Circulation 2008;118: 1881–4.

15. Dias E, Larnaja FS, Miranda A, et al. Chagas' disease: a clinical, epidemiologic, and pathologic study. Circulation 1956;14:1035–60.

16. Park DS, Fishman GI. The cardiac conduction system. Circulation 2011;123:904–15.

17. Smits JP, Veldkamp MW, Wilde AA. Mechanisms of inherited cardiac conduction disease. Europace 2005;7:122–37.

18. Amin AS, Asghari-Roodsari A, Tan HL. Cardiac sodium channelopathies. Pflugers Arch 2010;460:223–37.

19. Friedman DM, Rupel A, Buyon JP. Epidemiology, etiology, detection, and treatment of autoantibody-associated congenital heart block in neonatal lupus. Curr Rheumatol Rep 2007;9:101–8.

20. Khairy P, Balaji S. Cardiac arrhythmias in congenital heart diseases. Indian Pacing Electrophysiol J 2009; 9:299–317.

21. Epstein A, DiMarco JP, Ellenbogen KA, et al. 2012 ACCF/AHA/HRS focused update incorporated into the ACCF/AHA/HRS 2008 guidelines for device-based therapy of cardiac rhythm abnormalities: a report of the American College of Cardiology Foundation/American Heart Association Task Force on Practice Guidelines and the Heart Rhythm Society. Circulation 2013;127:e283–352.

22. Brignole M, Auricchio A, Baron-Esquivias G. 2013 ESC guidelines on cardiac pacing and cardiac resynchronization therapy: the Task Force on Cardiac Pacing and Resynchronization Therapy of the European Society of Cardiology (ESC). Developed in collaboration with the European Heart Rhythm Association (EHRA). Eur Heart J 2013;34: 2281–329.

Electrocardiographic Characteristics of Focal Atrial Tachycardias

Haris M. Haqqani, MBBS(Hons), PhD[a,b,1],
Gwilym M. Morris, BmBCh, PhD[c,d,1],
Peter M. Kistler, MBBS, PhD[e],
Jonathan M. Kalman, MBBS, PhD[c,e,*]

KEYWORDS

- Ventricular tachycardia • Electrocardiograph • Myocardial infarction

KEY POINTS

- Focal atrial tachycardia (AT) is an uncommon form of supraventricular tachycardia that most often occurs in structurally normal hearts.
- Focal AT is characterized by centrifugal activation of the atria from a point source.
- The sites of origin of AT are not randomly distributed throughout the atria but instead cluster around stereotypical sites of anatomic and electrophysiologic heterogeneity.
- The P-wave morphology on the surface ECG in focal AT is generally a reliable guide to the site of origin in the absence of significant structural heart disease or previous ablation.

INTRODUCTION AND DEFINITION

Focal atrial tachycardia (AT) is an uncommon form of supraventricular tachycardia (SVT) defined by its characteristic centrifugal pattern of atrial activation from a focal site of origin. It accounts for 5% to 15% of adults being referred for evaluation of SVT.[1,2] Unlike other forms of SVT, AT requires activation of neither AV nodal or ventricular tissue for tachycardia continuation. Patients may present with palpitations, dyspnea, or, rarely, syncope. Incessant AT is a well-recognized phenomenon that may lead to the development of tachycardia-mediated cardiomyopathy.[3]

PATHOPHYSIOLOGY

Multiple electrophysiologic mechanisms may be responsible for focal AT. These include abnormal automaticity, triggered activity, and microreentry. The absence of a definitive gold standard for in vivo diagnosis of each of these mechanisms means that each is inferred from a combination of observations. Triggered activity and microreentry may be induced by programed stimulation, although triggered activity can also be induced with burst pacing. Automatic focal AT frequently has spontaneous onsets and terminations. In the absence of spontaneous activity it is likely to only

The authors have nothing to disclose.
[a] School of Medicine, University of Queensland, Queensland, Australia; [b] Department of Cardiology, The Prince Charles Hospital, Rode Road, Brisbane, QLD 4032, Australia; [c] Department of Cardiology, The Royal Melbourne Hospital, Melbourne 3050, Australia; [d] Institute of Cardiovascular Sciences, University of Manchester, Manchester, UK; [e] Department of Medicine, University of Melbourne, Royal Parade, Parkville, Victoria 3052, Australia
[1] Dr H.M. Haqqani and Dr G.M. Morris contributed equally to the drafting of this article.
* Corresponding author. Department of Cardiology, The Royal Melbourne Hospital, Melbourne 3050, Australia.
E-mail address: jon.kalman@mh.org.au

be initiated with the use of isoproterenol and only transiently suppressed with adenosine. Abrupt termination of AT with adenosine suggests triggered activity.[4] Adenosine unresponsiveness may indicate microreentry as the mechanism, particularly if long-duration fractionated electrograms are found at the site of origin.[5]

Focal ATs do not occur randomly throughout the right and left atrial chambers. Instead, they arise from stereotypical sites of anatomic and electrophysiologic heterogeneity.[6] In the right atrium, the crista terminalis is most frequent, followed by the tricuspid annulus, coronary sinus (CS) ostium, right atrial appendage, and perinodal region.[7–10] The pulmonary veins, mitral annulus (usually the aortomitral continuity), left atrial appendage, CS body, and left septal region are the most common sites of origin in the left atrium.[11–15] The septal, perinodal region is particularly complex because several structures are located in close proximity, including the AV annuli, fossa ovalis, and the noncoronary aortic sinus of Valsalva. Some focal ATs arise from or may be ablated via the latter structure.[16] Multiple focal ATs may be seen in the same patient.[17]

ECG CHARACTERISTICS OF FOCAL AT

The P wave on the surface ECG during focal AT commences when a sufficient mass of atrial myocardium has been depolarized and continues until both atria are fully activated. Unlike macroreentrant ATs (atrial flutters), there is a diastolic period of quiescent atrial activity that accounts for most of the tachycardia cycle length. The vector, duration, and sequence of atrial depolarization determine the P-wave morphology (PWM) on the ECG. These are, in turn, determined by the location of the focus of origin and by the centrifugal wavefront propagation characteristics away from that focus. Additional factors that can influence the PWM include ECG electrode positioning, antiarrhythmic drugs, surgical or spontaneous atrial scars, and translational, rotational, or attitudinal variation in the normal cardio-thoracic anatomic relationship. In the absence of structural heart disease, the PWM represents a reliable guide to the general region of AT origin.[18]

GENERAL PRINCIPLES SURROUNDING THE ECG IN FOCAL AT

- Focal AT presents as a narrow complex tachycardia on the surface ECG.
- Spontaneous or induced AV block excludes orthodromic reciprocating tachycardia (ORT) mediated by a bypass tract and makes the diagnosis of AV nodal reentrant tachycardia (AVNRT) less likely.
- The sinus rhythm ECG is likely to be normal with no preexcitation.
- The PWM in tachycardia is described as positive, negative, or isoelectric, and is monophasic or multiphasic. Notching is also described.
- The initial P-wave vector is a vital component of the overall PWM and every effort should be made to induce an isoelectric interval following the preceding T wave by the use of carotid sinus massage, intravenous adenosine, or transient ventricular burst pacing before analyzing the P wave (**Fig. 1**).

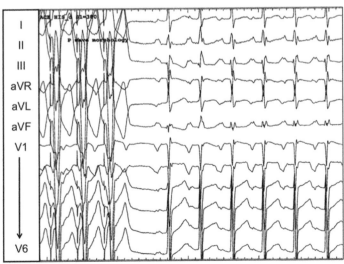

Fig. 1. Ventricular burst pacing causing retrograde AV nodal concealment and increased AV block during AT. This maneuver can be used to ensure an adequate preceding isoelectric interval that does not distort the initial P-wave vector.

- The first task is to distinguish right from left atrial origin. The V1 PWM was found to be most reliable for this purpose in the large study by Kistler and colleagues.[18] Negative or biphasic positive-negative P waves in V1 indicate a right atrial origin, whereas a positive or negative-positive V1 P wave suggests a left atrial focus (**Fig. 2**).
- Septal sites of origin produce narrow P waves that are of shorter duration than the sinus P waves due to synchronous rather than sequential right and left atrial activation.
- Anterior or annular structures tend to have late transitions to positive P waves across the precordium, whereas posterior atrial structures such as the pulmonary veins or crista terminalis usually have positive precordial concordance.
- Craniocaudal sites of origin may be distinguished by their frontal plane P-wave axis with cranial sites of origin such as the superior pulmonary veins and atrial appendages displaying positive P waves in the inferior leads.

ECG CHARACTERISTICS OF RIGHT ATRIAL SITES OF ORIGIN
Crista Terminalis

- The crista terminalis is the most common site of origin of focal AT and accounts for two-thirds of right ATs.[7]

- Most cristal ATs arise from the superior or midcristal region and have similar PWM to sinus rhythm (**Fig. 3**).
- Regarding positive-negative P wave in V1, in 10% of cases the P wave will be monophasic positive in tachycardia. However, in these cases, the sinus rhythm V1 PWM will also be positive. This is in contrast to the positive V1 P wave of nearby right superior pulmonary vein tachycardia in which the sinus rhythm P wave is biphasic positive-negative.
- Positive in I and II, and negative in aVR with positive/negative in V1: 93% sensitivity and 95% specificity for cristal tachycardia.[18]

Tricuspid Annulus

- Tricuspid annulus is the second-most common focal, right AT location.
- AT can arise from around the circumference of the annulus but is usually from the posterolateral (7–9 o'clock as viewed from the ventricle) aspect.[8] This affects frontal plane axis such that caudal sites on the annulus have negative P waves in the inferior leads (and vice versa).
- However, all tricuspid annular foci have broad, negative P waves in V1 and V2, often with a notch.[8]
- There is a late precordial transition, or negative precordial P-wave concordance.

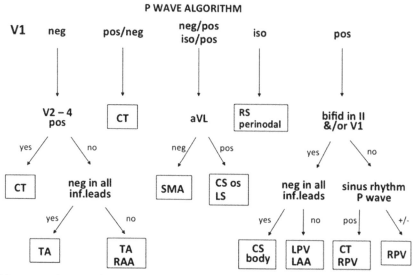

P WAVE ALGORITHM

Fig. 2. Algorithm to predict site of origin of focal AT from surface PWM. Systematic analysis of V1, precordial, and frontal plane axis allows for reliable discrimination between sites in the absence of structural heart disease. CS, coronary sinus; CT, crista terminalis; LPV, left pulmonary vein; LS, left septum; RAA, right atrial appendage; RPV, right pulmonary veins; RS, right septum; SMA, superior mitral annulus; TA, tricuspid annulus. (*From* Kistler PM, Roberts-Thomson KC, Haqqani HM, et al. P-wave morphology in focal atrial tachycardia: development of an algorithm to predict the anatomic site of origin. J Am Coll Cardiol 2006;48(5):1010–7.)

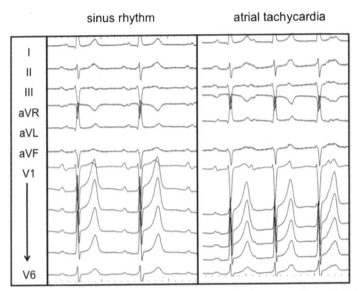

sinus rhythm   atrial tachycardia

Fig. 3. Electrocardiographic appearance of superior cristal tachycardia demonstrating a PWM very similar to that of sinus rhythm.

Right Atrial Appendage

- Most right atrial appendages arise from the base, near the tricuspid annulus but tip origins are also described.
- All are characterized by broad, negative, notched P waves in V1 with an inferior frontal plane axis and may be indistinguishable from superior tricuspid annular tachycardia (**Fig. 4**).[10]

CS Ostium

- Most AT in the CS arise from the superior, annular lip of the CS os.[9]
- The PWM is nearly identical to the P wave in typical counterclockwise isthmus-dependent atrial flutter. The latter can be thought of as activating the atrium from a point source after the wavefront exits the protected cavotricuspid isthmus in the immediate vicinity of the CS os.
- The P, wave is deeply negative in the inferior leads and is isoelectric-positive in V1 (sometimes negative-positive). The precordial transition to negativity is variable but the aVR and aVL are usually equally positive.[9]

Septal and Perinodal Region

- Owing to the anatomic proximity of several structures, the PWM is variable for focal AT arising from this region.[18,19]
- An isoelectric V1 P wave is helpful when present but only seen in 50% of cases.

- Generally, the P wave is narrow and biphasic but variable, depending on the precise site of origin.
- A negative-positive biphasic P wave in V1 is also commonly seen for right perinodal ATs but is a nonspecific finding. Left septal, left perinodal, noncoronary cusp, and aortomitral continuity foci frequently have the same V1 morphology.

ECG CHARACTERISTICS OF LEFT ATRIAL SITES OF ORIGIN
Pulmonary Veins

- Pulmonary veins are the most common sites of origin of left ATs.[11]
- PWM is invariably positive in V1 with positive precordial concordance.
- Left-sided pulmonary veins have broader, notched P waves in V1 and in the inferior leads compared with right-sided pulmonary veins. The latter are often positive in lead I.
- The superior pulmonary veins have an inferior frontal plane axis but the inferior pulmonary veins have variable PWM, which is usually isoelectric or low-amplitude positive.

Left Atrial Appendage

- The left atrial appendage is separated from the left superior pulmonary vein (LSPV) only by the Coumadin ridge and, therefore, can have a similar PWM.
- Most origins are at the base but foci of AT have also been described from the tip.

A

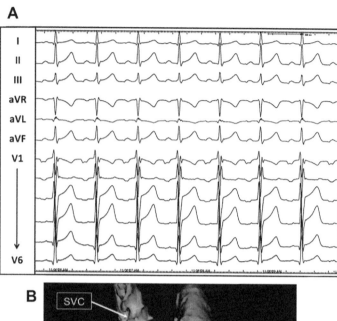

B

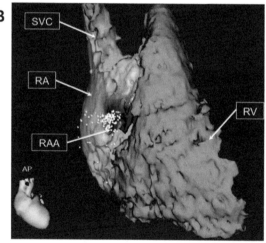

Fig. 4. (*A*) Typical ECG appearance of a focal AT arising from the right atrial appendage (RAA) with a notched, broad negative P wave in V1 and inferior frontal plane axis. (*B*) Electroanatomic map with CT image integration showing earliest activation breakout at the lateral base of the RAA. AP, anteroposterior; RA, right atrium; RV, right ventricle; SVC, superior vena cava.

- It is broad, positive, and notched in V1 and inferior leads (such as LSPV) but has a deeply negative P wave.[13,18] The latter suggests an appendage origin rather than the LSPV.

Mitral Annulus

- Almost all mitral annular ATs arise from the aortomitral continuity, adjacent to the left fibrous trigone.[12]
- The adjacent aortic root forces atrial activation to initially proceed leftward away from V1 before activating the left, then right, atria toward V1.[12,18] Hence, there is a biphasic negative-positive V1 PWM, analogous to the qR morphology of ventricular tachycardia

arising from the ventricular aspect of the aortomitral continuity.[20]
- The inferior leads are usually isoelectric or low-amplitude positive.

Noncoronary Aortic Sinus of Valsalva

- Focal AT may arise from the myocardial sleeves investing the aortic root or noncoronary aortic sinus of Valsalva ablation may eliminate tachycardias arising from closely apposed septal structures.
- The PWM is narrow owing to initial midline septal activation and may appear similar to aortomitral continuity and left perinodal ATs but is usually negative in V1 and V2 and positive in lead I and aVL (**Fig. 5**).[16,19]

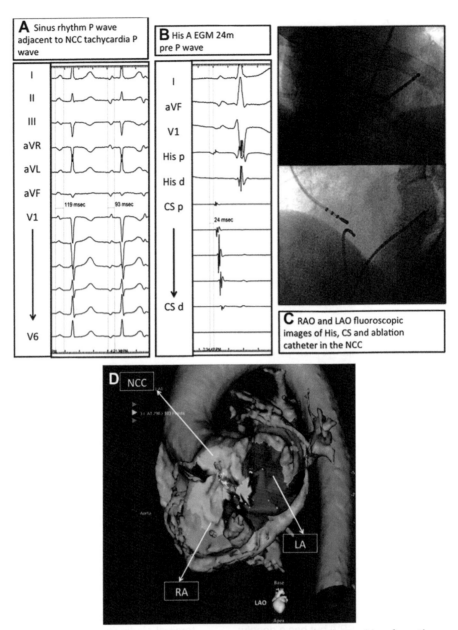

Fig. 5. A 76-year-old woman presented with frequent palpitations and focal AT arising from the noncoronary cusp (NCC). (*A*) The sinus rhythm PWM adjacent to the tachycardia P wave with a typical biphasic negative-positive V1. Significant narrowing of the P-wave duration can be seen during tachycardia. (*B*) The atrial electrogram on the His catheter is 24 ms pre-P wave, which is consistent with a perinodal origin. (*C*) Fluoroscopic right anterior oblique (RAO) and left anterior oblique (LAO) views shows the relative proximity of the ablation catheter within the NCC to the His catheter. (*D*) The relationship between the site of earliest activation breakout in the nadir of the NCC and the subjacent interatrial septum. LA, left atrium; LAO, left anterior oblique; RA, right atrium.

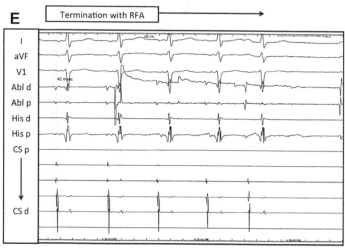

Fig. 5. (*continued*). (*E*) Ablation catheter signal 40 ms pre-P wave with termination of tachycardia within 1.5 seconds of radiofrequency energy application. A far-field His electrogram on the ablation catheter. RFA, radiofrequency ablation.

- The inferior leads are characteristically small biphasic negative-positive.

CS Body

- A CS body arises from 3 to 4 cm inside the CS ostium, from the myocardial coat of the CS.[14]
- It has a broad, positive V1 PWM with deeply negative inferior leads and an aVR to aVL ratio greater than 1.

Left Septal Region

- The left septal region is an infrequent left atrial site of origin of AT but important to distinguish from adjacent right and left atrial structures.
- PWM is biphasic negative-positive in V1 and in the precordium, and negative or biphasic negative-positive in the inferior leads (**Fig. 6**).[15]

DIFFERENTIAL DIAGNOSIS

Focal AT needs to be differentiated from other forms of SVT, from macroreentrant forms of ATs (atrial flutters) and, occasionally, from sinus tachycardia.

Focal AT is distinguished from reentrant forms of SVT (AVNRT and ORT) by the following observations:

1. There is a variable R-P relationship during stable tachycardia, either spontaneously or during pacing maneuvers. AVNRT may have slight RP wobble at its onset and, rarely, ORT may have RP variability due to decremental or multiple bypass tracts. However, a constant RP interval is integral to the mechanism of reentrant SVT but is not an actual conduction interval in AT.

2. An inferior frontal plane P-wave axis essentially excludes AVNRT (but not ORT).
3. Tachycardia persistence during AV block essentially excludes ORT (but not AVNRT).
4. Reproducible termination of tachycardia with AV block (ie, ending with a P wave rather than a QRS) excludes focal AT.
5. Ventricular extrastimuli or burst pacing that terminates tachycardia without conducting to the atrium excludes AT.
6. During entrainment of tachycardia with overdrive pacing from the ventricle with resumption of tachycardia on cessation of pacing, an A-A-H-V response is diagnostic of AT.[21]

The surface ECG morphology may not always adequately discriminate between focal and macroreentrant AT tachycardia. Although an isoelectric baseline between discrete P waves is characteristic of focal AT, rapid tachycardias occurring in atria with slow conduction may display baseline undulation. Conversely, although most macroreentrant ATs exhibit continuous undulation on the surface ECG (the flutter wave), significant scarring may result in long isoelectric segments between focal P waves. An electrophysiology (EP) study may be required to make the definitive distinction. This may be clinically important in assessing thromboembolic risk because this is essentially negligible in focal AT but may be high in patients with atrial flutter. During an EP study, the ability to record atrial activation throughout the tachycardia cycle length is largely diagnostic of a macroreentrant arrhythmia.

Some ATs can also be confused with sinus tachycardia but are distinguished by

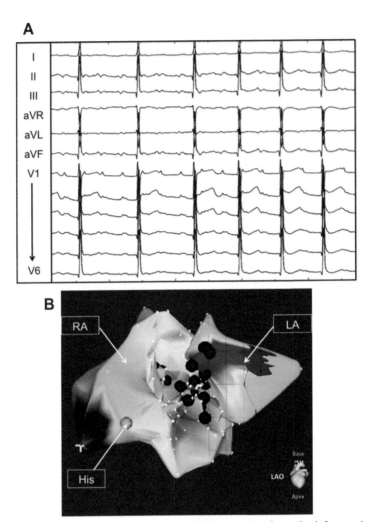

Fig. 6. (A) Surface electrocardiographic appearance of a focal AT arising from the left septal region. (B) Electro-anatomic activation map demonstrating earliest activation depicted in red in septal region of the left atrium (LA). LAO, left anterior oblique; RA, right atrium.

1. Sudden onset and offset, abruptly or more than three or four beats in AT, compared with gradual increases and decreases in rate over several minutes with sinus tachycardia
2. Induction with programed stimulation or burst pacing
3. Increase in rate of AT with isoproterenol with identical activation breakout (in sinus tachycardia, in addition to increasing rate, isoproterenol also causes migration of the earliest breakout site higher up the crista terminalis).

PHARMACOLOGIC MANAGEMENT

- There are no large-scale datasets to establish efficacy of particular agents, hence treatment is often empiric.
- Beta blockers and calcium blockers are commenced first because of their excellent

safety profile; however, evidence for efficacy is limited.
- Only around one-third of patients may find an effective antiarrhythmic drug option to suppress recurrences of focal AT.[22]

OUTCOMES OF EP STUDY AND ABLATION

At EP study, multipolar catheters are advanced transvenously to various sites, including the CS, the His recording position, the crista terminalis, and/or the tricuspid annulus. Tachycardia induction is attempted with pacing maneuvers with or without isoproterenol. Induced tachycardias are studied using these techniques to exclude other forms of SVT. Once AT has been diagnosed, every effort is made to obtain a noise-free, unencumbered P wave with preceding isoelectric line off the T wave. This is usually achieved with transient ventricular burst pacing. With the use of fluoroscopy alone or assisted by electroanatomic mapping systems, point-by-point activation mapping is commenced near the site of origin as suggested by the PWM. Multipolar catheters at the crista or tricuspid annulus can assist this process greatly. Transseptal access is obtained to map left atrial foci. Regardless of any surrogate intracardiac references used, all activation times are eventually referenced back to the P-wave onset. Sites of origin of focal AT are usually 20 to 30 ms pre–P-wave onset but this is variable. In most cases, a unipolar QS signal is likely to be seen at the successful ablation site.[23]

Noninducibility is a recognized problem in AT ablation. Minimizing sedation and local anesthesia, avoiding general anesthesia, ensuring adequate washout of antiarrhythmic drugs are important strategies to minimize this problem. Nonsustained ATs may be targeted with the use of noncontact mapping arrays.[24]

Catheter ablation is usually performed with radiofrequency energy but cryoablation may also be considered for perinodal tachycardias or in children.[25] Solid-tip ablation electrodes are generally sufficient for most right atrial sites of origin, although irrigated ablation may be required for thick myocardial tissue such as at the base of the atrial appendages. Open-irrigated catheters may reduce char formation and thromboembolic risk when ablation is performed in the left atrium and are required to achieve sufficient power for CS body tachycardia ablation.

The published success rates of focal AT catheter ablation vary between 70% and 100% with a recurrence rate of between 0% and 33%, depending on the site of origin.[18,26–28] Chen and colleagues[29] reported a recurrence rate of 7% in a systematic review of 16 studies. Of note, long-term follow-up of pulmonary vein tachycardia patients does not suggest any signal of increased risk of late atrial fibrillation.[30]

The overall complication rate is low, between 0% and 2%, and is usually vascular access related. However, major complications such as AV block, cardiac perforation with pericardial tamponade, phrenic nerve palsy, and pulmonary vein stenosis have been described. Stroke and systemic embolism are potential complications with left atrial ablations.

SUMMARY

Focal AT is an uncommon form of SVT that is defined by centrifugal atrial activation from a discrete site of origin. It occurs mostly in structurally normal hearts and arises from stereotypical locations of anatomic heterogeneity throughout both atria. Consequently, the PWM on the surface ECG is a reliable and helpful guide to mapping these arrhythmias. Catheter ablation can achieve successful acute and long-term clinical cure of these patients.

REFERENCES

1. Rodriguez LM, de Chillou C, Schlapfer J, et al. Age at onset and gender of patients with different types of supraventricular tachycardias. Am J Cardiol 1992;70:1213–5.
2. Wellens HJ. Atrial tachycardia. How important is the mechanism? Circulation 1994;90:1576–7.
3. Medi C, Kalman JM, Haqqani H, et al. Tachycardia-mediated cardiomyopathy secondary to focal atrial tachycardia: long-term outcome after catheter ablation. J Am Coll Cardiol 2009;53:1791–7.
4. Markowitz SM, Stein KM, Mittal S, et al. Differential effects of adenosine on focal and macroreentrant atrial tachycardia. J Cardiovasc Electrophysiol 1999;10:489–502.
5. Markowitz SM, Nemirovksy D, Stein KM, et al. Adenosine-insensitive focal atrial tachycardia: evidence for de novo micro-re-entry in the human atrium. J Am Coll Cardiol 2007;49:1324–33.
6. Roberts-Thomson KC, Kistler PM, Kalman JM. Focal atrial tachycardia I: clinical features, diagnosis, mechanisms, and anatomic location. Pacing Clin Electrophysiol 2006;29:643–52.
7. Kalman JM, Olgin JE, Karch MR, et al. "Cristal tachycardias": origin of right atrial tachycardias from the crista terminalis identified by intracardiac echocardiography. J Am Coll Cardiol 1998;31:451–9.
8. Morton JB, Sanders P, Das A, et al. Focal atrial tachycardia arising from the tricuspid annulus: electrophysiologic and electrocardiographic characteristics. J Cardiovasc Electrophysiol 2001;12:653–9.
9. Kistler PM, Fynn SP, Haqqani H, et al. Focal atrial tachycardia from the ostium of the coronary sinus: electrocardiographic and electrophysiological characterization and radiofrequency ablation. J Am Coll Cardiol 2005;45:1488–93.
10. Roberts-Thomson KC, Kistler PM, Haqqani HM, et al. Focal atrial tachycardias arising from the right atrial appendage: electrocardiographic and electrophysiologic characteristics and radiofrequency ablation. J Cardiovasc Electrophysiol 2007;18:367–72.
11. Kistler PM, Sanders P, Fynn SP, et al. Electrophysiological and electrocardiographic characteristics of focal atrial tachycardia originating from the pulmonary veins: acute and long-term outcomes of radiofrequency ablation. Circulation 2003;108:1968–75.
12. Kistler PM, Sanders P, Hussin A, et al. Focal atrial tachycardia arising from the mitral annulus: electrocardiographic and electrophysiologic characterization. J Am Coll Cardiol 2003;41:2212–9.

13. Yamada T, Murakami Y, Yoshida Y, et al. Electrophysiologic and electrocardiographic characteristics and radiofrequency catheter ablation of focal atrial tachycardia originating from the left atrial appendage. Heart Rhythm 2007;4:1284–91.

14. Badhwar N, Kalman JM, Sparks PB, et al. Atrial tachycardia arising from the coronary sinus musculature: electrophysiological characteristics and long-term outcomes of radiofrequency ablation. J Am Coll Cardiol 2005;46:1921–30.

15. Wong MC, Kalman JM, Ling LH, et al. Left septal atrial tachycardias: electrocardiographic and electrophysiologic characterization of a paraseptal focus. J Cardiovasc Electrophysiol 2013;24:413–8.

16. Ouyang F, Ma J, Ho SY, et al. Focal atrial tachycardia originating from the non-coronary aortic sinus: electrophysiological characteristics and catheter ablation. J Am Coll Cardiol 2006;48:122–31.

17. Hillock RJ, Kalman JM, Roberts-Thomson KC, et al. Multiple focal atrial tachycardias in a healthy adult population: characterization and description of successful radiofrequency ablation. Heart Rhythm 2007;4:435–8.

18. Kistler PM, Roberts-Thomson KC, Haqqani HM, et al. P-wave morphology in focal atrial tachycardia: development of an algorithm to predict the anatomic site of origin. J Am Coll Cardiol 2006;48:1010–7.

19. Teh AW, Kistler PM, Kalman JM. Using the 12-lead ECG to localize the origin of ventricular and atrial tachycardias: part 1. Focal atrial tachycardia. J Cardiovasc Electrophysiol 2009;20:706–9 [quiz: 705].

20. Dixit S, Gerstenfeld EP, Lin D, et al. Identification of distinct electrocardiographic patterns from the basal left ventricle: distinguishing medial and lateral sites of origin in patients with idiopathic ventricular tachycardia. Heart Rhythm 2005;2:485–91.

21. Knight BP, Zivin A, Souza J, et al. A technique for the rapid diagnosis of atrial tachycardia in the electrophysiology laboratory. J Am Coll Cardiol 1999;33: 775–81.

22. Prager NA, Cox JL, Lindsay BD, et al. Long-term effectiveness of surgical treatment of ectopic atrial tachycardia. J Am Coll Cardiol 1993;22:85–92.

23. Poty H, Saoudi N, Haissaguerre M, et al. Radiofrequency catheter ablation of atrial tachycardias. Am Heart J 1996;131:481–9.

24. Higa S, Tai CT, Lin YJ, et al. Focal atrial tachycardia: new insight from noncontact mapping and catheter ablation. Circulation 2004;109:84–91.

25. Wong T, Segal OR, Markides V, et al. Cryoablation of focal atrial tachycardia originating close to the atrioventricular node. J Cardiovasc Electrophysiol 2004; 15:838.

26. Goldberger J, Kall J, Ehlert F, et al. Effectiveness of radiofrequency catheter ablation for treatment of atrial tachycardia. Am J Cardiol 1993;72:787–93.

27. Kay GN, Chong F, Epstein AE, et al. Radiofrequency ablation for treatment of primary atrial tachycardias. J Am Coll Cardiol 1993;21:901–9.

28. Anguera I, Brugada J, Roba M, et al. Outcomes after radiofrequency catheter ablation of atrial tachycardia. Am J Cardiol 2001;87:886–90.

29. Chen SA, Tai CT, Chiang CE, et al. Focal atrial tachycardia: reanalysis of the clinical and electrophysiologic characteristics and prediction of successful radiofrequency ablation. J Cardiovasc Electrophysiol 1998;9:355–65.

30. Teh AW, Kalman JM, Medi C, et al. Long-term outcome following successful catheter ablation of atrial tachycardia originating from the pulmonary veins: absence of late atrial fibrillation. J Cardiovasc Electrophysiol 2010;21:747–50.

Right and Left Atrial Macroreentrant Tachycardias

Shih-Lin Chang, MD, PhD, Shih-Ann Chen, MD*

KEYWORDS

- ECG • Macroreentrant tachycardias • Atrial flutter • Circuit • Mapping • Algorithm

KEY POINTS

- A 12-lead electrocardiogram (ECG) during tachycardia provides important information in the initial strategy for the physician or specialized cardiologist.
- Catheter ablation of the cavotricuspid isthmus can eradicate typical and reverse typical atrial flutter (AFL) with a high success rate and few complications.
- For atypical AFL, catheter ablation of the isthmus between the boundaries using electroanatomic mapping can eliminate these arrhythmias.

Atrial macroreentrant tachycardia is a common tachycardia in clinical practice and its incidence is increasing because of the aging population.[1–6] It can result from structural heart disease or scarring from previous cardiac surgery/ablation but also can be found in patients without obvious heart disease.[2,3,7] Macroreentrant atrial tachycardia is characterized by an atrial tachycardia driven by a large reentry circuit around a central obstacle with fixed and/or functional barriers.[8] Entrainment is possible in most macroreentrant atrial tachycardias. Numerous forms of macroreentrant atrial tachycardia have been reported, and the surface electrocardiogram (ECG) patterns could correlate with the reentrant circuits. Atrial flutter (AFL) is defined by an undulating F wave in the ECG with a sawtooth appearance, which represents macroreentrant atrial tachycardia in surface ECG. Therefore, the 12-lead ECG provides important information for the location of the reentrant circuit location and mechanism.

It is crucial to understand how to determine a macroreentrant tachycardia origin based on the 12-lead ECG morphology of the flutter wave. A period of at least 3:1 AV block during tachycardias is suitable for flutter wave analysis. The widest flutter wave of any lead is used to define the onset and the offset of flutter wave in all other leads.[9] The schemas of variable flutter wave morphologies on 12-lead ECGs are shown in **Fig. 1**.

ELECTROPHYSIOLOGY STUDY AND ECG CHARACTERISTICS OF MACROREENTRANT TACHYCARDIAS

Typical and Reverse Typical AFL

Typical AFL is the most common type of macroreentrant atrial tachycardia, even in patients with prior cardiac surgery/ablation.[8,10] The cavotricuspid isthmus (CTI), defined as a path bounded by the orifice of the inferior vena cava, eustachian valve/ridge, coronary sinus ostium, and tricuspid annulus, is a protected zone of slow conduction during typical AFL.[7] Activation mapping has shown that the activation wave front goes downward in the right atrial (RA) free wall, travels

The authors have nothing to disclose.
Department of Medicine, Taipei Veterans General Hospital, 201 Section 2, Shih-Pai Road, Taipei, Taiwan
* Corresponding author.
E-mail address: epsachen@ms41.hinet.net

cardiacEP.theclinics.com

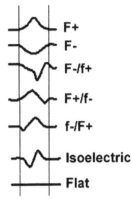

Fig. 1. The schemas of variable flutter wave morphologies on 12-lead ECGs. The first 2 waves are monophasic positive (F+) and negative (F−) flutter waves. The third to sixth waves are biphasic flutter waves, consisting of dominant negative with small terminal positive (F−/f+), dominant positive with small terminal negative (F+/f−), small initial negative with dominant terminal positive (f−/F+), and the equal amplitude of negative and positive waves (isoelectric). Flat polarity is amplitude less than 0.01 mV and more than −0.01 mV. (*From* Yuniadi Y, Tai CT, Lee KT, et al. A new electrocardiographic algorithm to differentiate upper loop re-entry from reverse typical atrial flutter. J Am Coll Cardiol 2005;46:525; with permission.)

through the CTI, spreads upward in the septal wall, and crosses the crista terminalis to complete the reentrant circuit (**Fig. 2**). Reverse slow conduction and rate-dependent conduction delay in the CTI is

mechanistically important for the development of typical AFL (**Fig. 3**). The activation sequence of reverse typical AFL is the opposite of typical AFL.

Slow conduction in the CTI may be mechanistically important for the development of typical and reverse AFL (CTI-dependent AFL). The tricuspid annulus is the anterior and fixed barrier. The crista terminalis and eustachian ridge form the posterior barrier in typical AFL. Split potentials can be recorded along the length of the crista terminalis during pacing from the low posterior right atrium at a long cycle length in patients with clinical AFL, suggesting that poor transverse conduction property in the crista terminalis may be the requisite substrate for the clinical occurrence of typical AFL.[11]

Typical AFL has positive F waves in lead V1; negative F waves in lead V6; and negative F waves in leads II, III, and aVF.[8] Low-amplitude flutter waves can be seen in leads I and aVL (**Fig. 4**A). Reverse typical AFL has wide, negative P waves in lead V1; positive P waves in lead V6; and broad, positive P waves in leads II, III, and aVF (see **Fig. 4**B).[12] However, it may present with different ECG patterns that need activation mapping to define the exact circuit.

RA Upper Loop Reentry and Lower Loop Reentry

Atypical RA flutters could arise from single-loop or double-loop figure-of-eight reentry.[13,14] The activation wave front circulates around the

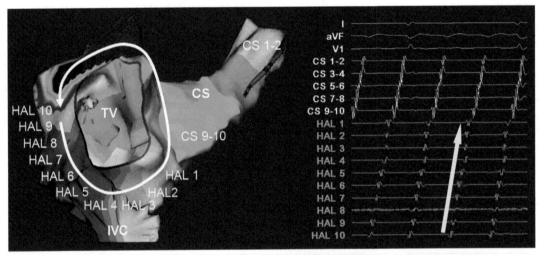

Fig. 2. Activation mapping during typical AFL. Left panel shows that the activation wave front goes downward in the free wall, travels through the cavotricuspid isthmus, spreads upward in the septal wall, and crosses the crista terminalis. Right panel reveals the intracardiac electrogram during typical AFL. Electrodes of halocatheter (HAL) 10 to 4 are located in the free wall, and electrodes of HAL 3 to 1 are located in the CTI. The wave front (*yellow arrow*) activates from HAL 10 to HAL 1 with passive conduction in the coronary sinus (CS). IVC, inferior vena cava; TV, tricuspid valve.

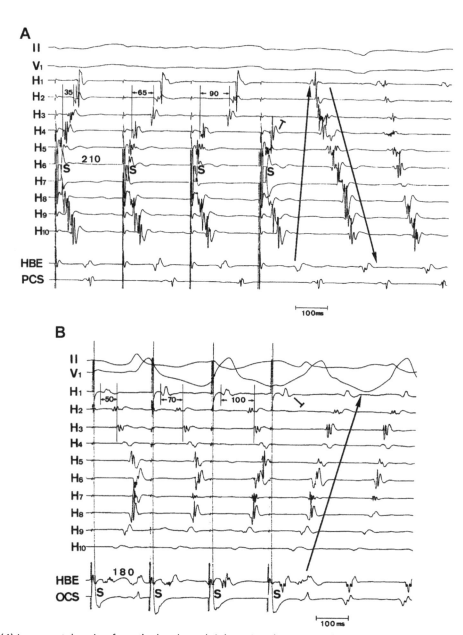

Fig. 3. (*A*) Incremental pacing from the low lateral right atrium (near H6 and H7) using a cycle length of 210 milliseconds produced gradual conduction delays and block in the isthmus (between H4 and H2) of the counterclockwise wave front and initiated clockwise atrial flutter. (*B*) Incremental pacing from the coronary sinus ostium (OCS) using a cycle length of 180 milliseconds produced gradual conduction delays and block in the isthmus (between H1 and H2) of the clockwise wave front and initiated counterclockwise atrial flutter. HBE, recordings at the His bundle area; PCS, recordings at the proximal coronary sinus. (*From* Tai CT, Chen SA, Chiang CE, et al. Characterization of low right atrial isthmus as the slow conduction zone and pharmacological target in typical atrial flutter. Circulation 1997;96:2606; with permission.)

central obstacle composed of a functional block area, and through a gap in the crista terminalis. The conduction channel between the crista terminalis and central obstacle and/or the crista terminalis gap are critical pathways for maintenance of AFL.

Using a noncontact, three-dimensional mapping technique, the wave front of upper loop reentry (ULR) had counterclockwise (CCW) activation (descending activation sequence in the free wall anterior to the crista) or clockwise (CW) activation (ascending activation sequence in the free wall anterior to the crista) around the central obstacle, which was composed of the crista terminalis, the area of functional block and the superior vena cava (SVC)

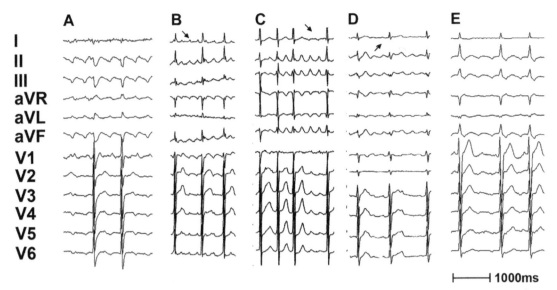

Fig. 4. Surface ECG of RA macroreentrant tachycardias. Typical AFL is characterized by negative waves in inferior leads and positive waves in V1 (*A*). Reverse typical AFL shows positive waves in inferior leads, negative waves in V1, and prominent positive polarity in lead I (*arrow*) (*B*). During upper loop reentry (ULR), lead I shows either negative flat (*arrow*) (*C*) or small positive (*arrow*) (*D*) polarity. Note the similarities of flutter waves in inferior leads between reverse typical and ULR AFL. The surface ECG pattern of lower loop reentry (LLR) is similar to the pattern of typical AFL with negative waves in inferior leads and positive waves in V1 (*E*). (*From* Yuniadi Y, Tai CT, Lee KT, et al. A new electrocardiographic algorithm to differentiate upper loop re-entry from reverse typical atrial flutter. J Am Coll Cardiol 2005;46:526; with permission.)

(**Fig. 5**).[9] During CCW ULR, there might be variable activation of the left atrium by the wave front from the mid or low interatrial septum. Therefore, the polarity of flutter waves in lead I can be flat, negative, or low-amplitude positive. The surface ECG morphology of lower loop reentry (LLR) resembles typical AFL. The differences are characterized by diminished amplitude of the late positive waves in the inferior leads, which may be contributed from wave front collision over the lateral RA wall.

ULR has negative P waves in lead V1 and positive flutter waves in inferior leads, which is analogous to the ECG pattern of atypical AFL (see **Fig. 4**C and D). Negative or flat flutter wave polarity in lead I can differentiate ULR from reverse typical AFL.[9] The surface ECG pattern of LLR is similar to the pattern of typical AFL (see **Fig. 4**E), except for the shorter cycle length and the lower amplitude of the inferior limb leads.[15]

Left Atrial Macroreentrant Tachycardias

Various circuits were reported in left atrial (LA) macroreentrant tachycardias by electroanatomic mapping. The circuits commonly rotate around the mitral annulus, pulmonary veins, or a scar area.[2] LA muscular bundles or a scar area can provide a conduction block line and barrier, which is important for the formation of LA flutter (**Fig. 6**).[16]

The ECG morphology of LA macroreentrant tachycardia shows inhomogeneous and variable patterns resembling atrial tachycardia (discrete P waves and isoelectric baseline) or typical or atypical AFL, and mostly reveals a positive flutter wave in lead V1.[2,8,15,17]

Mitral Annular AFL

The circuit of mitral flutter rotates around the mitral annulus, either CCW or CW. The boundaries of the critical isthmus include the mitral annulus anteriorly, and low-voltage zone or scars in the posterior wall of the LA posteriorly.[2,3,16] CCW mitral annular AFL has positive flutter waves in V1 and low amplitude in the inferior leads.[15] Gerstenfeld and colleagues[18] reported detailed surface ECG pattern for CW and CCW mitral annular AFL in patients after pulmonary vein isolation. CCW mitral annular AFL has positive flutter wave in the inferior and precordial leads, and presents prominent negative flutter waves in leads I and aVL. In contrast, CW mitral annular AFL reveals a negative flutter wave in the inferior leads and positive flutter wave in leads I and aVL (**Fig. 7**A).

LA Septal Flutter

In LA septal flutter, the macroreentrant circuit rotates around the left septum primum, either CCW or CW.[2,13,17] The critical isthmus is located

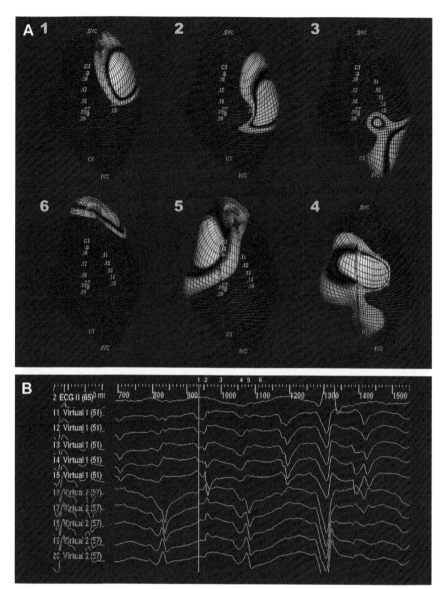

Fig. 5. (A) Isopotential maps showing the activation sequence (frames 1–6) of counterclockwise ULR in the right posterior oblique view. Color scale for each isopotential map has been set so that white indicates the most negative potential. The activation wave front propagates down the anterolateral RA near the SVC (frame 1) to the middle and inferior anterolateral RA (frame 2), then splits into 2 wave fronts (frame 3); one passes around the area of functional block, and the other passes through the cavotricuspid isthmus. The wave front in the lateral RA continues through the gap in the crista terminalis (CT) (frame 4) to the superior posterior RA (frame 5) and activates the atrial wall surrounding the SVC before reactivation of the anterolateral RA. (B) The virtual electrograms from the area of functional block (virtuals 11–15) and the CT (virtuals 16–20) including the conduction gap (virtuals 16–18) show double potentials. The numbers 1 to 6 represent the time points at which the isopotential maps are displayed in panel A. (From Tai CT, Huang JL, Lin YK, et al. Noncontact three dimensional mapping and ablation of upper loop reentry originating in the right atrium. J Am Coll Cardiol 2002;40:749; with permission.)

between the septum primum and the pulmonary veins or between the septum primum and the mitral annulus ring. LA septal AFL reveals prominent, large, positive waves in V1 with almost flat waves in other leads, suggesting that this morphology could be the result of a septal circuit with anterior-posterior forces projecting on V1 and cancellation of caudocranial forces.

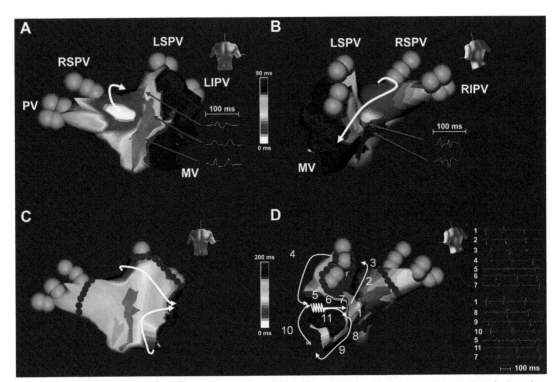

Fig. 6. LA macroreentrant tachycardia with double circuits. (*A, B*) The typical activation pattern during sinus rhythm in the LA. The wave fronts propagate around the gray zone, where isochrone lines are crowded together and double potentials were recorded during sinus rhythm in the anteroposterior and left posteromedial view, respectively. (*C, D*) Activation of a figure-of-eight LA flutter with a cycle length of 199 milliseconds. Arrows indicate circuit loop(s). The brown lesion indicates the pulse of circumferential ablation. One loop rotates around the mitral annulus and the other rotates around the left pulmonary veins with a common channel conducted through the mitral isthmus. The reentrant circuits of atrial flutter were bordered anteriorly and posteriorly by lines of conduction block (*gray zone*), which were in similar locations during sinus rhythm (*A, B*). (*D*) The local bipolar electrograms along the circuit of double-loop reentry. Recording positions are shown in the isochrones map. During LA flutter, clockwise atrial activation around the mitral annulus was manifested by atrial electrograms in the middle posterior wall (site 1), lower posterior wall (site 8), medial mitral isthmus (site 9), and lower anterior wall (site 10), followed by activation in the lateral mitral isthmus (sites 5, 11, and 7). A slow conduction zone with fractionated electrograms was recorded at site 5. Another counterclockwise atrial activation around the left pulmonary vein was manifested by atrial electrograms in the middle posterior wall (site 1), upper posterior wall (site 2), roof (site 3), and upper anterior wall (site 4), followed by activation in the lateral mitral isthmus (sites 5, 6, and 7). Labeled anatomic locations include the mitral valve (MV), right superior pulmonary vein (RSPV), right inferior pulmonary vein (RIPV), left superior pulmonary vein (LSPV), left inferior pulmonary vein (LIPV). (*From* Chang SL, Tai CT, Lin YJ, et al. The role of left atrial muscular bundles in catheter ablation of atrial fibrillation. J Am Coll Cardiol 2007;50:967; with permission.)

CCW septal flutter shows a prominent positive flutter wave in lead V1 and flat flutter or low-amplitude positive wave in the limb leads (see **Fig. 7**B). CW septal flutter has a prominent negative deflection in lead V1 and flat flutter or low-amplitude positive F wave in limb leads.[17]

Other LA Flutters

Macroreentrant circuits can rotate around one or more pulmonary veins and a scar in the posterior wall or roof of LA.[2,3] These circuits may have multiple loops (see **Fig. 6**). In LA posterior flutter, the circuit rotates around low-voltage or scarred areas on the LA posterior wall.[17]

The ECG pattern of pulmonary vein flutter is characterized by a positive wave in V1 with positive wave in lead I and isoelectric wave in aVL for right pulmonary vein flutter; and an isoelectric P wave in lead I and negative wave in aVL for left pulmonary vein flutter (see **Fig. 7**C). LA posterior wall AFL is less commonly seen, and its ECG morphology resembles typical AFL with diminished amplitude in the inferior leads.[15]

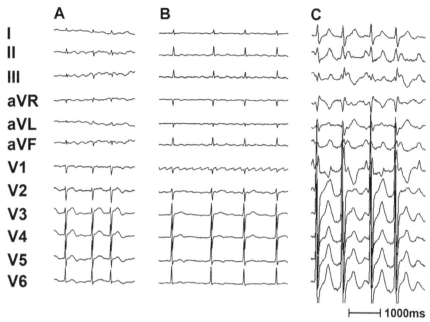

Fig. 7. Surface ECG of LA macroreentrant tachycardias. Clockwise mitral annular AFL reveals a negative flutter wave in the inferior leads and positive flutter wave in leads I and aVL (*A*). Counterclockwise septal flutter shows a prominent positive flutter wave in lead V1 and low amplitude of positive wave in limb leads (*B*). Left pulmonary vein flutter shows a positive wave in V1 with an isoelectric P wave in lead I and negative wave in aVL (*C*).

DIFFERENTIAL DIAGNOSIS IN 12-LEAD ECG

Several diagnostic criteria of surface ECGs have been proposed to localize the flutter circuit. Understanding the origin of macroreentrant tachycardia can facilitate radiofrequency ablation. Distinguishing typical from atypical AFL in advance is helpful, because these two tachycardias require different mapping and ablation techniques. LA AFL has more inhomogeneous patterns compared with RA AFL. A positive flutter wave in the inferior leads has been found in LA, ULR, and reverse typical AFL. Scheinman and colleagues[15] reported that there was a decreased voltage of the flutter waves in the inferior leads for LA flutter compared with RA flutter. Left AFL can be distinguished from right AFL by the lower amplitude of flutter wave in the inferior ECG leads.

Our laboratory proposed an ECG algorithm to further differentiate ULR from reverse typical AFL (**Fig. 8**).[9] The polarity and amplitude of a flutter wave in lead I of the 12-lead ECG could discriminate ULR from reverse typical AFL. During reverse typical AFL, the RA free wall is electrically silent when the LA, including the atrial septum, is activated in the leftward and downward directions, similar to activation during sinus rhythm.[19] Therefore, the polarity of flutter waves in lead I is positive because the activation direction faces toward lead I. In contrast, during CW ULR, the right atrium,

including its free wall, is activated in the rightward direction via the gap in the crista terminalis and the upward direction when the left atrium is activated in the leftward and downward directions. These two oppositely directing and simultaneously propagating wave fronts seem to offset the polarity of each other, resulting in a flat, negative, or low-amplitude positive wave in lead I. During CCW ULR, there might be variable activation of the left atrium by the wave front from the mid or low interatrial septum. Therefore, the polarity of flutter waves in lead I can also be flat, negative, or low-amplitude positive.

Atrial tachyarrhythmias, including focal and macroreentrant atrial tachycardia, are commonly observed following catheter ablation of atrial fibrillation (AF) with a varied incidence of 3% to 29%.[3–6,20] Our laboratory had provided a diagnostic algorithm for differentiating the macroreentrant and focal atrial tachycardias, and localizing the origin of the circuit after pulmonary vein isolation.[21] **Fig. 9** shows that the amplitude of the flutter or P waves in V6 and tachycardia cycle length can distinguish macroreentrant from focal atrial tachycardia with sensitivity of 88%, specificity of 96%, and accuracy of 94%. Furthermore, negative flutter waves in any of the precordial leads could differentiate an RA macroreentrant tachycardia from an LA macroreentrant tachycardia with a

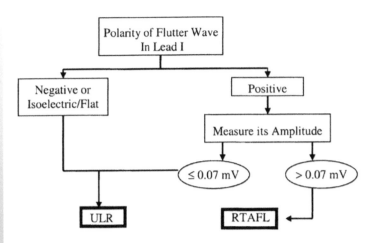

Fig. 8. Diagnostic algorithm to differentiate between ULR and reverse typical atrial flutter (RTAFL). Flat polarity is defined as polarity of less than 0.01 mV but more than −0.01 mV. Isoelectric is defined as biphasic polarity in which negative and positive deflection have equal amplitude. (*From* Yuniadi Y, Tai CT, Lee KT, et al. A new electrocardiographic algorithm to differentiate upper loop re-entry from reverse typical atrial flutter. J Am Coll Cardiol 2005;46:527; with permission.)

sensitivity and specificity of 83% and 100% (**Fig. 10**), respectively, and an accuracy of 98%. Opposite polarity of flutter wave could be found clinically in V1 and V6 in cavotricuspid isthmus–dependent AFL. Precordial negativity may represent an RA origin. Regarding the LA macroreentrant tachycardia, most macroreentrant atrial tachycardias were terminated during the ablation of the mitral isthmus and roof.[3,21] Prominent positive flutter waves in V1 were more commonly seen in roof/mitral isthmus–dependent than non–roof/mitral isthmus–dependent macroreentrant atrial tachycardias, suggesting that V1 is useful for differentiation (**Figs. 11** and **12**). The sensitivity and specificity were 80% and 83%,

respectively, with an accuracy of 81%.[21] Gerstenfeld and colleagues[18] showed that mitral annular AFL following pulmonary vein isolation had a positive P wave in V1 with a small initial negative depolarization in the other precordial leads. Positive flutter waves in leads I and aVL can differentiate CW mitral AFL from CCW RA flutter and left pulmonary vein atrial tachycardia after AF ablation.

MANAGEMENT

Three methods of treatment can be used to convert AFL to sinus rhythm: antiarrhythmic drugs, electrical cardioversion, or catheter ablation. Catheter ablation has a higher success rate in

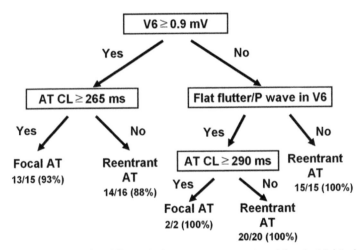

Fig. 9. A new diagnostic algorithm for differentiating macroreentrant and focal atrial tachycardia (AT). A flat wave is defined as a polarity of the flutter or P wave of less than or equal to 0.05 and greater than or equal to −0.05 mV. Numbers indicates numbers of patients with accurate prediction/total number of patients; percentage indicates the percentage of patients with accurate prediction/total number of patients in the study by Chang and colleagues.[21] CL, cycle length. (*From* Chang SL, Tsao HM, Lin YJ, et al. Differentiating macroreentrant from focal atrial tachycardias occurred after circumferential pulmonary vein isolation. J Cardiovasc Electrophysiol 2011;22:753; with permission.)

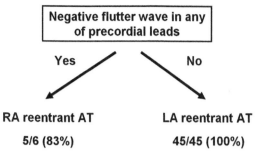

RA reentrant AT   LA reentrant AT

5/6 (83%)   45/45 (100%)

Fig. 10. Diagnostic algorithm for differentiating RA and LA macroreentrant AT. Number indicates number of patients with accurate prediction/total number of patients; percentage indicates the percentage of patients with accurate prediction/total number of patients in the study by Chang and colleagues.[21] (*From* Chang SL, Tsao HM, Lin YJ, et al. Differentiating macroreentrant from focal atrial tachycardias occurred after circumferential pulmonary vein isolation. J Cardiovasc Electrophysiol 2011;22:753; with permission.)

elimination of AFL and maintenance of sinus rhythm.[2,3,6,8] The CTI is the target for radiofrequency ablation of typical and reverse typical AFL, in which it is easiest to obtain complete bidirectional isthmus block via a venous approach. However, atypical AFL could arise from the RA or LA. Electroanatomic mapping and transseptal approach are sometimes needed. Radiofrequency ablation of the isthmus between the boundaries can eliminate these arrhythmias. It is more time consuming and difficult to eliminate atypical AFL compared with typical AFL. Therefore, it is important to identify the origin of reentrant tachycardias

using 12-lead ECG in management of AFL. Recognizing the location of macroreentrant tachycardia from the 12-lead ECG is useful for (1) determining an initial treatment (pharmacologic or ablation therapy), (2) facilitating mapping and navigating ablation, and (3) monitoring and understanding the possible mechanism of recurrence from prior catheter ablation of tachyarrhythmias.

INTERVENTION OUTCOME

The acute and long-term outcomes of macroreentrant atrial tachycardia are shown in **Table 1**. Radiofrequency ablation of the CTI can eliminate typical and reverse AFL with low recurrence and complication rates.[22–24] However, AF continues to be a long-term risk for patients undergoing this procedure, with incidence of 20% to 50%.[22,25] The presence of structural heart disease and prior spontaneous or inducible sustained AF increases the risk of developing AF. For atypical RA AFL, radiofrequency ablation of the free-wall channel and/or the crista terminalis gap is effective in eliminating these macroreentrant tachycardias.[14]

Regarding LA macroreentrant tachycardia, the protected isthmus between 2 anatomic barriers is amenable to radiofrequency ablation. Identifying the conduction block line and further creating additional line(s) crossing the isthmus of the reentry barrier may contribute to a better clinical outcome.[2,20,26]

With increasingly aggressive treatments of AF, postablation macroreentrant atrial tachycardias are expected to increase in number and complexity in daily clinical practice. Detailed

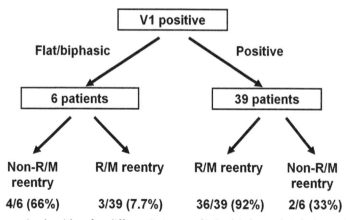

Fig. 11. A new diagnostic algorithm for differentiating roof/mitral isthmus (R/M)–dependent from non–R/M-dependent macroreentrant AT. Number indicates number of patients with accurate prediction/total number of patients; percentage indicates the percentage of patients with accurate prediction/total number of patients in the study by Chang and colleagues.[21] (*From* Chang SL, Tsao HM, Lin YJ, et al. Differentiating macroreentrant from focal atrial tachycardias occurred after circumferential pulmonary vein isolation. J Cardiovasc Electrophysiol 2011;22:754; with permission.)

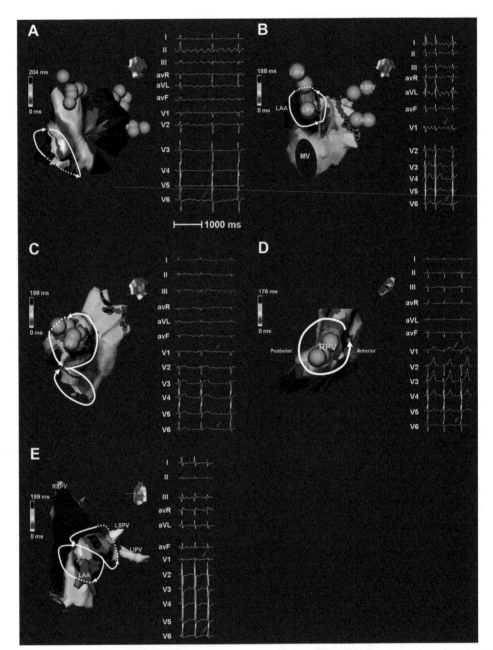

Fig. 12. Three-dimensional activation map and surface ECG of macroreentrant atrial tachycardias. The white arrow indicates the activation circuit, and red arrowhead the P or flutter wave of the macroreentrant atrial tachycardias. (*A*) A mitral macroreentrant atrial tachycardia (CL, 225 milliseconds) rotating clockwise around the mitral annulus. The surface ECG of the tachycardia shows positive flutter waves in V1 and V6. The amplitude of the flutter waves in V6 is 0.5 mV. (*B*) A left pulmonary vein (LPV) macroreentrant atrial tachycardia rotating around the LPV with a CL of 205 milliseconds. The surface ECG of the tachycardia shows positive flutter waves in V1 and V6. The amplitude of the flutter waves in V6 is 0.6 mV. (*C*) A double macroreentrant atrial tachycardia rotating around the LPV and mitral annulus with a CL of 236 milliseconds. The surface ECG of the tachycardia shows positive flutter waves in V1 and flat waves in V6. (*D*) A right pulmonary vein (RPV) macroreentrant atrial tachycardia rotating around the RPV with a CL of 199 milliseconds. The surface ECG of the tachycardia shows positive flutter waves in V1 and V6. The amplitude of the flutter waves in V6 is 0.1 mV. (*E*) A double macroreentrant atrial tachycardia rotating around the LPV and LA appendage (LAA) with a CL of 237 milliseconds. The surface ECG of the AT shows flat flutter waves in V1 and positive waves in V6. The amplitude of the flutter waves in V6 is 0.25 mV. LVZ, low-voltage zone. (*From* Chang SL, Tsao HM, Lin YJ, et al. Differentiating macroreentrant from focal atrial tachycardias occurred after circumferential pulmonary vein isolation. J Cardiovasc Electrophysiol 2011;22:751; with permission.)

Table 1
Acute and long-term outcome of macroreentrant atrial tachycardia in published studies

First Author, Reference Number	Type of AFL	Number of Cases	Acute Success Rate (%)	Long-term Success Rate Without AAD (%)	Follow-up (mo)
Pérez et al,[23] 2009	Cavotricuspid isthmus–dependent AFL	10,719	94.3	89	13.8 ± 0.3
Hsieh et al,[24] 2002	Typical AFL	333	97	96	29 ± 17
Tai et al,[14] 2004	Atypical RA flutter	15	87	87	16.8 ± 3.8
Jais et al,[2] 2000	LA flutter	22	91	73	15 ± 7
Ouyang et al,[20] 2002	LA flutter	28	89	93	$1 - 31$
Fiala et al,[26] 2007	RA and LA atypical flutter	26	85	73	37 ± 15
Chae et al,[4] 2007	Organized atrial tachycardia after AF ablation	78	85	77	13 ± 10
Chang et al,[3] 2009	LAMRT after AF ablation	35	87.5	97	21 ± 8
Coffey et al,[27] 2013	LAMRT after AF ablation	91	90	77	16 ± 12

Abbreviations: AAD, antiarrhythmic drug; LAMRT, LA macroreentrant tachycardia.

mapping to identify the reentrant circuit or foci with radiofrequency ablation is still the most effective approach to eliminate macroreentrant atrial tachycardias.[3,4,27]

DISCUSSION
Distinguishing Typical AFL from Atypical AFL

Differentiating typical from atypical AFL is crucial because the treatment strategies for these macro-reentrant tachycardias may differ. Typical and reverse typical AFL, as a macroreentrant circuit originated in the right atrium, can be eliminated with a high success rate and a low incidence of complication by radiofrequency catheter ablation of CTI. Typical AFL manifests positive P waves in lead V1; negative P waves in lead V6; and prominent negative P waves in leads II, III, and aVF, which is easily distinguished from 12-lead ECG. Milliez and colleagues[28] showed that a positive flutter wave in the inferior leads during CCW typical AFL is related to an increased likelihood of structural heart disease and AF. Chugh and colleagues[10] reported atypical ECG patterns in CTI-dependent AFL after AF ablation. These atypical ECG features, including upright flutter waves in the inferior leads and negative flutter waves in lead aVL, could mimic a tachycardia arising from the LA.

Catheter-based therapeutic techniques for atypical AFL are more complicated than for CTI-dependent AFL. Various forms of atypical AFL have been shown, and several diagnostic criteria to differentiate them have been proposed to facilitate cardiac mapping and catheter ablation. Positive flutter wave in inferior leads could be found in LA, ULR, and reverse typical AFL. Polarity and voltage measurement of flutter wave in lead I can differentiate reverse typical AFL from ULR.[9] Left AFL can be distinguished from right AFL from the amplitude of flutter wave in the inferior ECG leads. Understanding the mechanisms of AFL would allow better advanced planning, because typical and atypical AFL require different mapping and ablation techniques.

Macroreentrant Atrial Tachycardias Following AF Ablation

Macroreentrant atrial tachycardias can occur during catheter ablation of AF or after the procedure. Varying prevalence has been reported in previous studies and was associated with the ablation technique. Large low-voltage zones from the underlying atrial substrate and/or prior ablation make the mapping and ablation more challenging. It is important to predict the origin of the macroreentrant atrial tachycardias before the catheter ablation. Entrainment and electroanatomic mapping are the optimal approaches to differentiating and localizing the macroreentrant atrial tachycardias; however, they are sometimes time consuming and laborious because of the extensive low-voltage areas. Our laboratory developed an ECG algorithm allowing rapid identification of the mechanism of atrial tachyarrhythmias after circumferential pulmonary vein isolation.[21] A lower voltage of the flutter or P waves with a shorter tachycardia cycle length in V6 could differentiate macroreentrant from focal atrial tachycardias. A negative polarity in at least 1 precordial lead can differentiate RA from LA macroreentrant atrial tachycardias.

This novel algorithm can accurately diagnose the mechanism and origin of atrial tachyarrhythmias after pulmonary vein isolation. To facilitate the mapping and ablation, simple and accurate algorithms using the surface ECG are always welcome.

SUMMARY

With improved mapping techniques and more aggressive treatment in management of macroreentrant atrial tachycardias, a 12-lead ECG during tachycardia provides important information in the initial strategy for the physician or specialized cardiologist. Catheter ablation of CTI can eradicate typical and reverse typical AFL with a high success rate and few complications. For atypical AFL, catheter ablation of the isthmus between the boundaries using electroanatomic mapping can eliminate these arrhythmias.

REFERENCES

1. Granada J, Uribe W, Chyou PH, et al. Incidence and predictors of atrial flutter in the general population. J Am Coll Cardiol 2000;36:2242–6.

2. Jais P, Shah DC, Haissaguerre M, et al. Mapping and ablation of left atrial flutters. Circulation 2000; 101:2928–34.

3. Chang SL, Lin YJ, Tai CT, et al. Induced atrial tachycardia after circumferential pulmonary vein isolation of paroxysmal atrial fibrillation: electrophysiological characteristics and impact of catheter ablation on the follow-up results. J Cardiovasc Electrophysiol 2009;20:388–94.

4. Chae S, Oral H, Good E, et al. Atrial tachycardia after circumferential pulmonary vein ablation of atrial fibrillation: mechanistic insights, results of catheter ablation, and risk factors for recurrence. J Am Coll Cardiol 2007;50:1781–7.

5. Gerstenfeld EP, Callans DJ, Dixit S, et al. Mechanisms of organized left atrial tachycardias occurring after pulmonary vein isolation. Circulation 2004;110: 1351–7.

6. Gerstenfeld EP, Callans DJ, Sauer W, et al. Reentrant and nonreentrant focal left atrial tachycardias occur after pulmonary vein isolation. Heart Rhythm 2005;2:1195–202.

7. Tai CT, Chen SA, Chiang CE, et al. Characterization of low right atrial isthmus as the slow conduction zone and pharmacological target in typical atrial flutter. Circulation 1997;96:2601–11.

8. Saoudi N, Cosio F, Waldo A, et al. Classification of atrial flutter and regular atrial tachycardia according to electrophysiologic mechanism and anatomic bases: a statement from a joint expert group from the Working Group of Arrhythmias of the European Society of Cardiology and the North American Society of Pacing and Electrophysiology. J Cardiovasc Electrophysiol 2001;12:852–66.

9. Yuniadi Y, Tai CT, Lee KT, et al. A new electrocardiographic algorithm to differentiate upper loop re-entry from reverse typical atrial flutter. J Am Coll Cardiol 2005;46:524–8.

10. Chugh A, Latchamsetty R, Oral H, et al. Characteristics of cavotricuspid isthmus-dependent atrial flutter after left atrial ablation of atrial fibrillation. Circulation 2006;113:609–15.

11. Tai CT, Chen SA, Chen YJ, et al. Conduction properties of the crista terminalis in patients with typical atrial flutter: basis for a line of block in the reentrant circuit. J Cardiovasc Electrophysiol 1998;9: 811–9.

12. Tai CT, Chen SA, Chiang CE, et al. Electrophysiologic characteristics and radiofrequency catheter ablation in patients with clockwise atrial flutter. J Cardiovasc Electrophysiol 1997;8:24–34.

13. Tai CT, Lin YK, Chen SA. Atypical atrial flutter involving the isthmus between the right pulmonary veins and fossa ovalis. Pacing Clin Electrophysiol 2001;24:384–7.

14. Tai CT, Liu TY, Lee PC, et al. Non-contact mapping to guide radiofrequency ablation of atypical right atrial flutter. J Am Coll Cardiol 2004;44:1080–6.

15. Bochoeyer A, Yang Y, Cheng J, et al. Surface electrocardiographic characteristics of right and left atrial flutter. Circulation 2003;108:60–6.

16. Chang SL, Tai CT, Lin YJ, et al. The role of left atrial muscular bundles in catheter ablation of atrial fibrillation. J Am Coll Cardiol 2007;50:964–73.

17. Marrouche NF, Natale A, Wazni OM, et al. Left septal atrial flutter: electrophysiology, anatomy, and results of ablation. Circulation 2004;109:2440–7.

18. Gerstenfeld EP, Dixit S, Bala R, et al. Surface electrocardiogram characteristics of atrial tachycardias occurring after pulmonary vein isolation. Heart Rhythm 2007;4:1136–43.

19. Ndrepepa G, Zrenner B, Weyerbrock S, et al. Activation patterns in the left atrium during counterclockwise and clockwise atrial flutter. J Cardiovasc Electrophysiol 2001;12:893–9.

20. Ouyang F, Ernst S, Vogtmann T, et al. Characterization of reentrant circuits in left atrial macroreentrant tachycardia: critical isthmus block can prevent atrial tachycardia recurrence. Circulation 2002; 105:1934–42.

21. Chang SL, Tsao HM, Lin YJ, et al. Differentiating macroreentrant from focal atrial tachycardias occurred after circumferential pulmonary vein isolation. J Cardiovasc Electrophysiol 2011;22:748–55.

22. Tai CT, Chen SA, Chiang CE, et al. Long-term outcome of radiofrequency catheter ablation for typical atrial flutter: risk prediction of recurrent arrhythmias. J Cardiovasc Electrophysiol 1998;9: 115–21.

23. Pérez FJ, Schubert CM, Parvez B, et al. Long-term outcomes after catheter ablation of cavo-tricuspid isthmus dependent atrial flutter: a meta-analysis. Circ Arrhythm Electrophysiol 2009;2:393–401.

24. Hsieh MH, Tai CT, Chiang CE, et al. Recurrent atrial flutter and atrial fibrillation after catheter ablation of the cavotricuspid isthmus: a very long-term follow-up of 333 patients. J Interv Card Electrophysiol 2002;7:225–31.

25. Mittal S, Pokushalov E, Romanov A, et al. Long-term ECG monitoring using an implantable loop recorder for the detection of atrial fibrillation after cavotricuspid isthmus ablation in patients with atrial flutter. Heart Rhythm 2013;10:1598–604.

26. Fiala M, Chovancik J, Neuwirth R, et al. Atrial macro-reentry tachycardia in patients without obvious structural heart disease or previous cardiac surgical or catheter intervention: characterization of arrhythmogenic substrates, reentry circuits, and results of catheter ablation. J Cardiovasc Electrophysiol 2007;18:824–32.

27. Coffey JO, d'Avila A, Dukkipati S, et al. Catheter ablation of scar-related atypical atrial flutter. Europace 2013;15:414–9.

28. Milliez P, Richardson AW, Obioha-Ngwu O, et al. Variable electrocardiographic characteristics of isthmus-dependent atrial flutter. J Am Coll Cardiol 2002;40:1125–32.

Paroxysmal Supraventricular Tachycardias:
Atrioventricular Nodal Reentrant Tachycardia and Atrioventricular Reentrant Tachycardias

Mohammad Shenasa, MD[a,b,*],
Hossein Shenasa, MD, MsC[a,b], Hamid Assadi, MD[a],
Mona Soleimanieh, RN[a]

KEYWORDS

- Accessory pathways • Atrioventricular node • Atrioventricular nodal reentry tachycardia
- Atrioventricular reentry tachycardia • Catheter ablation • Tachycardias
- Wolff-Parkinson-White syndrome

KEY POINTS

- Atrioventricular nodal reentrant tachycardia (AVNRT) and A-V reentrant tachycardia (AVRT) are the foundation of rhythmology.
- Detailed electrocardiographic and electrophysiologic evaluation of AVNRT and AVRT leads to accurate diagnosis.
- Catheter ablation is a curative procedure that has proved to be safe and effective (>95%).
- Electrocardiograms play an important role in diagnosis and deductive mechanism(s) of the arrhythmias.

INTRODUCTION

The paroxysmal supraventricular tachycardias (PSVT), atrioventricular (A-V) nodal reentrant tachycardia (AVNRT) and A-V reentrant tachycardia (AVRT), are two arrhythmias that have fascinated rhythmologists and electrophysiologists for many decades. A wealth of information has been gained from them from electrophysiology, intracardiac investigations, and intraoperative mapping, as well as recently catheter ablation. These arrhythmias represent microreentry (AVNRT) and macroreentry (AVRT). This article discusses the electrocardiogram (ECG) and electrophysiologic studies (EPS) aspects of these two arrhythmias.

This article discusses the electrocardiographic and electrophysiologic correlation of AVNRT and AVRT, but does not provide a detailed discussion of mapping and ablation of these arrhythmias.

HISTORY OF AVNRT

Denes and colleagues[1] first reported the presence of dual A-V nodal pathways as possible mechanisms of AVNRT in humans. Moe and colleagues[2]

Disclosures: None.
[a] Heart & Rhythm Medical Group, 105 N Bascom Ave, St 204, San Jose, CA 95128, USA; [b] Department of Cardiovascular Services, O'Connor Hospital, 2105 Forest Ave, San Jose, CA 95128, USA
* Corresponding author. Heart & Rhythm Medical Group, 105 North Bascom Avenue, San Jose, CA 95128.
E-mail address: mohammad.shenasa@gmail.com

also showed the presence of dual A-V nodal conduction in animal experiments.

AVNRT is the most common form of PSVT in adolescence and adults (slightly more common in women). The reentry circuit is confined in the region of the A-V junction, anatomically at the apex of the triangle of Koch, which consists of the tendon of Todaro (superiorly and anteriorly) and the coronary sinus (posteriorly) and tricuspid annulus (inferiorly), called the compact A-V node.[3–9]

The atrial input to the A-V node consists of at least 2 atrionodal connections (**Fig. 1**). The compact A-V node compromises multiple pathways with different anterograde and retrograde conduction times and refractory periods producing dual or more A-V nodal physiology. The cellular electrophysiologists have classified the A-V nodal region into 3 distinct parts:

1. Transitional region, where atrial myocardium emerges into the A-V nodal tissue
2. Midnodal regions or typical A-V nodal cells
3. Distal A-V nodal tissue or NH (nodal-His), which connects to the His bundle

The nodal region is responsible for most of the delay of the A-V nodal conduction, whereas the fast pathway bypasses the nodal region. It is thought that this is an oversimplification of the A-V nodal anatomy and physiology of the A-V node. The A-V nodal fibers constitute a family of fibers with different A-V nodal conductions and refractory periods, which are heterogonous and anisotropic. **Fig. 2** shows the interconnection of the A-V nodal tissue.

CLINICAL PRESENTATION

Most patients with PSVT describe a recurrent, sudden onset of rapid palpitations, often during exercise. Patients occasionally complain of chest pain, shortness of breath, dizziness, and rarely syncope. They also describe their palpitations stopping abruptly. Duration of each episode varies and may last from a few seconds to several hours. Patients with AVNRT do worse hemodynamically compared with patients with AVRT.

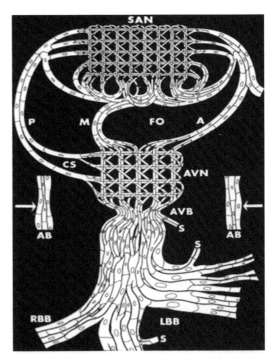

Fig. 2. Cardiac conduction system. The geometric organization, cell diameters, and intercalated discs are shown in the sinoatrial node (SAN), A-V node (AVN), A-V bundle (AVB), left bundle branch (LBB), and right bundle branch (RBB). Atrial muscle cells form an anterior (A), middle (m), and posterior (P) intermodal bundle. Note relations of these bundles to the fossa ovalis (FO) and ostium of the coronary sinus (CS). Accessory A-V muscle bridges or bundles of Kent (AB) may persist and cross the A-V junction (*arrows*) in some adult hearts. Septal cells known as paraspecific fibers of Mahiam(s) may leave the A-V bundle and left bundle branch to enter the upper portion of the human interventricular septum. (*Adapted from* Truex RC. Structural basis of atrial and ventricular conduction. Cardiovasc Clin 1974;6(1):1–24; with permission.)

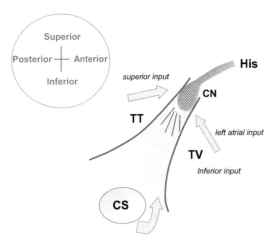

Fig. 1. The triangle of Koch and A-V nodal inputs (*arrows*) in right anterior oblique (RAO) projection. Landmarks are the tendon of Todaro (TT) at the posterior superior aspect, the coronary sinus ostium (CS) at the base, and the tricuspid annulus (TA) located anteriorly. The apex of the triangle is formed by the compact A-V node (CN). (*From* Willems S, Daniel S, Lutomsky B, et al. Mapping and ablation of AV NRT and its Subtypes. In: Shenasa M, Hindricks G, Borggrefe M, et al, editors. Cardiac mapping. 3rd edition. Chichester (United Kingdom): Blackwell; 2009; with permission.)

ELECTROCARDIOGRAPHIC CHARACTERISTICS OF AVNRT

The first step in ECG diagnosis of regular supraventricular tachycardias (SVTs) is to determine the relationship between P-wave and QRS complexes. When encountering an absence of P waves (no P wave) or P waves obscured within the QRS, the differential diagnosis should be AVNRT (**Fig. 3**A, B), atrial flutter, atrial tachycardia with first degree A-V block, and less often junctional tachycardias. The next step is timing of P waves in relation to the R wave (**Fig. 4**A, B). An important differential diagnosis of AVNRT is orthodromic (OT) tachycardias with septal or posteroseptal accessory pathways (APs) in which the retrograde conduction time is short and the P

wave may be registered at the end of the QRS or within the ST segment. Patients with common-type AVNRT show short RPs and those with un-common forms show long RP intervals (discussed further later in the article).

In most cases of typical AVNRT the ECG is of narrow QRS complex morphology and a clear P wave is not visible. Because of the short RP interval the P wave may be seen at the end of QRS, giving rise to an RSr' pattern in V1 or a small S wave in V2. There may be some degree of ST segment depression in precordial leads, which is nonspecific and does not reflect myocardial ischemia (see **Fig. 3**B). The onset of AVNRT with right bundle branch block (RBBB) (rate related) may be present and often subside spontaneously. Neither the RBBB nor the left bundle branch block

A

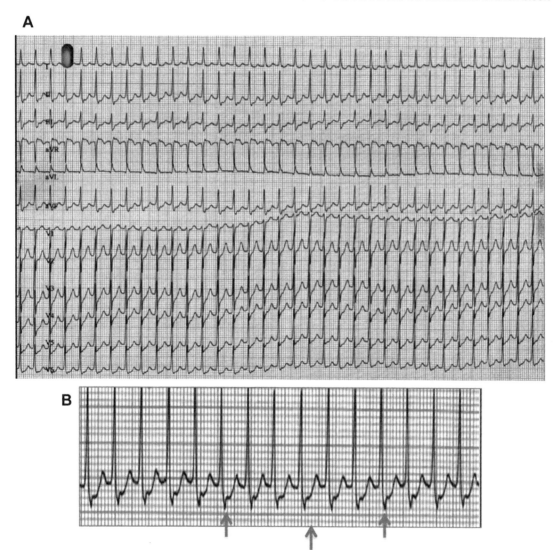

B

Fig. 3. (*A*) Twelve-lead ECG of a patient with AVNRT. (*B*) Enlarged view of (*A*) Arrows denote retrograde P wave with short RP interval (P-waves are at the end of QRS).

A   Short R-P

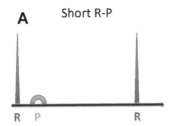

R   P   R

B   Long R-P

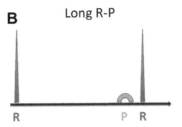

R   P   R

Fig. 4. Short R-P (*A*) long R-P (*B*) relationship.

(LBBB) affect the rate of tachycardia or the RR interval because the AVNRT circuit is within the compact A-V node. QRS alternans may be seen when tachycardia rates are fast. This phenomenon is more common in AVRT than AVNRT. Cycle length (CL) alternans may be seen in AVNRT especially before its spontaneous termination, which occurs after the long cycle. The site block is often in the anterograde A-V node.

In fast/slow AVNRT the RP interval is longer than PR interval, whereas in slow/slow AVNRT the RP interval is usually shorter or equal to the PR interval. The differential diagnosis in this case is AVRT.

DUAL A-V NODAL PHYSIOLOGY

Dual A-V nodal physiology is commonly observed during atrial extrastimulation studies to initiate the tachycardia; however, it is not an absolute requirement.[1,5,6] Presence of dual A-V nodal physiology is caused by different effective refractory periods of slow and fast A-V nodal pathways. Dual retrograde A-V nodal physiology can similarly be shown during ventricular extrastimulation.

Dual A-V nodal physiology can usually be shown in 80% to 85% of patients with AVNRT. In a small percentage of patients triple A-V or multiple nodal physiology (or curves) can be shown when using multiple atrial drive cycles or multiple atrial stimuli.[6]

TYPES OF AVNRT

Depending on the electrophysiologic properties of the slow and fast pathways that are used in anterograde or retrograde directions during AVNRT, the reentry circuits are described as common and uncommon types (**Fig. 5**A–C).[6] The most common form, also called typical AVNRT, is slow anterograde and fast retrograde pattern (slow/fast type) (see **Fig. 5**A).

Typical forms of AVNRT are seen in about 80% to 90% of cases. The fast pathway is located more anterior and superior to the A-V node, whereas the slow pathway is inferior and posterior in the triangle of Koch. Early studies during surgical mapping of patients with AVNRT, and later studies during transcatheter mapping and ablation, have verified

the presence of anatomically distinct slow and fast pathways.[10] In the slow/fast type AVNRT the earliest retrograde atrial activation is registered at the interatrial septum behind the tendon of Todaro with long A-H and short H-A interval.[11–14]

UNCOMMON OR ATYPICAL FORMS OF AVNRT

Variant forms of anterograde slow and retrograde fast pathways exist and depend on the interplay of the pathways.

Slow/slow-type AVNRT involves anterograde slow and retrograde slow pathways (see **Fig. 5**B). In this case the retrograde P waves are visible after the QRS and earliest retrograde atrial activation is usually detected at the proximal end of the coronary sinus.

Another rare form is a fast-slow type in which reentry circuit uses a anterograde fast pathway and retrograde slow pathway (see **Fig. 5**C). Otomo and colleagues[15] reported on 435 patients on 4 types of AVNRT as follows:

1. Slow/fast AVNRT, 329 (76%)
2. Left variant slow/fast, 8 (2%)
3. Slow/slow AVNRT, 53 (12%)
4. Fast/slow AVNRT, 45 (10%)

ELECTROPHYSIOLOGIC CHARACTERISTICS OF AVNRT

Typical AVNRT accounts for more than 80% to 90% cases of AVNRT. The reentry circuit uses a slow pathway in the anterograde direction with conduction time of (depending on tachycardia CL) usually more than 200 milliseconds, and a fast pathway in the retrograde direction with conduction time (H-A) of less than 70 milliseconds. Typical AVNRTs are easily inducible during incremental atrial pacing as well as atrial extrastimulation techniques (**Fig. 6**A, B).

AVNRTs are also inducible (less commonly) during incremental ventricular pacing, as shown in **Fig. 7**. In **Fig. 7** the first 3 beats of the tachycardia are with RBBB and then normalizes to the narrow QRS morphology. A retrograde P wave is registered at the end of QRS in V1.

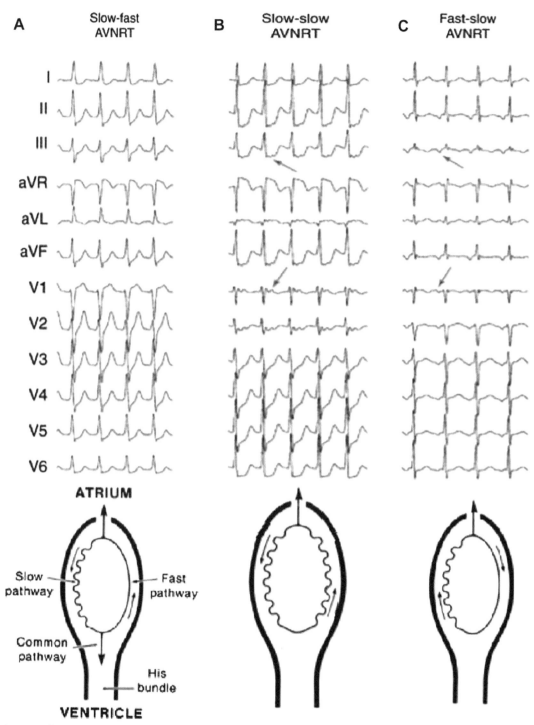

Fig. 5. Surface ECG and the different types of AVNRT. Arrows mark the P waves. (*A*) In slow-fast (typical) AVNRT, the P wave may lie within the QRS (not shown). (*B*) In slow-slow AVNRT, the P wave lies outside the QRS in the ST-T wave, and the RP interval is longer than that in slow-fast AVNRT. (*C*) In fast-slow AVNRT, the P wave lies before the QRS with a long RP interval. In all varieties of AVNRT, the P wave is narrow, negative in the inferior leads, and positive in V1. (*Adapted from* Issa ZF, Miller JM, Zipes DP. Atrioventricular nodal reentrant tachycardia. In: Issa ZF, Miller JM, Zipes DP, editors. Clinical arrhythmology and electrophysiology; a companion to Braunwald's heart disease. Philadelphia: Elsevier; 2009.)

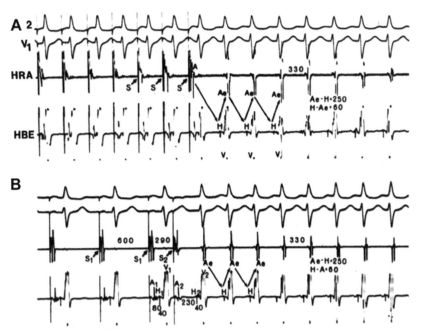

Fig. 6. Induction of typical A-V nodal reentrant tachycardia during incremental atrial pacing (*A*) and during atrial extrastimulation (*B*). Note the long A-H and short H-Ae intervals. Also the long A2-H2 during atrial extrastimulation suggests conduction over the slow pathway. HBE, His bundle; HRA, high right atrium. S (*arrows*) denotes stimulus artifact.

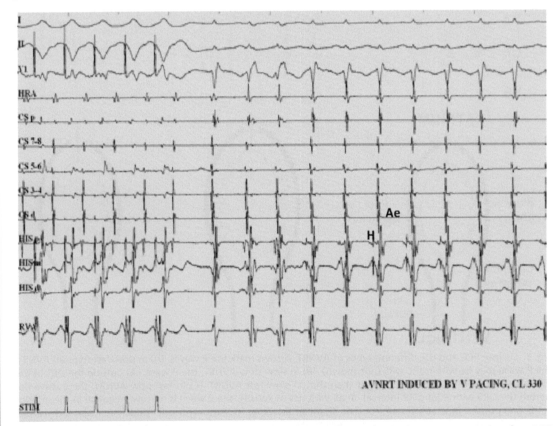

Fig. 7. Induction of AVNRT by ventricular pacing at a CL of 330 milliseconds. Tracings are arranged surface ECG leads I, II, V1, HRA, CSP (Coronary Sinus Proximal), CS electrogram, HBE, and RV₁, simulation artifact; Ae, atrial echo; HBS, His bundle electrogram; RV, right ventricle.

In the typical form of AVNRT, atrial and ventricular activation are almost simultaneous. The ventricles are not necessarily part of the reentry circuit, and in rare cases of AVNRT with 2:1 A-V block is occasionally observed. **Fig. 8A, B** confirms that the His-Purkinje system is not part of the reentrant circuit.[16,17]

Other evidence obtained during electrophysiologic studies that support the lower common pathway being confined within the compact A-V node includes longer retrograde Wenckebach CL during ventricular pacing than the tachycardia CL, longer H-A interval during ventricular pacing than during AVNRT, and programmed ventricular extrasystole during AVNRT that changes His bundle activation without changing the

tachycardia CL. Whether atria tissue is a necessary part of the reentry circuit remains controversial and currently it is thought that upper common pathways are the necessary link in AVNRT.[18]

INVESTIGATION AND DIFFERENTIAL DIAGNOSIS OF AVNRT AND AVRT IN THE ELECTROPHYSIOLOGY LABORATORY
Timed Ventricular Premature Beats (Premature Ventricular Contractions) During SVT

Captured premature ventricular contraction (PVC) during SVT suggests AVNRT:

1. Retrograde atrial activation sequence changed but remained concentric

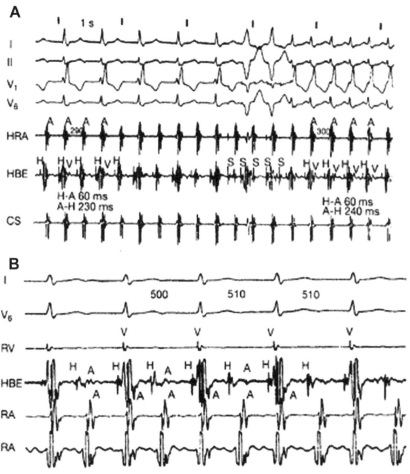

Fig. 8. (A) AVNRT with 2:1 A-V block distal to the His bundle. Conversion and 1:1 conduction after the delivery of 5 ventricular premature stimuli (capture of 2 stimuli) during sustained AVNRT. Normalization of conduction occurred presumably by retrograde concealment into the right and Hisian bundle. There is slight alteration of the A-A interval. Surface ECG leads I, II, V1. (B) 2:1 infra-Hisian block during sustained AVNRT. Note the alternans of the CL of the conducted and blocked beats. Surface ECG leads 1, V6. RA, right atrium; RV, right ventricle; S, ventricular stimulus. Local electrograms: A, right atrium; H, His bundle; V, right ventricle. (From Willems S, Shenasa M, Borggrefe M, et al. Atrioventricular nodal reentry tachycardia: electrophysiologic comparisons in patients with and without 2:1 infra-His block. Clin Cardiol 1993;16:883–8; with permission.)

2. Retrograde His and atrial activation is advanced; less than 10 to 15 milliseconds suggests typical AVNRT and more than 30 milliseconds suggests atypical AVNRT
3. PVCs reset the tachycardia when His is refractory
4. Retrograde atrial activation unchanged and remaining eccentric suggests AVRT
5. Reset tachycardia suggests AVRT
6. If there is no reset of the tachycardia, this may be related to bystander AP
7. Abolishment of SVT during radiofrequency ablation of tachycardia of retrograde slow or fast A-V nodal pathway

P-WAVE MORPHOLOGY

Because of retrograde activation of the atria via the fast or slow pathways, the P wave morphology during AVNRT is always negative in inferior leads. In cases with very short retrograde conduction or negative H-A interval in reference to the QRS the P wave may be seen at the onset of QRS producing Q waves in the inferior leads: pseudo-Q waves. A positive P wave in the inferior leads is almost always inconsistent with AVNRT (assuming it is normal cardiac anatomy).

MANAGEMENT OF AVNRT

If patients are hemodynamically stable clinicians should obtain 12-lead ECGs for analysis and comparison with previous ECGs. In hemodynamically unstable tachycardias cardioversion is safest.

MANAGEMENT OF PATIENTS WITH NARROW COMPLEX TACHYCARDIA

1. In AVNRT and AVRT, vagal maneuvers and administration of intravenous (IV) adenosine (usually 6-mg IV bolus) are used for acute termination of the tachycardias. Transient atrial fibrillation (AF) may be seen in 10% to 12% of cases following administration of adenosine. PVCs and rarely nonsustained ventricular tachycardia (VT) may similarly occur after adenosine. The slowing of tachycardia or increasing the A-V nodal responses (ie, 2:1 or higher A-V ratios) is useful to differentiate sinus tachycardia, atrial tachycardia, and flutter from AVNRT and AVRT. A-V nodal blocking agents such as verapamil, diltiazem, and β-blockers are second choices after adenosine for acute conversion. Anterograde fast pathway conduction is almost always blocked by 12 mg of adenosine, whereas retrograde fast pathway conduction is not blocked by adenosine in about 40% of patients with typical AVNRT, which may

suggest that anterograde and retrograde fast pathways are anatomically and or functionally distinct. Therefore, unresponsiveness of retrograde conduction to adenosine is not a reliable indicator of the presence of an APs. It has been reported that the effects of calcium antagonists and β-blockers may block the retrograde A-V nodal conduction in patients without AVNRT as well as those with AVNRT.[19,20]

Wide complex tachycardias are discussed in detail in the article by Das and colleagues elsewhere in this issue.

CATHETER ABLATION OF AVNRT

Catheter ablation of AVNRT is now considered as first-line therapy in patients, with more than a 95% success rate.[13,21–23] Most laboratories now use the slow pathway ablation that is anatomically located near the posterior-inferior base of the triangle of Koch between the coronary sinus and tricuspid valve. **Fig. 9** illustrates an electroanatomic mapping of the A-V junctional region during slow pathway ablation.

Some investigators think that the so-called slow pathway potentials that are detected during sinus rhythm are related to the anatomic sites of slow pathway location, and that ablation of slow pathways may eliminate these potentials. Delivery of radiofrequency (RF) currents to the slow pathway region is often associated with emergence of junctional rhythms with narrow QRS morphology. Ventriculoatrial (VA) conduction remains intact during these junctional rhythms. Atrial pacing at faster rates than the junctional rhythm is useful to show intact anterograde conduction during RF delivery. Absence of junction rhythm during RF ablation of the slow pathway region is often associated with unsuccessful target sites and AVNRT is often inducible or may occur spontaneously.

TWO APPROACHES HAVE BEEN USED FOR AVNRT ABLATION

1. Posterior approach: slow pathway ablation, inferoposterior region of Koch triangle between coronary sinus orifice and tricuspid annulus and tendon of Todaro
2. Anterior approach: fast pathway ablation

ADVANTAGES OF SLOW PATHWAY ABLATION

1. Significantly lower risk of complete A-V block
2. Maintenance of normal PR interval.

END POINTS OF SLOW PATHWAY ABLATION

1. Elimination of slow pathway conduction

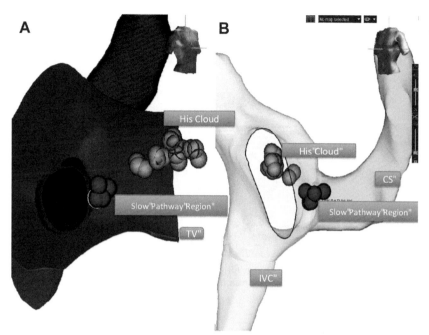

Fig. 9. Electroanatomic mapping of the A-V junctional region during slow pathway ablation. (*A*) Left anterior oblique (LAO) view. Red dots denote the slow pathway region; gold dots denote the His bundle region. Mapping of the His bundle region is done to avoid inadvertent ablation of the A-V node His bundle and induction of A-V block. (*B*) RAO view. CS, coronary sinus; IVC, inferior vena cava; TV, tricuspid valve.

2. Modification or complete elimination of dual or multiple A-V nodal physiology
3. Elimination of slow pathway potential (if present before ablation)
4. Increase in the effective refractory period of A-V node
5. Demonstration of intact anterograde and retrograde conduction over the fast pathway
6. Most importantly, noninducibility of AVNRT

Single A-V nodal echo beats (in up to 50% to 75%) of cases may persist, but sustained AVNRT remains noninducible. In clinical practice all the requirements discussed earlier may not be necessary. In patients with documented AVNRT that is noninducible during electrophysiologic studies, anatomically guided slow pathway ablation is sufficient.

IMAGING DURING AVNRT ABLATION

Because catheter ablation of AVNRT is mostly based on anatomic landmarks, advanced imaging technologies are not needed to improve the success rate of the slow pathway ablation. However, in certain cases it may help to identify the His region and also identify the slow pathway region to avoid inadvertent induction of A-V block. **Fig. 9** illustrates mapping of the slow pathway region.

Because radiation exposure is of concern, especially in young patients, advanced mapping technologies that reduce radiation exposure or are radiation free are appealing. **Fig. 10** shows use of three-dimensional mapping of the slow pathway in the region of the triangle of Koch. The slow pathway can be visualized by a low-voltage area in the triangle of Koch.

ELECTROPHYSIOLOGIC EFFECTS OF SLOW PATHWAY ABLATION

1. Increase in the shortest atrial pacing CL that maintains a 1:1 anterograde conduction
2. Prolongs A-V nodal refractory period
3. No change in A-H interval
4. No change in retrograde conduction via A-V node (fast pathway)
5. Shortening of fast pathway effective refractory period (ERP) in the presence of autonomic blockade probably caused by electrotonic effects of slow pathway conduction
6. Reduction in ventricular rate during AF

ELECTROPHYSIOLOGIC EFFECTS OF FAST PATHWAY ABLATION

1. Prolongation of PR and A-H interval
2. Retrograde block via A-V node

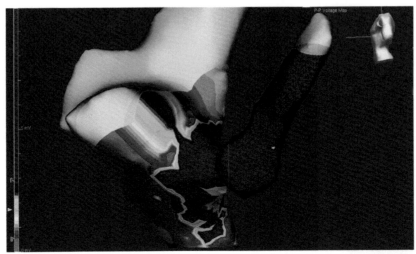

Fig. 10. Radiation-free ablation of AVNRT using voltage mapping to evaluate the slow pathway. (*From* Von Bergen NH, Law IH. A-V nodal reentrant tachycardia in children: current approaches to management. Progress Pediatr Cardiol 2013;35:25–32; with permission.)

CRYOMAPPING AND ABLATION OF AVNRT

The advantage of cryomapping is to identify target sites for ablation. Cryomapping is done at temperatures around −30°C, at which the cryolesion is reversible. Once the appropriate target site is identified, cryoablation at temperatures of −70° to −80° C for up to 4 minutes generally creates permanent ablation (**Fig. 11**A, B).[24]

END POINTS AND OUTCOMES OF CRYOABLATION IN AVNRT

End points in cryoablation of AVNRT are the same as for RF ablation, as described earlier. Compared with the RF technique, the outcome of successful cryoablation is slightly lower AVNRT at 80% to 90% versus 95% to 98%. During long-term follow-up the recurrence rate of cryoablation is slightly lower than that of RF ablation of AVNRT. There is an ongoing trial comparing RF ablation with cryoablation in a randomized fashion (FIRE and ICE ABLATION TRIAL).[25]

SUBTHRESHOLD STIMULATION MAPPING OF AVNRT

The technique of subthreshold stimulation (STS) mapping has been well described. STS provides a unique method to identify target sites for ablation.[26] Willems and colleagues[27] reported the usefulness of this method to identify target sites in AVNRT in a randomized fashion. **Fig. 12** shows termination of typical AVNRT during STS and **Fig. 13** shows the distribution of successful

ablation sites according to the termination of tachycardia by STS.

COMPLICATIONS OF AVNRT ABLATION

The induction of permanent A-V block (incidence is about 0.2% to 0.6%). The incidence is higher with fast pathway ablation because it is closer to the compact A-V node.

AVRT

AVRTs are seen in patients with either manifest ventricular preexcitation (Wolff-Parkinson-White [WPW] syndrome) or concealed APs and are the second most common type of PSVTs after AVNRT. APs connect the atria to the ventricle and create a substrate for reentry to occur. Most APs are located epicardially around the A-V groove. These APs have the capacity to conduct bidirectionally, retrogradely only, or rarely anterogradely only. The typical ECG characteristics of manifest preexcitation is a short PR interval, presence of delta wave, and broad QRS that is caused by ventricular activation via AP.

The ECG localization of AP is beyond the scope of this article. Issa and colleagues[28] proved an excellent review.

CLINICAL PRESENTATION

Most patients with WPW syndrome and concealed AP remain asymptomatic for several years and the WPW-type ECG often is discovered incidentally during routine physical examination for other causes.

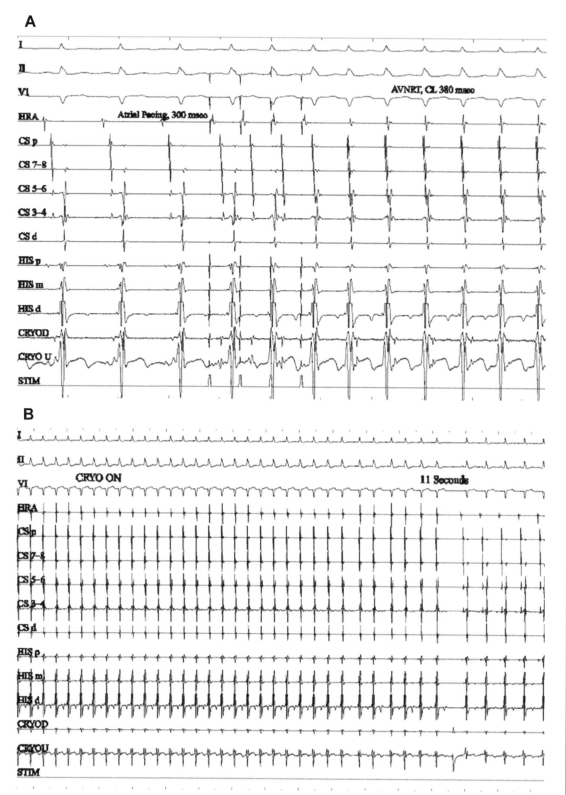

Fig. 11. Cryomapping and cryoablation of typical AVNRT. Tracings from top to bottom are: surface ECG leads I, II, and V1; HRA; CS from proximal (p) to distal (d); His bundle electrogram (His) from proximal to distal; electrograms obtained from the ablation catheter (CRYO), distal (D) and unipolar (U) recordings; and the stimulation marker (STIM). (*A*) AVNRT initiation by a short burst of rapid atrial pacing at 300 milliseconds delivered during sinus rhythm. The CL of AVNRT is 380 milliseconds. Also note that the PR greater than or equal to RR feature is present during rapid atrial pacing. (*B*) AVNRT is terminated when the last atrial impulse blocks antegradely in the slow pathway approximately 11 seconds after initiations of cryomapping. (*From* Jazayeri MR. Transcatheter cryomapping in AV nodal reentrant tachycardias. In: Shenasa M, Hindricks G, Borgreffe M, et al, editors. Cardiac mapping. 3rd edition. Chichester (United Kingdom): Blackwell; 2009; with permission.)

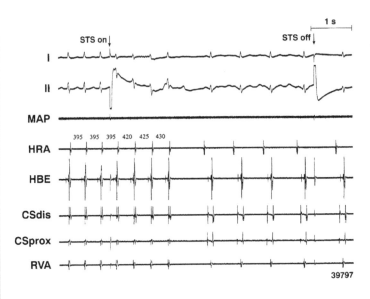

Fig. 12. Subthreshold stimulation (STS) during AVNRT at a posteroseptal mapping position. After induction of sustained AVNRT (CL, 395 milliseconds), STS is applied for 5 seconds (*arrows*). The tachycardia is interrupted by selective block within the slow anterograde pathway after 1.5 seconds, and normal sinus rhythm is established. Note that no apparent capture is visible at surface ECG or intracardiac recordings. The termination of the tachycardia is preceded by discrete prolongation of the CL from 395 to 430 milliseconds, which suggests the slowing of conduction within the slow pathway because the A-H interval, but not the H-A interval, is prolonged. CSdis, coronary sinus, distal; CSprox, coronary sinus, proximal; HBE, His bundle ECG; HRA, high right atrium; MAP, mapping catheter; RVA, right ventricular apex. (*From* Willems S, Weiss C, Shenasa M, et al. Optimized mapping of slow pathway ablation guided by subthreshold stimulation: a randomized prospective study in patients with recurrent A-V nodal re-entrant tachycardia. J Am Coll Cardiol 2001;37(6):1645–50; with permission.)

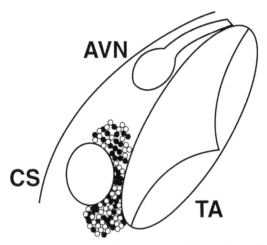

Fig. 13. Distribution of successful ablation sites. All target sites with subsequent abolition of AVNRT in patients undergoing the conventional approach (group A, open circles) and STS-guided ablation strategy (group B, solid circles). There is a well-balanced distribution of target sites from the posteroseptal aspect around the CS ostium up to the lower midseptal region in both groups. Solid circle (STS), n = 50; open circle (conventional), n = 50. AVN, A-V node; CS, coronary sinus; TA, tricuspid annulus. (*From* Willems S, Weiss C, Shenasa M, et al. Optimized mapping of slow pathway ablation guided by subthreshold stimulation: a randomized prospective study in patients with recurrent A-V nodal re-entrant tachycardia. J Am Coll Cardiol 2001;37(6):1645–50; with permission.)

In symptomatic patients, palpitations are the most common symptom either at rest or during exercise. Most patients describe palpitations of sudden onset and sudden termination. Other symptoms are shortness of breath, chest discomfort, light-headedness, neck pulsation, and presyncope. Syncope is rare except with AF and rapid conduction over AP, which may rarely degenerate into ventricular fibrillation (VF) and cardiac arrest. The incidence of VF and sudden cardiac death (SCD) in WPW syndrome is 0.1% to 0.4%.

TACHYCARDIAS IN WPW SYNDROME

1. OT using the A-V node, His-Purkinje system in the anterograde direction, and AP in the retrograde direction. These tachycardias usually have a narrow QRS morphology or may have RBBB or LBBB morphology either caused by rate-related phenomena or with preexisiting bundle branch block. **Fig. 14**A shows an example of 12-lead ECG in a patient with recurrent palpitations. In **Fig. 14**B the ECG of the same patient shows sinus rhythm and ventricular preexcitation.

2. Preexcited tachycardias:
   a. Antidromic AVRT is less common and uses AP in the anterograde direction and His-Purkinje, A-V nodal system in the retrograde

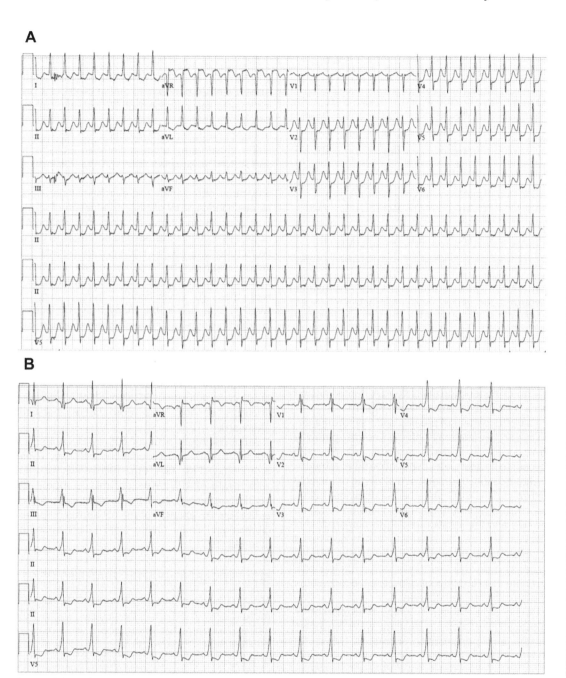

Fig. 14. (*A*) Twelve-lead ECG of orthodromic tachycardia (OT). (*B*) Twelve-lead ECG shows sinus rhythm and preexcitation of the same patient shown in (*A*), showing the presence of ventricular preexcitation.

direction (**Fig. 15**), and is always a wide complex morphology because the ventricular activation is exclusively via AP.

b. Atrial tachycardias including AF, atrial flutter, sinus tachycardia, sinus node reentrant tachycardias, AVNRT, and permanent junctional reciprocating tachycardia.

ELECTROCARDIOGRAPHIC CHARACTERISTICS OF WPW SYNDROME AND RELATED TACHYCARDIAS

In patients with manifest preexcitation, intracardiac recording during sinus rhythm reveals short H-V interval of less than 35 milliseconds. H-V interval may be zero or even negative in patients with

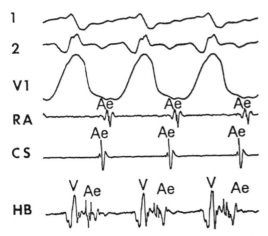

Fig. 15. Antidromic tachycardia with wide complex morphology in a patient with WPW syndrome. Note that the retrograde activation via the A-V node is concentric; the earliest retrograde activation is on His bundle electrogram (HB), then on CS, followed by right atrium (RA). Tracings arranged as electrocardiographic lead I, II, V1. Ae, atrial echo; V, ventricular electrogram.

A-V nodal conduction delay (long A-H interval) and more pronounced preexcitation **Fig. 16**.

The ECG pattern of preexcitation syndrome depends on the interplay between normal pathway (A-V node, His-Purkinje system) and AP with respect to its heart rate, conduction time, refractoriness, location, and presence of single or multiple pathways. The ECG patterns during sinus rhythm are caused by the magnitude of fusion between the two and the location of AP. In some patients preexcitation may be intermittent; that is, present at certain times or on alternate beats **Fig. 17**A, B. Depending on the heart rate, AP refractoriness, and other neurohormonal variables, the magnitude of preexcitation may change.

During atrial pacing in which preexcitation is increased, the stimulus to delta wave becomes shorter and preexcitation increases. Most AP shows 1:1 conduction during atrial pacing;

however, some AP may show decremental conduction.

Retrograde atrial activation during ventricular pacing and OT shows eccentric atrial activation. Absence of VA conduction during ventricular pacing makes the diagnosis of OT unlikely, but patients with manifest preexcitation are still at risk of other preexcited tachycardias such as AF, atrial flutter, atrial tachycardia, antidromic tachycardia, and AVNRT (discussed later). OT may be induced during incremental atrial and ventricular pacing, and atrial and ventricular extrastimulation techniques. During atrial pacing, conduction block occurs over AP and impulses travel through the A-V node, His-Purkinje system and conducts to the atria retrogradely via AP. Eccentric retrograde activation suggests participation of an extranodal pathway. Ventriculoatrial (VA) conduction time of less than 70 milliseconds strongly suggests AVNRT. Changes in the tachycardia CL and VA conduction time during ipsilateral BBB also suggest OT.

Fig. 18 is from a patient with WPW syndrome who also had established LBBB pattern. OT was inducible with LBBB pattern and concentric retrograde atrial activation. RF ablation of AP revealed abolition of the APs and LBBB persisted afterward.

Atrial pacing at a CL of 500 milliseconds produced maximal preexcitation with an RBBB morphology **Fig. 19**A. **Fig. 19**B shows slow OT with a rate of 125 beats per minute (bpm) with LBBB morphology. Note the concentric retrograde activation. RF ablation of the AP abolished preexcitation and sinus rhythm with LBBB appeared (see **Fig. 19**C).

ELECTROCARDIOGRAPHIC FEATURES OF OT

Most OT tachycardias are of narrow QRS complex morphology. The heart rate usually ranges from 140 to 250 bpm. The retrograde P wave may not be identifiable; however, in most cases careful examination of the 12-lead ECG reveals a retrograde

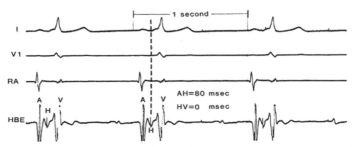

Fig. 16. Intracardiac recording of a patient with WPW syndrome. The dotted line represents the onset of the delta wave to the His bundle recording (HBE), which measured zero. Tracings are arranged as lead I, V1, RA, and HBE.

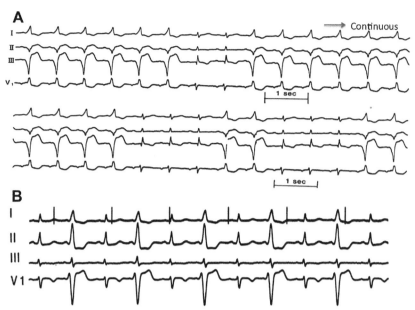

Fig. 17. Electrocardiographic leads I, II, III, and V1 show intermittent preexcitation (*A*) and preexcitation alternating with normal QRS (*B*).

P wave within the ST segment with an RP interval of more than 100 milliseconds (**Fig. 20**A, B).

Functional (rate-related) BBB is frequently observed during OT, mostly at the onset of the tachycardia. ST segment depressions may be present; however, like AVNRT, it is a nonspecific finding and does not reflect ischemic changes.

QRS alternans may be present during OT, as shown in **Fig. 21**. CL alternans may also be present, but is less common than AVNRT.

Effect of BBB During OT

Because the His-Purkinje system and ventricular myocardium are part of the tachycardia circuit, conduction delays produced by BBB are ipsilateral to the location of AP with induced conduction delay in the retrograde pathway (**Fig. 22**). As a result, the VA conduction time increases. Magnitude of VA conduction prolongation during ipsilateral BBB depends on the location of the AP. OT with left lateral location shows longer VA

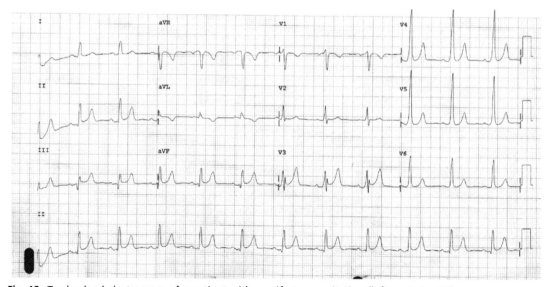

Fig. 18. Twelve-lead electrogram of a patient with manifest preexcitation (left posterior AP).

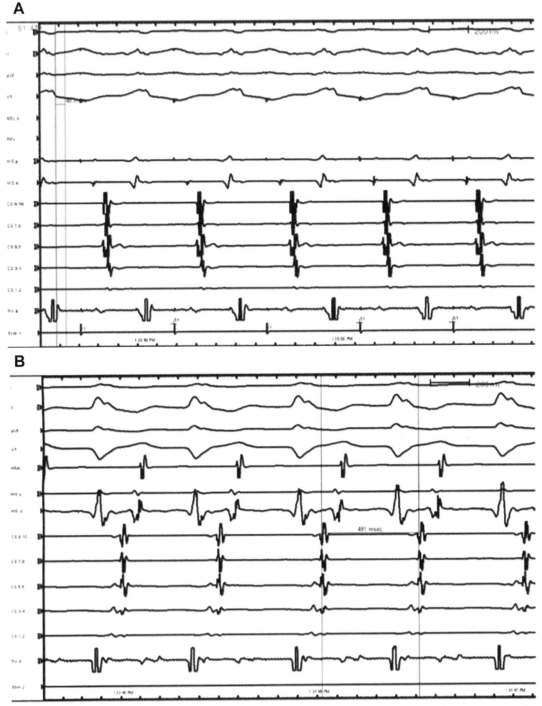

Fig. 19. (*A*) Atrial pacing at a CL of 500 milliseconds showing maximal preexcitation. Tracings are arranged at electrocardiographic I, II, III, V1, HRA, His bundle posterior (HiSp), His bundle distal (Hisd), CS, right ventricular distal (RVD), stimulation channel (Stim 1). (*B*) Orthodromic tachycardia with a rate of 125 beats per minute with an LBBB morphology and concentric retrograde activation. Tracings are arranged as in (*A*). (*C*) Radiofrequency ablation of APs. Left part of the tracing shows atrial tracing rhythm with preexcitation and, on the right, atrial tracing with LBBB is seen. Tracings are arranged as in (*A*) and (*B*).

C

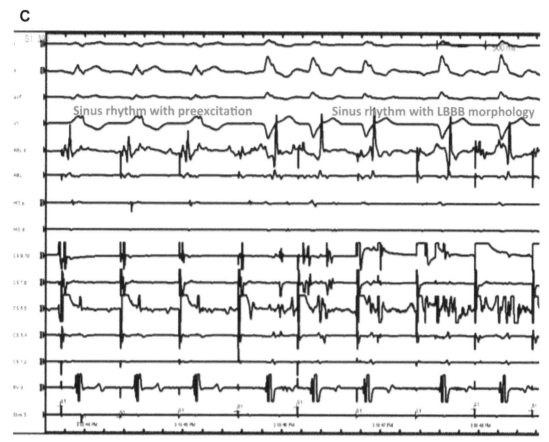

Sinus rhythm with preexcitation   Sinus rhythm with LBBB morphology

Fig. 19. (*continued*)

prolongation time (generally more than 35 milliseconds) than those with septal AP (generally <25 milliseconds). Compared with AVNRT, BBB is more common during OT.

The P wave morphology during OT depends on the location of AP and, in general, a negative P wave in lead I suggests a left lateral AP, whereas a positive P wave indicates a right lateral AP. A positive P wave in V_1 similarly suggests right lateral AP. Left posterior and posteroseptal AP show a negative P-wave morphology in II, III, and AVF.

ELECTROCARDIOGRAPHIC FEATURES OF PREEXCITED TACHYCARDIAS

In antidromic tachycardia the reentry circuit uses the AP in the antegrade direction and A-V node pathway in the retrograde direction. Antidromic tachycardias therefore are always of wide complex morphology and should resemble the maximal preexcitation pattern during sinus rhythm. The wide complexes in antidromic tachycardias are not similar to those of typical RBBB or LBBB. During intracardiac recording, because the ventricular activation is exclusively via AP, no

His recording is detectable before each QRS. Furthermore because retrograde activation is via the normal A-V conduction system, the retrograde atrial activation shows a concentric pattern (see **Fig. 15**).

In antidromic tachycardia the anterograde conduction is exclusively via the AP and the retrograde conduction is via the normal pathway (AVN) or another AP.

In summary, preexcited tachycardias can be categorized as:

1. AP part of tachycardia circuit
   a. Antidromic reentry (including atriofascicular type; see **Fig. 15**)
   b. Reciprocating tachycardias using 2 or more APs (AP-to-AP) reentry
   c. Nodoventricular or nodofascicular reentry
2. AP not part of tachycardia circuit (bystander conduction)
   a. AF (**Fig. 23**)
   b. Atrial flutter (**Fig. 24**)
   c. Sinus node reentry
   d. Atrial tachycardia
   e. AVNRT

A

B

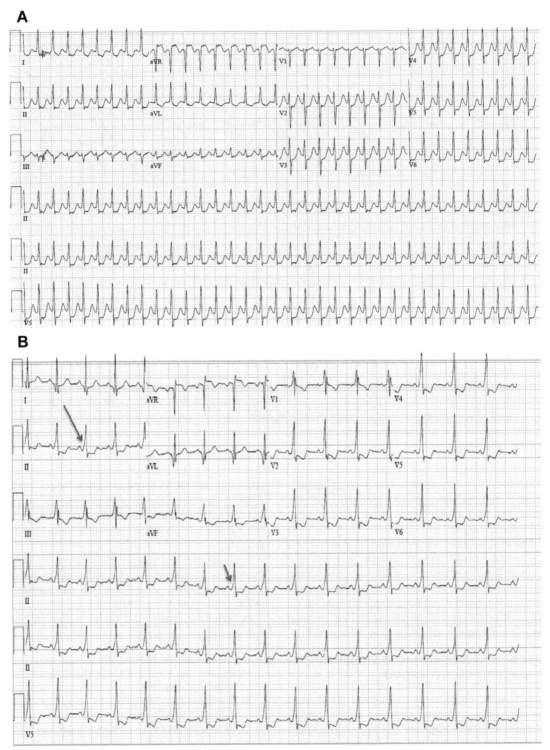

Fig. 20. (*A*) Twelve-lead ECG of an orthodromic tachycardia. Note the ST segment depression in leads II and III, which are nonspecific. (*B*) Twelve-lead electrogram of the same patient showing preexcitation. Arrows denote the delta wave.

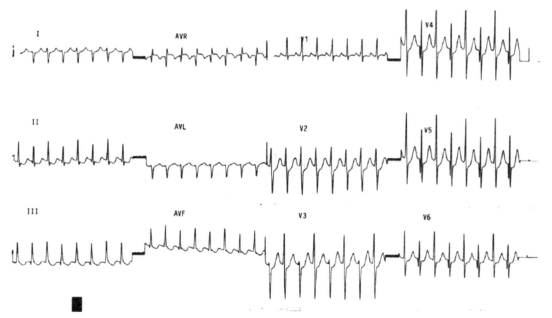

Fig. 21. Twelve-lead ECG of a 12-year-old boy with orthodromic tachycardia. Note significant QRS alternans seen in precordial leads.

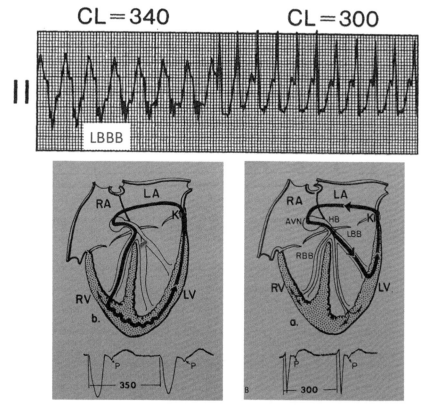

Fig. 22. Effect of LBBB on the tachycardia CL. Top tracing shows lead II ECG of an orthodromic tachycardia (OT) with an LBBB with a CL of 340 milliseconds. The tachycardia morphology normalizes on the right with a narrow QRS complex morphology with a CL of 300 milliseconds. Lower panels show the schematic route of impulse propagation during LBBB and narrow QRS complex OT. HB, His bundle; K, Kent bundle; LBB, left bundle branch; RBB, right bundle branch. (*Courtesy of* Mark E. Josephson, MD, Boston, MA.)

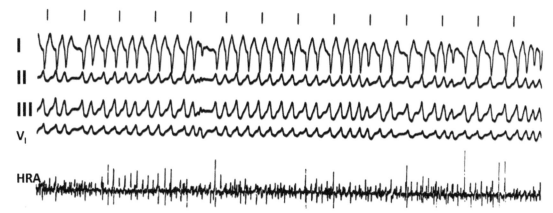

Fig. 23. AF in a patient with WPW syndrome with rapid ventricular response, which degenerated into VF. Tracings are arranged at ECG leads I, II, III, V_1, and intracardiac ECG of HRA.

In cases of antidromic tachycardias and preexcited tachycardia with A-V nodal reentry, retrograde atrial activation is concentric, whereas in preexcited tachycardias caused by antidromic tachycardia and tachycardias using another AP retrogradely the retrograde atrial activation is eccentric.

PATIENTS WITH MULTIPLE APs

In 10% to 15% of patients multiple APs may be present, and detailed intracardiac electrophysiologic studies and mapping are necessary to delineate the exact location and participation of the pathways in the reentry circuit. **Fig. 25A–C** shows

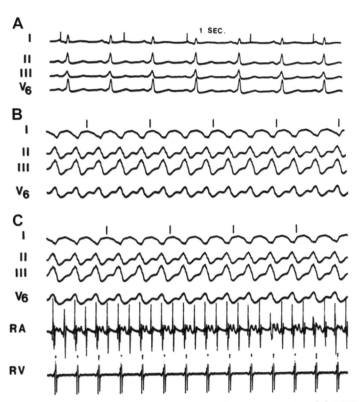

Fig. 24. Atrial flutter with 2:1 conduction in a patient with manifest preexcitation. (*A*) WPW syndrome in sinus rhythm. (*B*) Wide complex tachycardia (preexcited tachycardia). (*C*) Atrial flutter with 2:1 A-V conduction. Tracings are arranged at electrocardiographic leads I, II, III, V_6, RA, and right ventricle (RV).

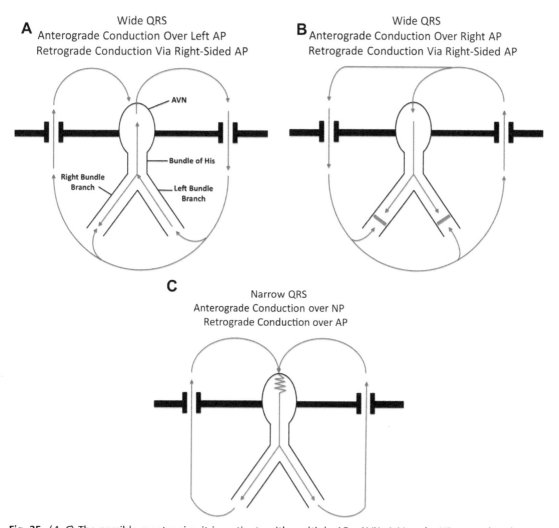

Fig. 25. (*A–C*) The possible reentry circuit in patients with multiple APs. AVN, A-V node; NP, normal pathway.

the potential reentry circuits in patients with multiple AP.

Induction of AF is a useful technique to detect multiple APs, because the QRS morphology changes according to conduction over each AP.[29] **Fig. 26** shows AF in a patient with 2 distinct lateral APs (right and left). In our series changed morphology of QRS was a useful criterion for identification of patients with multiple APs (see **Fig. 26**).

ELECTROCARDIOGRAPHIC CLUES TO MULTIPLE APs

1. Variation in preexcited QRS morphology especially during AF
2. Atypical patterns of preexcitation

3. Antidromic AVRT using a posterior septal accessory bypass tract
4. OT (AVRT) with changing retrograde P-wave morphologies
5. Antidromic AVRT with varying degrees of antegrade fusion

AF AND ATRIAL FLUTTER IN WPW SYNDROME

AF in WPW syndrome is common and at times is the first arrhythmia manifestation. AF in WPW syndrome when the effective refractory period of the AP is short can conduct very quickly and degenerates into VF and cardiac arrest. **Fig. 27A** shows an example of OT with a left-sided AP in which, after ablation of the AP, AVNRT was inducible, and

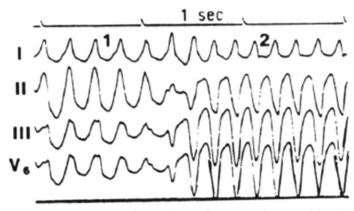

Fig. 26. AF in a patient with 2 APs. Note the distinct change in the morphology of the QRS.

Fig. 27B shows that AVNRT was inducible after transient ablation of the APs, which degenerated to AF with conduction over the AP.

Ablation of AP is reported to reduce the incidence of AF in these patients. The incidence of AF is lower in patients with concealed AP compared with manifest preexcitation. The fastest ventricular response during AF has prognostic implications and is related to the effective refractory period of AP. Patients with short AP effective refractory periods conduct faster. These findings may be useful to consider AP ablation in such cases.

Atrial flutter in the presence of manifest preexcitation can produce wide complex tachycardia as shown in **Fig. 24**.

OTHER ARRHYTHMIAS IN AVRT

AVNRT may coexist in patients with AVRT, so a complete electrophysiologic evaluation in patients with SVT is mandatory. AVNRT in patients with manifest preexcitation may cause a preexcited tachycardia. Ablation of AP in these cases may unmask the AVNRT. **Fig. 28** shows induction of AVNRT in a patient with WPW syndrome; note that the atrial pacing produces maximal preexcitation. However, with extra stimuli, AVNRT is induced.

In a preexcited tachycardia caused by AVNRT, ablation of the AP caused the AP to disappear. However, AVNRT persisted. Ablation of a slow pathway further abolished AVNRT (**Fig. 29**).

OT is shown in **Fig. 30**. A short burst of atrial pacing has converted AVRT to AVNRT; note that the blood pressure has significantly reduced during AVNRT, probably because of simultaneous closure of the A-V valves during tachycardia.

MAPPING AND ABLATION OF APs

Abolition of anterograde and retrograde conduction of AP pathways is mandatory in the WPW syndrome. Complete loss of function of concealed AP is similarly necessary for a successful procedure. In patients with manifest preexcitation mapping is usually done during sinus rhythm or atrial pacing to achieve maximal preexcitation. The shortest A-V interval and AP potential are good markers for ablation target sites.

Several maneuvers are used to show efficacy of ablation, including atrial pacing, induction of AF, attempts to induce AVRT, and ventricular pacing to show VA block and pharmacologic challenges such as administration of isoproterenol or adenosine. **Figs. 31**A and **32** are from a patient after RF ablation of AP. Induction of AF did not manifest preexcitation; however, IV adenosine administration (6 mg) produced significant bradycardia and intermittent preexcitation emerged (see **Fig. 31**B).

Mapping during OT or ventricular pacing to identify the shortest VA interval and presence of AP potential are also good markers for target sites. Care is needed in the interpretation of retrograde activation mapping during ventricular pacing because fusion of activation via the A-V conduction system and AP may occur, especially in free wall locations.

Two ablation approaches are used, depending on the experience of operators and mapping techniques used:

1. Anterograde transseptal approach
2. Retrograde transaortic approach

For anterolateral, lateral, and posterolateral APs the transseptal approach is technically easier,

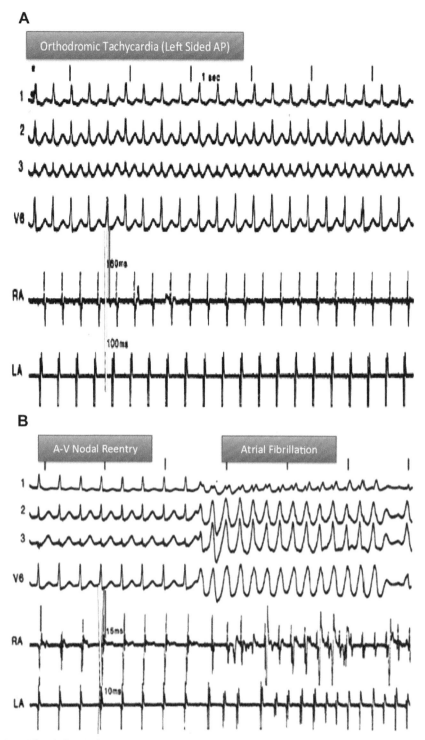

Fig. 27. (*A*) OT with a left-sided AP. Note that the left atrial activation is 60 milliseconds earlier than the right atrial activation. (*B*) AVNRT in the same patient with a very short retrograde atrial activation of 10 to 15 milliseconds from the left and right atrial activation respectively. Note that AVNRT degenerates to AF with rapid ventricular response over the APs. Atrial electrogram confirms the presence of AF.

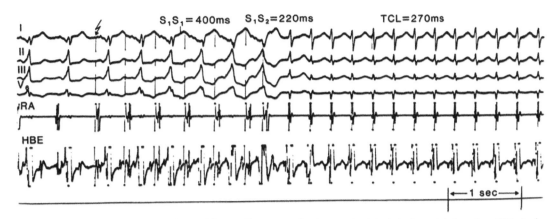

Fig. 28. Induction AVNRT in a patient with manifest preexcitation as depicted during atrial pacing. TCL, tachycardia CL. *Arrows* indicate pacing artifact.

whereas in posterolateral and posterior AP locations the retrograde aortic approach is easier.

For experienced clinicians in high-volume centers the overall success rate of AP ablation is more than 98%,[30] with complication rates of less than 1%. With complex anatomy (ie, congenital heart disease with or without surgical interventions) and multiple APs the success rate may be lower and a redo procedure may be needed.

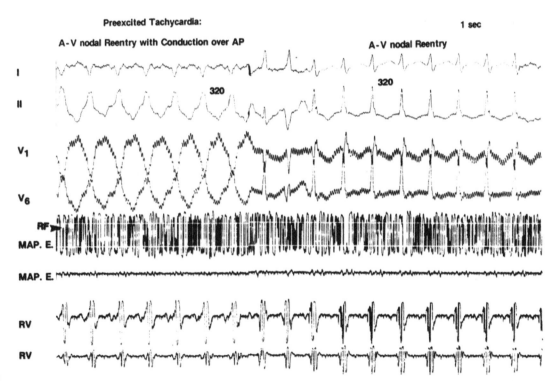

Fig. 29. Preexcited tachycardia with maximal preexcitation in a patient with left lateral AP. Ablation of the AP revealed abolition of AP; however, tachycardia persisted and revealed A-V nodal reentrant tachycardia. Ablation of the slow pathway (not shown here) abolished the AVNRT.

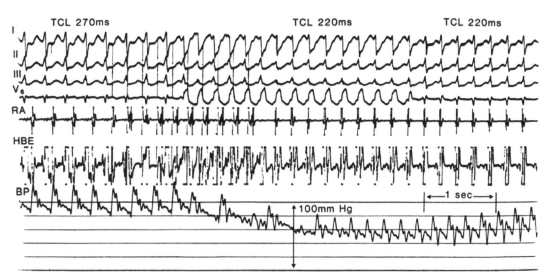

Fig. 30. AVRT with a TCL of 270 milliseconds. Atrial pacing induced AVNRT, initially with an RBBB pattern, which normalized, and later AVNRT converted to narrow QRS complex morphology. Note that the CL of AVNRT is 220 milliseconds and the systolic blood pressure (BP) is significantly lower during AVNRT compared with OT, as shown in the lower panel.

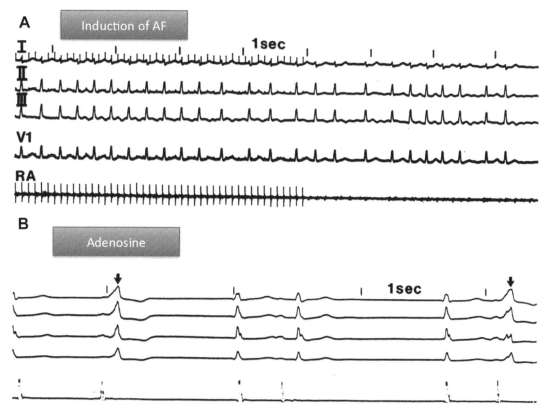

Fig. 31. (*A*) Induction of AF with rapid burst pacing after ablation (note no preexcited beats). (*B*) In the same patient, administration of IV adenosine induced significant bradycardia, and 2 preexcited beats emerged (*arrows*).

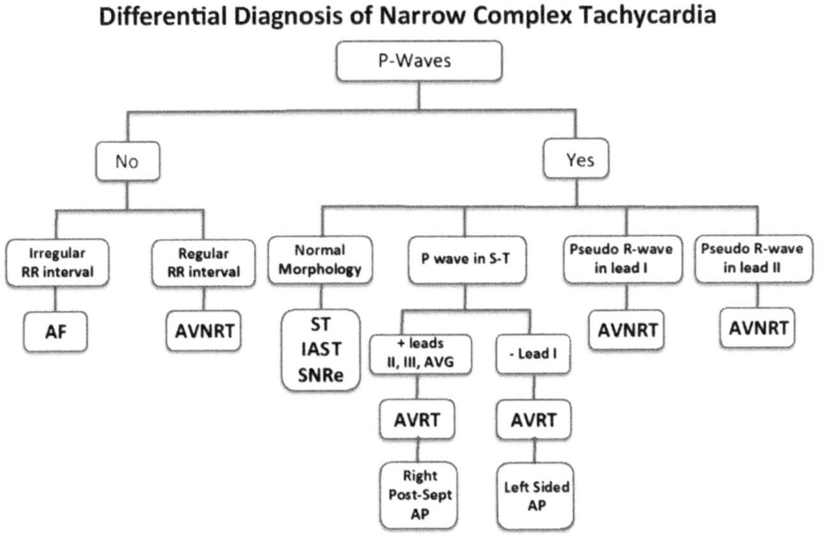

Differential Diagnosis of Narrow Complex Tachycardia

Fig. 32. Algorithm for differential diagnosis of narrow complex tachycardia. IAST, inappropriate sinus tachycardia; SNRe, sinus node reentrant.

SUMMARY

AVNRT and AVRT are the foundation of rhythmology. Detailed electrocardiographic and electrophysiologic evaluation of these arrhythmias leads to accurate diagnosis. There is now a curative procedure (ie, catheter ablation) that has proved to be safe and effective (more than 95%). ECGs play an important role in diagnosis and deductive mechanism(s) of the arrhythmias (**Fig. 32**).

REFERENCES

1. Denes P, Wu D, Dhingra RC, et al. Demonstration of dual A-V nodal pathways in patients with paroxysmal supraventricular tachycardia. Circulation 1973;48(3):549–55.
2. Moe GK, Preston JB, Burlington H, et al. Physiologic evidence for a dual A-V transmission system. Circ Res 1956;4(4):357–75.
3. Delacretaz E. Supraventricular tachycardia. N Engl J Med 2006;354:1039–51.
4. Link MS. Evaluation and initial treatment of supraventricular tachycardia. N Engl J Med 2012;367:1438–48.
5. Akhtar M, Jazayeri MR, Sra J, et al. Atrioventricular nodal reentry: clinical, electrophysiological, and therapeutic considerations. Circulation 1993;88:282–95.
6. Katritsis DG, Camm J. Atrioventricular nodal reentrant tachycardia. Circulation 2010;122:831–40.
7. Inoue S. Posterior extensions of the human compact atrioventricular node. Circulation 1998;97:188–93.
8. McGuire M, Bourke J, Robotin M. High resolution mapping of Koch's triangle using sixty electrodes in humans with atrioventricular junctional (AV nodal) reentrant tachycardia. Circulation 1993;88(5):2315–28.
9. Willems S, Daniel S, Lutomsky B, et al. Mapping and ablation of AV NRT and its subtypes. In: Shenasa M, Hindricks G, Borggrefe M, et al, editors. Cardiac mapping. 3rd edition. Chichester (United Kingdom): Blackwell; 2009. p. 199–211.
10. Issa ZF, Miller JM, Zipes DP. Clinical arrhythmology and electrophysiology; a companion to Braunwald's heart disease. Chapter 13. Philadelphia: Elsevier; 2009.
11. Keim S, Werner P, Jazayeri M, et al. Localization of the fast and slow pathways in atrioventricular nodal reentrant tachycardia by intraoperative ice mapping. Circulation 1992;86(3):919–25.
12. Pritchett E, Anderson R, Benditt D, et al. Reentry within the atrioventricular node: surgical cure with preservation of atrioventricular conduction. Circulation 1979;60(2):440–6.
13. Jackman WM, Beckman KJ, McClelland JH, et al. Treatment of supraventricular tachycardia due to atrioventricular nodal reentry by radiofrequency catheter ablation of slow-pathway conduction. N Engl J Med 1992;327(5):313–8.
14. Tai C, Chen S, Chiang C, et al. Complex electrophysiological characteristics in atrioventricular nodal reentrant tachycardia with continuous atrioventricular node function curves. Circulation 1997;95(11):2541–7.
15. Otomo K, Wang Z, Lazzara R, et al. Atrioventricular nodal reentrant tachycardia: electrophysiological characteristics of four forms and implications for the reentrant circuit. In: Zipes DP, Jalife J, editors. Cardiac electrophysiology: from cell to bedside. Third edition. Philadelphia: W.B. Saunders; 2000. p. 504–21.

16. Willems S, Shenasa M, Borggrefe M, et al. Atrioventricular nodal reentry tachycardia: electrophysiologic comparisons in patients with and without 2:1 infra-his block. Clin Cardiol 1993;16:883–8.

17. Mahajan T, Berul CI, Cecchin F, et al. Atrioventricular nodal reentrant tachycardia with 2:1 block in pediatric patients. Heart Rhythm 2008;5:1391–5.

18. Jazayeri MR, Moghaddam M, Deshpande S, et al. Penetration of atrioventricular nodal reentrant circuit during atrial extrastimulation without resetting tachycardia cycle length: further insights into the anatomic boundary of reentry. J Am Coll Cardiol 1994;23:367A.

19. Shenasa M, Denker S, Mahmud R, et al. Effect of verapamil on retrograde atrioventricular nodal conduction in the human heart. J Am Coll Cardiol 1983;2:545.

20. Shenasa M, Lacombe P, Coté MA, et al. Depressant effect on the retrograde atrial ventricular nodal conduction of beta-adrenergic block by propanolol in humans. Can J Cardiol 1987;3:281–7.

21. Jazayeri MR, Sra JS, Deshpande SS, et al. Electrophysiologic spectrum of atrioventricular nodal behavior in patients with atrioventricular nodal reentrant tachycardia undergoing selective fast or slow pathway ablation. J Cardiovasc Electrophysiol 1993;4:99–111.

22. Jazayeri MR, Hempe SL, Sra JS, et al. Selective transcatheter ablation of the fast and slow pathways using radiofrequency energy in patients with atrioventricular nodal reentrant tachycardia. Circulation 1992;85:1318–28.

23. Haissaguerre M, Gaita F, Fischer B, et al. Elimination of atrioventricular nodal reentrant tachycardia using discrete slow potentials to guide application of radiofrequency energy. Circulation 1992;85:2162–75.

24. Jazayeri MR. Cryomapping of the perinodal region: a safe and effective technique for ablation of the AV nodal reentrant tachycardia. In: Shenasa M, Hindricks J, Borggrefe M, et al, editors. Cardiac Mapping. 3rd edition. Oxford(UK): Wiley-Blackwell; 2009. p. 183–98.

25. FIRE AND ICE: comparative study of two ablation procedures in patients with atrial fibrillation. Available at: http://clinicaltrials.gov/ct2/show/NCT01490814.

26. Fromer M, Shenasa M. Ultrarapid subthreshold stimulation for termination of atrioventricular nodal reentry tachycardia. J Am Coll Cardiol 1992;20:879–83.

27. Willems S, Weis C, Shenasa M, et al. Optimized mapping of slow pathway ablation guided by subthreshold stimulation: a randomized prospective study in patients with recurrent atrioventricular nodal re-entrant tachycardia. J Am Coll Cardiol 2001;37(6):1645–50.

28. Issa ZF, Miller JM, Zipes DP. Atrioventricular nodal reentrant tachycardia. In: Issa ZF, Miller JM, Zipes DP, editors. Clinical arrhythmology and electrophysiology; a companion to Braunwald's heart disease. Philadelphia: Saunders Elsevier; 2009. p. 293–318.

29. Shenasa M, Cardinal R, Savard P, et al. Cardiac mapping. Part I. Wolff-Parkinson-White syndrome. Pacing Clin Electrophysiol 1990;13:223–30.

30. Morady F. Catheter ablation of supraventricular arrhythmias: state of the art. J Cardiovasc Electrophysiol 2004;15:124–34.

Wide Complex Tachycardia

Mithilesh Kumar Das, MD[a,b,*], Archana Rajdev, MD[a], Vikas Kalra, MBBS[a]

KEYWORDS

- Wide complex tachycardia • Ventricular tachycardia • Supraventricular tachycardia with aberrancy
- Catheter ablation

KEY POINTS

- A patient with a wide complex tachycardia needs immediate attention because it is often a life-threatening arrhythmia, especially in the presence of structural heart disease.
- Common electrocardiographic (ECG) criteria for ventricular tachycardia (VT) include wide QRS, right superior axis, positive QRS concordance, atrioventricular dissociation, capture beat, fusion beat, and absence of typical bundle branch block pattern.
- Supraventricular tachycardia with aberrancy (SVT-A) has a typical BBB pattern, and a baseline ECG may be helpful. When doubt exists, patients should be treated for VT, especially those with structural heart disease.
- Hemodynamically unstable rhythm is treated with DC shock, and stable rhythm due to SVT-A can be terminated with intravenous adenosine and atrioventricular nodal blocking agents.
- Preexcited atrial fibrillation or flutter should be treated with intravenous procainamide or amiodarone.
- SVT-A and VT are treated effectively with catheter ablation.

A patient with a wide complex tachycardia (WCT) needs immediate attention because it is often a life-threatening arrhythmia, especially in the presence of structural heart disease. Therefore, physicians must have a good understanding of the differential diagnosis of WCT so that a malignant arrhythmia, such as ventricular tachycardia (VT), can be differentiated from a benign arrhythmia, such as supraventricular tachycardia with aberrancy (SVT-A) (**Box 1**). A hemodynamically stable VT in a patient with structural heart disease mistaken for a benign arrhythmia such as SVT-A is one of the most common errors in the interpretation of WCT. This error in the judgment may be life threatening when these patients are treated with an intravenous calcium blocker, which may lead to hemodynamic instability. The quick and correct diagnosis not only helps in prompt treatment, but also helps in the optimal long-term management of these patients. This review discusses the differential diagnosis of WCT using various electrocardiographic (ECG) criteria, correlation with intracardiac findings during electrophysiology (EP) study, and its management in brief.

MECHANISM OF WCT

In adults, normal QRS is usually less than 110 ms and mostly is between 60 and 80 ms, because the ventricular activation is rapid via the His-Purkinje system (HPS; His bundle, bundle branches, and fascicles).[1] During a normal

The authors have nothing to disclose.
[a] Krannert Institute of Cardiology, Indiana University Health, Indianapolis, IN, USA; [b] Cardiac Arrhythmia Service, Roudebush Veterans Affairs Medical Center, Indianapolis, IN, USA
* Corresponding author. Cardiac Arrhythmia Service, Roudebush Veterans Affairs Medical Center, Indianapolis, IN.
E-mail address: midas@iupui.edu

Card Electrophysiol Clin 6 (2014) 511–523
http://dx.doi.org/10.1016/j.ccep.2014.05.002
1877-9182/14/$ – see front matter Published by Elsevier Inc.

Box 1
Terminology

Wide-complex tachycardia (WCT): A wide QRS complex on tachycardia on electrocardiogram is defined as rhythm with QRS duration ≥120 ms and rate ≥100 beats per minute.

Ventricular tachycardia: tachycardia with a focus or reentrant circuit in the ventricle below the bundle of His

Supraventricular tachycardia: tachycardia requiring participation of structures above bundle of His

Left bundle branch block (LBBB) configuration[1]:

1. QRS duration ≥120 ms with predominantly negative terminal portion of lead V1.

2. Broad-notched or slurred R wave in leads I, aVL, V5, and V6 and an occasional RS pattern in V5 and V6 attributed to displaced transition of QRS complex.

3. Absent q waves in leads I, V5, and V6, but in the lead aVL, a narrow q wave may be present in the absence of myocardial pathology.

4. R peak time greater than 60 ms in leads V5 and V6 but normal in leads V1, V2, and V3, when small initial r waves can be discerned in the above leads.

5. ST and T waves usually opposite in direction to QRS.

Right bundle branch block (RBBB) configuration (positive T wave in leads with upright QRS may be normal [positive concordance])[1]:

1. QRS duration ≥120 ms with predominantly positive terminal portion of lead V1

2. Rsr′, rsR′, or rSR′ in leads V_1 or V_2. The R′ or r′ deflection is usually wider than the initial R wave. In a minority of patients, a wide and often notched R-wave pattern may be seen in lead V1 and/or V2.

3. S wave of greater duration than R wave or greater than 40 ms in leads I and V6.

4. Normal R peak time in leads V5 and V6 but greater than 50 ms in lead V1.

---

myocardial conduction, QRS can widen when one of the bundle branches fails to conduct due to anatomic block at baseline or functional block during a rapid rate (aberrancy) during SVT. This is because the ventricular activation is transmyocardial from the nonblocked portion of the HPS (conducting bundle branch or fascicle) to the contralateral ventricle with a nonconducting bundle branch. The QRS also may widen when the major part of ventricular activation is transmyocardial, such as during VT, antidromic atrioventricular tachycardia (ART) via a manifest pathway, paced rhythm, electrolyte imbalance, or with the use of antiarrhythmic therapy.

VT

VT is the most common cause of WCT, accounting for 70% to 80% of cases, which occurs mostly in the presence of significant structural heart disease, such as coronary artery disease (CAD) or cardiomyopathy and less commonly in the presence of normal heart. The QRS complex has a left bundle branch block (LBBB) or a right bundle branch block (RBBB) pattern during VT depending on the origin of the VT (right vs left ventricle). As a general rule, the LBBB-pattern VT arises from the right ventricle (RV) or septal aspect of the left ventricle (LV), and the RBBB pattern VT arises from the LV.

SVT-A

SVT-A is the second most common cause of WCT. Patients with permanent BBB will have a similar QRS morphology during sinus tachycardia or an SVT, whereas rate-related BBB during SVT resembles VT, and needs a closer look by using diagnostic criteria for differentiation.

Antidromic AV Reentrant Tachycardia (ART)

In Wolff-Parkinson-White (WPW) syndrome, abnormal ventricular activation occurs via an accessory pathway (AP) that almost always inserts into the epicardial aspect of the ventricular muscle near the atrioventricular (AV) groove. This results in preexcitation (delta waves). During ARTs, ventricular activation initially occurs transmyocardially when the impulse reaches the ventricle from the atria via the AP, and the transmyocardial impulse conduction continues till it reaches the HPS to return to the atrium again via the AV node. The initial portion of the QRS deflection (delta wave) during ART is similar to the sinus rhythm QRS. Therefore,

QRS is slurred (delta waves) due to relatively slow epicardial to endocardial conduction during sinus rhythm, which becomes more pronounced during ART.

Nonspecific Intraventricular Conduction Delays

Various QRS morphologies without any typical bundle branch pattern are included in the definition of nonspecific intraventricular conduction delays (IVCDs). They can occur in electrolyte imbalance, antiarrhythmic therapy, and myocardial diseases, such as CAD and various cardiomyopathies.

Paced Ventricular Rhythm

Ventricular paced rhythm with a wide QRS complex at a rate greater than 100 beats per minute (bpm) can be recorded during sinus tachycardia, atrial tachycardia, or pacemaker-mediated tachycardia. It can be easily recognized by the presence of pacemaker stimulus artifacts ("spikes"), which are easily recognized, and the underlying rhythm is often evident. However, in some cases, pacemaker artifacts may be filtered by the ECG machine and may be of a very low amplitude and even unrecognizable.

ECG CRITERIA FOR DIFFERENTIAL DIAGNOSIS OF A WCT

The major differential diagnosis of WCT is between VT and SVT-A, because VT accounts for up to 80% of WCT and the next largest group is SVT-A. Other causes are less common. The diagnostic approach in differentiating is to ask the question "is the QRS complex compatible with some form of aberration?" If the answer is yes, then the rhythm is most likely an SVT-A and if not, then VT is the more likely diagnosis. The fundamental rule is that a WCT not mimicking aberrancy in the presence of structural heart disease is VT unless proven otherwise (**Table 1**). However, possible diagnoses should be put into the context with the patient's history and clinical scenario, such as the presence of a pacemaker, preexcitation, electrolyte imbalance, or continued antiarrhythmic drug therapy.

To evaluate the accuracy of the established criteria, we studied 650 patients with WCT in which the correct diagnosis was confirmed by EP study.[2] ECGs were obtained from 385 patients (279 [73%] men), aged 9 to 89 years (mean 53 ± 19 years), among whom structural heart disease was present in 54% patients (prior myocardial infarction [MI] in 38%, cardiomyopathy in 13%, and repaired congenital heart disease in 2%). Among these, 73% of WCTs were VT, 20% were SVT-A, 6% were preexcited SVT, and fewer than 1% were SVT with abnormal baseline QRS complex and fewer than 1% were ventricular pacing with poorly evident stimulus artifacts.

QRS Duration

Usually in SVT-A, the QRS duration is 140 ms or less in RBBB aberration, and 160 ms or less in LBBB aberration. Therefore, QRS complexes wider than these are more likely to be VT. However, it should be cautioned that QRS may widen further during SVT-A in the presence of severe myocardial disease, antiarrhythmic drugs, or electrolyte imbalance. Patients with VT originating from the interventricular septum may depolarize both ventricles relatively rapidly especially in a structurally normal heart, resulting in relatively narrow QRS complexes and can sometimes be less than 120 ms. Loss of aberrancy spontaneously or by a PVC may be diagnostic of SVT-A (see **Fig. 3**).

QRS Axis

QRS axis during WCT as well as deviation from the baseline during sinus rhythm may help in differentiating VT from SVT-A.

a. QRS axis is usually normal (−30° to +120°) or, can be right (+90° to +180°) or left (−0° to −90°) in most cases (94%) of SVT-A (due to the ventricular activation via the HPS), as compared with 80% of VTs.
b. Northwest QRS axis: 20% of VTs have a northwest axis (between −90° and 180°) versus 4% of SVT-As (sensitivity 20%, specificity 96%). Therefore, a northwest axis practically helps in identifying a VT from SVT-A.
c. Rightward inferior axis deviation in LBBB SVT-A is extremely rare because the LV activation (leftward) occurs from the RV. Thus, it should suggest VT. Whereas, RBBB-type VT rarely has a normal axis (0° to +90°), as the RBBB pattern VT usually arises away from the basal interventricular septum.
d. In patients with history of MI, specific QRS morphology in aVF and V1, and frontal plane axis deviation greater than 40° different from the baseline ECG correctly identified 90% of WCTs.

QRS Concordance

A concordant pattern is defined as predominant QRS deflection, which is either all positive or all negative across the precordial leads V1 to V6.

Table 1
Clinical and electrocardiographic criteria for differentiation between supraventricular tachycardia with aberrancy and ventricular tachycardia

	Differentiation Criteria	VT	SVT with Aberrancy
Clinical	Structural heart disease	CAD, MI, DCM	Normal heart
	Long history	Only with idiopathic VT	>3 y
	Syncope	Common	Not common
	Termination with Valsalva maneuvers, adenosine, beta-blocker, or calcium blocker	Idiopathic VT	Likely
	Terminate with calcium blocker (not beta-blocker)	Idiopathic left fascicular VT	Likely
ECG	Baseline QRS	Infarct, aberrancy, IVCD	Normal, aberrancy
	QRS duration	RBBB >140 ms[a] LBBB >160 ms[b]	
	QRS axis	−180 to −90 (northwest) Change of >40° from baseline RBBB + LAD ($\geq$−30°) LBBB + RAD ($\geq$+90°)	RBBB with normal QRS axis[c]
	QRS concordance in precordial leads	Positive or negative concordance (Sn >90%, Sp 20%)	Rarely positive concordance in antidromic SVT with left posteroseptal pathway
	>1 QRS configuration during WCT	Present in 50% VTs	Only in 8% of SVT
	AV relationship	AV ratio <1 AV dissociation (Sn 100%, Sp 20%–50%)[b] 1:1 VA relation (30%), 2:1 or Wenckeback (15%–20%) Fusion beat (diagnostic of VT)[d] Capture beat (diagnostic of VT)[d]	AV ratio $\geq$1 1:1 VA relation in AVNRT or AVRT with aberrancy, antidromic AVRT
	RBBB-like pattern	• Monophasic R, biphasic qR, or broad R (>40 ms) in lead V1[e] • Double-peaked R in lead V1 with the amplitude of left peak > the right peak • rS complex in lead V6	
	LBBB-like pattern (negative QRS polarity in lead V1)[f]	• R wave $\geq$40 ms in lead V1 or V2 favors VT • Slow descent to the nadir of the S wave (an RS interval >70 ms) in lead V1 or V2 • Notching in the downstroke of the S wave • Q or QS wave in lead V6 favors VT	• Absence of an initial R wave (or a small initial R wave <40 ms) in lead V1 or V2 • No Q wave in lead V6
	QRS morphology in lead aVR	Initial R wave R wave; q or R >40 ms Notching on the initial downstroke of a predominantly negative QRS complex $v_i/v_t \leq 1$	$v_i/v_t > 1$
	QRS duration (WCT vs baseline)	QRS during WCT narrower than the baseline QRS (septal VT)	QRS during WCT same or slightly more than the baseline QRS duration

Abbreviations: AV, atrioventricular; BBB, bundle branch block; CAD, coronary artery disease; DCM, dilated cardiomyopathy; ECG, electrocardiogram; IVCD, intraventricular conduction delays; LAD, left axis deviation; LBBB, left bundle branch block; MI, myocardial infarction; NSR, normal sinus rhythm; RAD, right axis deviation; RBBB, right bundle branch block; SVT, supraventricular tachycardia; v_i, voltage excursion in the initial 40 ms of QRS; v_t, voltage excursion in the last 40 ms of QRS; VT, ventricular tachycardia; WCT, wide-complex tachycardia.

[a] Fascicular VT or septal VT can be less than 140 ms.

[b] Greater than 95% chance for VT except in patients with preexisting BBB or preexcitation.

[c] Only 3% of VT have RBBB with normal QRS axis, v_i/v_t ratio less than 1 indicates VT and v_i/v_t ratio greater than 1 signifies SVT with aberrancy with positive predictive accuracy for SVT with aberrancy of 83.5%.

[d] Usually seen in a slower VT.

[e] Capital letter "R" indicates large-wave amplitude and/or duration, and the lower-case letter "r" indicates small-wave amplitude and/or duration.

[f] Presence of either slow descent to the nadir of the S wave or notching in the downstroke of the S wave, or an RS interval (from the onset of the QRS complex to the nadir of the S wave) of $\geq$70 ms in lead V1 or V2, favors VT with a likelihood greater than 50:1.

QRS concordance is usually not possible when the conduction occurs via the HPS, even in the presence of BBB (see **Fig. 2**, **Table 1**). Although relatively specific for VT, it occurs in only 15% of VTs.[2] RBBB-type QRS complex concordance ("positive" concordance) is reported in 18% of VTs with RBBB-type pattern and only 5% of RBBB-type SVT ($P<.005$, sensitivity 18%, specificity 95%). Positive concordance also can occur during an ART because APs activate the ventricles from base to apex. On the other hand, a negative concordant pattern discriminated poorly: only 12% of LBBB-type VTs showed negative concordance, whereas 10 of SVT-As had an LBBB pattern (P = NS [non significant]; sensitivity 12%, specificity 90%). Negative concordance also can occur during RV apical pacing. Although the specificity of a concordant pattern for VT is greater than 90%, its sensitivity is low. The QRS concordance is seen in only approximately 20% of all VTs with almost equal incidence of positive and negative patterns.

Atrioventricular Relationship

Approximately 30% of VTs have 1:1 retrograde ventriculoatrial (VA) conduction and, therefore, cannot be distinguished from SVT-A, whereas AV dissociation (AVD) is the most specific electrocardiographic feature for VT (see **Fig. 2**, **Table 1**). Complete AVD is seen in 20% to 50% of all VTs and almost in none of the SVT-As (sensitivity of 20%–50%, with specificity approaching 100%). The wide range of prevalence of AVD may be due to inability to identify P waves (which should be upright in inferior leads and lead I). Furthermore, it is more difficult to diagnose VT with AVD with AV ratio of greater than 1 in the presence of dual tachycardia, such as atrial tachycardia/flutter and VT.

Capture and Fusion QRS Complexes

A capture complex occurs when a supraventricular impulse propagates through the normal HPS system between VT QRS complexes and excites both ventricles completely. Therefore, capture complexes are narrow QRS complexes similar to sinus complexes, whereas fused QRS complexes are those in which the QRS is a combination of 2 sources of ventricular activation (supraventricular and ventricular during VT). Therefore, these complexes are wider than normal QRS complexes and narrower than the pure VT complexes. These are uncommon and occur in only 0.5% of VTs and are typically seen in a slow VT, when a supraventricular impulse travels via the AV node and HPS that have recovered from refractoriness

related to the prior QRS to be able to either capture the ventricles fully (capture beat) or partially (fusion beat) (see **Table 1**). Of note, fusion complexes can rarely occur during SVT-A when a premature ventricular complex occurs during SVT.

QRS Morphology

QRS morphologies in WCT can be divided into RBBB-like and LBBB-like patterns to aid in distinguishing VT from SVT (see **Box 1**, **Figs. 1–5**, see **Table 1**).

a. RBBB pattern:
   i. QRS morphology in lead V1: During the RBBB aberration, the septum and LV is depolarized normally via the left bundle, whereas the RV does not participate in initial ventricular depolarization. Therefore, the initial portion of the QRS complex is not affected during aberrancy. QRS patterns in V1 consistent with aberration include rSr′, rR′, Rsr′, and rSR′, and represent SVT-A (see **Box 1**, **Fig. 4**, **Table 1**). Lack of rapid upstroke in lead V1 with a broad (>30 ms) R wave with any following terminal negative QRS forces and a monophasic R wave is highly suggestive of VT. A qR pattern in lead V1 is incompatible with ventricular activation using the normal LBBB (unless it represents MI) and is suggestive of VT. These abnormal QRS patterns are reported in 88% of VT and in only 3% of SVT-A. The sensitivity of these patterns for recognizing VT is 97% and the specificity is 88%.
   ii. QRS morphology in lead V6: With RBBB aberration, there is typically a small S wave (qRs or Rs pattern) representing the depolarization of small RV muscle mass away from V6. As mentioned previously, all RBBB-type VTs originate in the LV that subsequently excites RV; therefore, all of the RV depolarization plus some LV depolarization (depending on the site of origin of VT) occurs away from V6, resulting in qRS, qrS, rS, or QS pattern and R/S less than 1 rule in V6 (see **Box 1**, **Table 1**). R/S less than 1 occurs in 74% of VT and in only 24% of SVT-A. The R/S ratio less than 1 has sensitivity of 73%, specificity of 79%, and positive predictive accuracy of 90% for diagnosing VT in a WCT.
b. LBBB pattern:
   i. QRS morphology in lead V1: In true LBBB aberration, the initial portion of the QRS in V1 shows rapid activation, with an R wave duration (if present) of 30 ms or less and interval from QRS onset to S-wave nadir of 70 ms or less (see **Box 1**, **Figs. 1** and **2**,

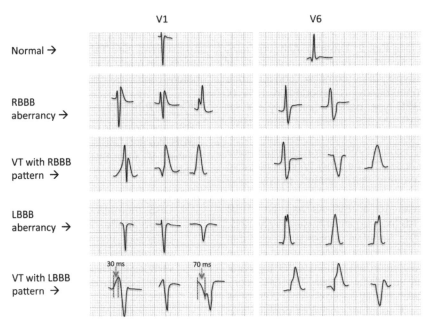

Fig. 1. Common QRS morphologies encountered in VT and SVT, with aberration in leads V1 and V6 for both LBBB and RBBB QRS patterns. QRS morphologies not typical of a bundle branch pattern suggest VT. Note the initial portions of the QRS complex in normal and aberrant QRS complexes, contrasted with the initial QRS forces in VT complexes. The RS configurations can be designated as an RBBB or an LBBB type. In LBBB-type morphology, a slow upstroke and a slow descent to the nadir of the S wave or notching in the downstroke of the S wave, or an RS interval (from the onset of the QRS complex to the nadir of the S wave) of ≥70 ms suggests VT.

Table 1). This pattern is reported in 85% of LBBB-type SVT-A ECGs, but in only 22% of LBBB-type VT ECGs. In contrast, a broad initial R wave (>30 ms) or longer interval from QRS onset to S-nadir (>70 ms) is more likely VT, and 97% of ECGs with such a pattern are VT. In addition, tall R/small S ("Rs"), "W" configuration in V1 and fragmentation of QRS (notching, which usually represents myocardial scar) strongly suggests VT, as these patterns are incompatible with any type of aberration.

ii. QRS morphology in lead V6: A monophasic R wave with a slow upstroke in lead V6 can occur in either LBBB aberrancy or VT. However, a qR or QS should not be seen in V6 with true LBBB aberration; therefore, these strongly suggest VT.

Brugada Criteria

The "precordial RS absent" criteria (Brugada criteria) studied the value of 4 criteria incorporated in a stepwise approach, which was prospectively analyzed in a total of 554 WCTs (170 SVT-A and 384 VT) (see **Fig. 5**; **Fig. 6**).[3] Because SVT-As have an RS complex in at least one precordial lead, whereas VT QRSs need not have an RS

complex, the absence of an RS in any precordial lead would allow a diagnosis of VT. This VT criterion was present in 15% of VTs. In the next step of the algorithm, the presence of an RS complex in a precordial lead was analyzed. An interval from R-wave onset to S-wave nadir greater than 100 ms was noted, which was present in 37% of WCTs and diagnosed VTs. These 2 criteria could make the correct diagnosis in 47% of patients. If the R-wave onset to the S-wave nadir was less than 100 ms, then AV dissociation was analyzed as the next step of the algorithm. If AV dissociation was present, the diagnosis of VT was made. If absent, the classic morphology criteria for VT are analyzed in leads V5 and V6. If both leads fulfilled the criteria for VT, the diagnosis of VT was made. The sensitivity of the 4 consecutive steps was 98.7%, and the specificity was 96.5% for diagnosing VT (see **Fig. 6**).

Lead aVR Criteria

Vereckei and colleagues,[4] analyzed various QRS morphologies in lead aVR and generated an algorithm to diagnose VT, which was later modified by them and compared with the Brugada criteria for diagnosing VT (see **Figs. 5** and **6**).[5] They analyzed lead aVR for (1) presence of an initial R wave, (2)

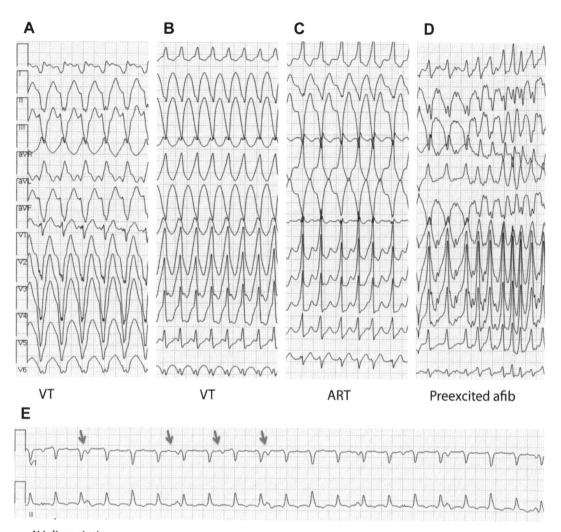

Fig. 2. Different QRS morphologies of WCT. (*A*) WCT with negative concordance on precordial leads. There is a notch in the nadir of the S wave and QRS onset to the nadir greater than 100 ms in lead V1. In addition, lead aVR morphology and northwest axis suggests VT. (*B*) Right bundle branch morphology VT with QRS duration of 200 ms and slurred peak of R wave suggests epicardial VT. (*C*) Antidromic atrioventricular tachycardia. (*D*) Preexcited atrial fibrillation (afib) with rapid ventricular response. (*E*) AV dissociation. The rhythm strip shows VT with AV dissociation. P waves are shown by *arrows*.

width of an initial r or q wave greater than 40 ms, (3) notching on the initial downstroke of a predominantly negative QRS complex, and (4) ventricular activation–velocity ratio (v_i/v_t), the vertical excursion (in millivolts) recorded during the initial (v_i) and terminal (v_t) 40 ms of the QRS complex. When any of criteria 1 to 3 was present, VT was diagnosed; when absent, the next criterion was analyzed. In step 4, v_i/v_t greater than 1 suggested SVT, and v_i/v_t of 1 or less suggested VT. The new aVR algorithm, as well as their previous algorithm, had greater sensitivity for VT diagnosis than did

the Brugada algorithm (96.5% and 95.7% vs 89.2%, *P*<.001 and *P* = .001, respectively). The negative predictive values of the new aVR and previous aVR algorithms were better than the Brugada algorithm (86.6% and 83.8% vs 67.2%). The v_i/v_t criterion applied in the fourth step of the new aVR had a significantly greater sensitivity for VT diagnosis (90.7% and 69.8%) compared with the fourth Brugada criterion (45.2%; *P*<.001 and *P* = .007, respectively), as well as negative predictive value for VT diagnosis (87.5% and 83.8% vs 67.2%).

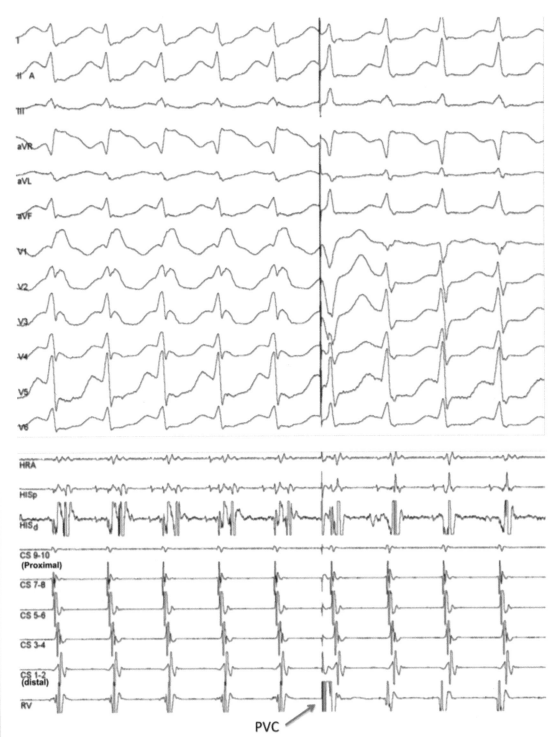

Fig. 3. A WCT changes to the narrow complex tachycardia during His refractory PVC. This is an AV nodal reentrant tachycardia with aberrancy, which, after introduction of a PVC the QRS, is narrow due to retrograde concealed conduction in the left bundle causing mild delay in antegrade conduction in the left bundle resulting in loss of right bundle branch aberrancy due to equal conduction time. Alternatively, the loss of aberrancy is because the PVC has caused peeling back of the refractoriness in the right bundle. CS 1,2, distal coronary sinus; CS 9-10, proximal coronary sinus; His$_d$, distal His; His$_p$, proximal His; HRA, high right atrium; PVC, premature ventricular contraction; RV, distal RV.

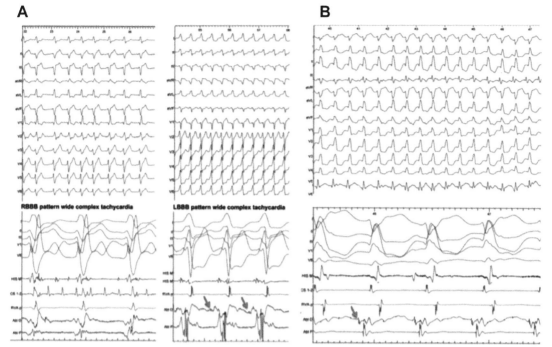

Fig. 4. (*Patient A*) The patient has history of atrial fibrillation and baseline RBBB and presented with LBBB pattern WCT suggestive of a VT. (*Patient B*) The RBBB pattern WCT has monophasic R wave in lead V1, and aVR morphology suggests VT. Both VTs were entrained and the distal ablation (Abl$_d$) electrodes show presystolic potential (*arrows*). Abl$_d$, ablation distal; Ablp, ablation proximal; CS 1,2, coronary sinus distal; CS 9-10, coronary sinus proximal; His M, His middle; HRA, high right atrium; RV, RV distal.

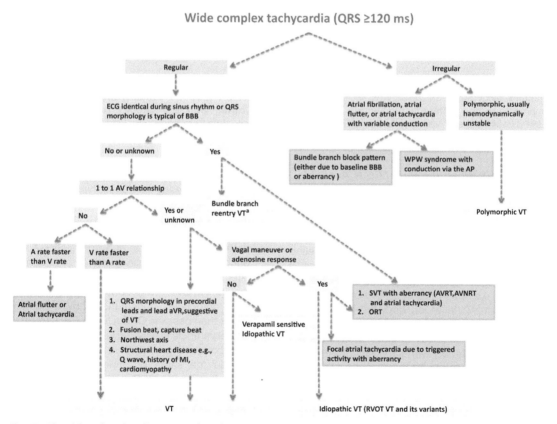

Fig. 5. Algorithm for the diagnosis of wide complex tachycardia. A rate, atrial rate; ORT, Orthodromic AV reenterant tachycardia; V rate, ventricular rate. [a] Bundle branch VT is usually LBBB (left bundle branch) pattern in patients with preexisting LBBB.

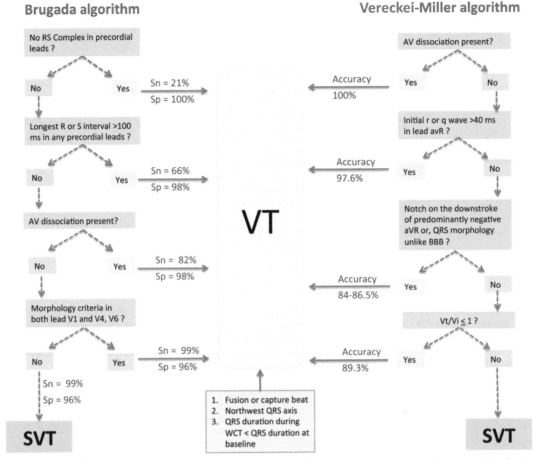

Fig. 6. Brugada algorithm and Vereckei-Miller algorithm using lead aVR, for differential diagnosis of wide QRS complex tachycardia. Sn, sensitivity; Sp, specificity. (*Data from* Brugada P, Brugada J, Mont L, et al. A new approach to the differential diagnosis of a regular tachycardia with a wide QRS complex. Circulation 1991;83:1649–59; and Vereckei A, Duray G, Szenasi G, et al. New algorithm using only lead aVR for differential diagnosis of wide QRS complex tachycardia. Heart Rhythm 2008;5:89–98.)

ECG Criteria When Baseline ECG Is Available

Baseline ECG available before or after the termination of a WCT may also help in differentiating VT from SVT-A.

a. Identical QRS configuration between baseline and WCT: If WCT complexes are identical to those of the baseline ECG, it is very likely an SVT-A, except in the case of bundle branch reentrant VT, in which both the resting ECG and VT have a LBBB pattern (see **Fig. 5**). It is because the VT circuit often involves RBBB antegradely with subsequent LV depolarization similar to baseline conduction due to LBBB.

b. Contralateral bundle branch block (BBB) patterns in baseline versus WCT: If a patient has resting LBBB in sinus rhythm and has an episode of RBBB-type tachycardia, it is unlikely to be SVT-A because the contralateral bundle branch is already nonfunctioning and cannot conduct at a faster rate. Therefore, it represents a VT (see **Fig. 4**). Rarely, there is a functional delay in one of the bundles resulting in a BBB pattern in sinus rhythm and during SVT-A that bundle starts conduction, whereas the contralateral bundle may develop delay in conduction resulting in SVT-A with contralateral aberrancy.

c. QRS complexes during the tachycardia narrower than baseline QRS: During BBB, the ipsilateral ventricle is depolarized from the ventricle with conducting HPS, thus QRS duration may remain the same or prolong further during SVT. A narrower QRS complex during tachycardia can occur during a VT only when it originates from the interventricular septum activating both ventricles nearly simultaneously or it engages the HPS early.

Miscellaneous Criteria

a. WCT in patients with IVCD (Pava criteria): Datino and colleagues[6] studied the QRS morphology during rapid atrial pacing and compared with the QRS morphology during VT at the time of EP study in the same patient. Most of the VT criteria had a low specificity in these patients. In these patients with IVCD, if the R-wave peak time (RWPT) is 50 ms or more, or when the algorithm was analyzed, the combination of RWPT of 50 ms or more in lead II, along with absence of RS patterns in precordial leads, were predictable for VT.

b. WCT slurred QRS: Wide and slurred QRS are unlikely to be an aberrancy and may represent WPW syndrome with antidromic SVT, VT in a patient with antiarrhythmic therapy, severe myocardial disease, an epicardial VT, or LV epicardial pacing.

c. WCT at a rate of approximately 150 bpm should arise the suspicion of atrial flutter with 2:1 AV conduction and ventricular aberrancy. Carotid sinus massage or vagal maneuver in a hemodynamically stable patient may unmask flutter wave by increasing AV block.

APPLICATION OF VARIOUS ECG CRITERIA

Correct application of established diagnostic criteria of WCT (which have varying diagnostic accuracy) is needed in emergency situations; however, it remains a significant problem in management of these patients. Incorrect diagnosis of SVT-A treated with an AV nodal blocker during a hemodynamically stable rhythm in a patient with structural heart disease and VT may be disastrous. It can cause persistent hypotension, which can result in rapid deterioration of clinical status of the patient and even can lead to ventricular fibrillation (VF) due to hypoxia. Baseline ECG before or after the termination WCT, if available, may help in determining the cause. WCT in a patient with history of MI or cardiomyopathy is most likely VT unless the ECG strongly favors an SVT-A, whereas WCT suggesting VT in a young patient without history of heart disease may represent an idiopathic VT. The accurate diagnosis mainly depends on the level of expertise of the physicians interpreting the ECG. When 2 cardiologists and 2 emergency physicians were asked to apply the Brugada algorithm to 157 WCTs, the diagnostic accuracy (sensitivity 98.7% and specificity 96.5%) was not as high as reported by Brugada and colleagues.[7] The sensitivity and specificity of diagnoses were 85% to 91% and 55% to 60%, respectively, for the cardiologists, and 79% to 83% and 43% to 70% for emergency physicians, respectively. The 2 studies suggest that the expert ECG interpreters who are focused on carefully applying the algorithm will have a higher yield than others; therefore, the "real-world" yield for diagnostic accuracy of WCT may not be as high as reported. However, if careful history is taken and clinical scenario is put in context, a simple guess of VT will be correct more than 70% of the time.

MANAGEMENT OF WCT

It is critical for clinicians to be able to differentiate a benign WCT from a malignant WCT because prompt intervention is needed if it is a potential life-threating arrhythmia, such as VT in structural heart disease or atrial fibrillation with rapid ventricular response via an AP. The common error is when physicians fail to recognize a potentially life-threatening arrhythmia in a patient with structural heart disease because the patient presents with hemodynamically stable rhythm and is treated for an SVT-A. To worsen it further, if these patients are treated with an intravenous calcium blocker, such as verapamil or diltiazem, hemodynamic collapse due to negative inotropy and peripheral vasodilation can occur.

Hemodynamically Unstable WCT

It is not uncommon for a WCT to present as, or transform quickly into, a hemodynamically unstable rhythm, regardless of the etiology. The mainstay of therapy in such patients is emergent DC cardioversion using 200 J to 360 J of biphasic shock. SVT-A or stable VT (refractory to antiarrhythmic drug therapy) may be treated initially with a lesser energy (50–100 J), which can be incrementally increased up to 360 J, if needed. Advanced cardiac life support algorithms should be initiated if a patient becomes pulseless or the VT degenerates into VF. Electrolyte correction, rapid ventricular pacing, and intravenous magnesium (2 g) are needed to treat torsade de pointes. Because most of sustained torsade are hemodynamically unstable, they require prompt defibrillation and discontinuation of offending drug and correction of electrolyte imbalance.

1. Hemodynamically stable WCT: As emphasized previously, hemodynamic stability does not rule out VT.
    a. Antiarrhythmic therapy:
        i. Adenosine and other AV nodal blocking drugs (digoxin, class II and IV antiarrhythmic drugs): For hemodynamically stable patients with WCT, if the history or ECG criteria suggests SVT-A, then

the use of intravenous adenosine provides a quick termination of the tachycardia. Adenosine can terminate AV node–dependent tachycardias, such as AVRT (Atrioventricular reenterant tachycardia), AVNRT (Atrioventricular nodal reenterant tachycardia), and atrial tachycardia, due to triggered activity, and unmasks other atrial arrhythmia by causing transient AV block. Additionally, it should be kept in mind that idiopathic VT originating from the right ventricular outflow tract (RVOT) and its variant may also terminate with adenosine. Of note, in patients with CAD, adenosine may induce myocardial ischemia by causing vasodilation and hypotension as well as by coronary artery "steal" syndrome during VT. Idiopathic fascicular VT responds to calcium channel blockers such as intravenous verapamil or diltiazem. The other word of caution is that AV nodal blockers are contraindicated in patients with WPW syndrome with atrial flutter and atrial fibrillation with a rapid ventricular response. Digoxin and verapamil enhance conduction down the accessory pathway, which can result in a higher ventricular rate, which can lead to VT/VF.

ii. Class I and class III antiarrhythmic drugs: Antiarrhythmic agents, such as procainamide or amiodarone, are reasonable choices for WCT, because they can treat both VT and SVT.[7] Amiodarone is supported as a first-line agent.[7] Amiodarone should be given 150 mg intravenous slowly over the period of 10 minutes followed by 1 mg/kg body weight. Procainamide (20 mg/min) is the treatment of choice for WCT with WPW syndrome; however, it is usually not expected to produce therapeutic blood levels for at least 40 to 60 minutes. Because it can also cause hypotension, amiodarone is a reasonable alternative. Furthermore, ibutilide also is shown to be very effective and safe in patients with preexcited AF.[8]

b. Catheter ablation:

i. SVT: Catheter ablation is the treatment of choice for all symptomatic SVTs and idiopathic VTs with success rates of approximately 90% to 95% and 80% to 85%, respectively. Patients with WPW syndrome who present with atrial fibrillation and rapid ventricular response are at a risk of sudden cardiac death due to potential risk for VT/VF. Catheter ablation

of the AP is recommended to eliminate the risk.

ii. VT: Patients with structural heart disease presenting with hemodynamically unstable or sustained VT require an implantable cardioverter defibrillator (ICD). Catheter ablation of monomorphic VT is usually performed in patients with idiopathic VT, and VT associated with structural heart disease with recurrent ICD shocks.[9] Catheter ablation has an acute success rate of 85%, but is lower in hemodynamically unstable rhythms induced during EP study. Prophylactic substrate-based catheter ablation in patients with a history of MI also has been studied and has shown to reduce the risk of ICD therapy.[10] The Ventricular Tachycardia Ablation in Coronary Heart Disease (VTACH) study randomized patients with stable VT, previous MI, and reduced LV ejection fraction of 50% or less.[11] A total of 110 patients were randomly allocated in a 1:1 ratio to receive catheter ablation and an ICD (ablation group) or ICD alone (control group). During a mean follow-up of 22.5 ± 9 months, the first recurrence of VT/VF was significantly longer in the ablation group than in the control group (median 18.6 months vs 5.9 months). At 2 years, estimates for survival free from VT/VF were 47% in the ablation group and 29% in the control group (hazard ratio 0.61; 95% confidence interval 0.37–0.99; $P = .045$). On further treatment analyses of this study, ablation markedly decreased VT/VF burden.[12]

SUMMARY

Careful history taking, quick clinical evaluation, and meticulous ECG evaluation is the cornerstone of accurate diagnosis and management of patients with WCT. Long-term history of palpitations in patients with a structurally normal heart usually suggests SVT-A or idiopathic VT, and careful use of ECG criteria helps in quick and effective management of these patients. Vagal maneuver or the use of adenosine is helpful in terminating these arrhythmias. In patients with history of MI or cardiomyopathy, a WCT most likely represents VT and can be confirmed by different VT algorithms with clinically acceptable accuracy. As a general rule, when in doubt, treat the WCT as VT, especially in patients with structural heart disease. Common ECG criteria for differentiating VT from

SVT-A have reasonable accuracy. Hemodynamically unstable VT requires urgent DC cardioversion and initiation of advanced life-support system protocol. Hemodynamically stable WCT due to VT can be treated with intravenous amiodarone. Preexcited tachycardias can be treated with procainamide, or preferably amiodarone because of less risk of hypotension. Catheter ablation of SVT-A, preexcited atrial fibrillation, and VT may be curative. The success of ablation in patients with VT depends on the substrate and site of origin of the focus or circuit.

REFERENCES

1. Surawicz B, Childers R, Deal BJ, et al. AHA/ACCF/HRS recommendations for the standardization and interpretation of the electrocardiogram: part III: intraventricular conduction disturbances: a scientific statement from the American Heart Association Electrocardiography and Arrhythmias Committee, Council on Clinical Cardiology; the American College of Cardiology Foundation; and the Heart Rhythm Society. Endorsed by the International Society for Computerized Electrocardiology. J Am Coll Cardiol 2009;53:976–81.
2. Miller JM, Das MK, Yadav AV, et al. Value of the 12-lead ECG in wide QRS tachycardia. Cardiol Clin 2006;24:439–51,. ix–x.
3. Brugada P, Brugada J, Mont L, et al. A new approach to the differential diagnosis of a regular tachycardia with a wide QRS complex. Circulation 1991;83:1649–59.
4. Vereckei A, Duray G, Szenasi G, et al. Application of a new algorithm in the differential diagnosis of wide QRS complex tachycardia. Eur Heart J 2007;28:589–600.
5. Vereckei A, Duray G, Szenasi G, et al. New algorithm using only lead AVR for differential diagnosis of wide QRS complex tachycardia. Heart Rhythm 2008;5:89–98.
6. Datino T, Almendral J, Avila P, et al. Specificity of electrocardiographic criteria for the differential diagnosis of wide QRS complex tachycardia in patients with intraventricular conduction defect. Heart Rhythm 2013;10:1393–401.
7. Isenhour JL, Craig S, Gibbs M, et al. Wide-complex tachycardia: continued evaluation of diagnostic criteria. Acad Emerg Med 2000;7:769–73.
8. Glatter KA, Dorostkar PC, Yang Y, et al. Electrophysiological effects of ibutilide in patients with accessory pathways. Circulation 2001;104:1933–9.
9. Aliot EM, Stevenson WG, Almendral-Garrote JM, et al, European Heart Rhythm Association, Registered Branch of the European Society of Cardiology, Heart Rhythm Society, American College of Cardiology, American Heart Association. EHRA/HRS expert consensus on catheter ablation of ventricular arrhythmias: developed in a partnership with the European Heart Rhythm Association (EHRA), a registered branch of the European Society of Cardiology (ESC), and the Heart Rhythm Society (HRS); in collaboration with the American College Of Cardiology (ACC) and the American Heart Association (AHA). Heart Rhythm 2009;6:886–933.
10. Reddy VY, Reynolds MR, Neuzil P, et al. Prophylactic catheter ablation for the prevention of defibrillator therapy. N Engl J Med 2007;357:2657–65.
11. Kuck KH, Schaumann A, Eckardt L, et al, VTACH Study Group. Catheter ablation of stable ventricular tachycardia before defibrillator implantation in patients with coronary heart disease (VTACH): a multicentre randomised controlled trial. Lancet 2010;375:31–40.
12. Delacretaz E, Brenner R, Schaumann A, et al, VTACH Study Group. Catheter ablation of stable ventricular tachycardia before defibrillator implantation in patients with coronary heart disease (VTACH): an on-treatment analysis. J Cardiovasc Electrophysiol 2013;24:525–9.

Ventricular Tachycardia in Coronary Artery Disease

Haris M. Haqqani, MBBS(Hons), PhD[a],*, David J. Callans, MD[b]

KEYWORDS

- Ventricular tachycardia • Electrocardiograph • Myocardial infarction • Reentry • Mapping
- Catheter ablation

KEY POINTS

- The mechanism of ventricular tachycardia (VT) in the setting of previous myocardial infarction is reentrant excitation within the infarct scar.
- The electrocardiograph (ECG) during VT shows a wide QRS tachycardia. The diagnosis is established by excluding aberrant supraventricular and preexcited tachycardias.
- The QRS complex in postinfarct VT is produced when the reentrant excitation wavefront exits the scar border and activates normal ventricular myocardium.
- The ECG is a vital tool in the initial assessment of both the underlying substrate as well as the exit site of scar-related VT.
- The surface ECG is necessary in pace mapping and entrainment mapping during localization and ablation of postinfarct VT.

PATHOPHYSIOLOGY OF SCAR-RELATED VENTRICULAR TACHYCARDIA

Multiple human mapping studies have confirmed that postinfarct monomorphic ventricular tachycardia (VT) is caused by scar-related reentry.[1–4] The anatomic substrate for VT consists of surviving, poorly coupled myocyte bundles within the dense healed infarct scar. Often, these scars are large and confluent with associated dyskinesis or frank aneurysm formation. Unidirectional conduction block and slow conduction through these bundles facilitate the development of macroreentrant VT circuits.[5] The activation wavefront through these regions during VT is constrained by both dense scar and functional barriers to form the protected diastolic isthmus, during which no electrical activity is recorded on the surface electrocardiograph (ECG). In sinus rhythm, such bundles can be defined by scar heterogeneity on magnetic resonance imaging, electroanatomic voltage mapping, or electrogram analysis.[6–8]

The QRS complex on the surface ECG is recorded when the wavefront exits the dense scar and activates the remaining ventricular myocardium. The vector, duration, and sequence of ventricular depolarization determine the VT morphology on the surface ECG, and these are in turn determined by the size, location, and electrophysiologic characteristics of the infarct substrate.[9] Additional factors such as antiarrhythmic drugs, ECG electrode positioning, surgical scars, and geometric variations in the normal cardiothoracic anatomic relationship can affect the VT morphology.[10] Polymorphic VT is seen predominantly in the acutely ischemic heart and is often caused by Purkinje cell irritability related to diastolic calcium overload, causing triggered activity.

The authors have nothing to disclose.

[a] Department of Cardiology, The Prince Charles Hospital, School of Medicine, University of Queensland, 627 Rode Road, Chermside, Brisbane 4032, Australia; [b] Cardiovascular Division, Hospital of the University of Pennsylvania, University of Pennsylvania, 3400 Spruce Street, Philadelphia, PA 19104, USA
* Corresponding author.
E-mail address: h.haqqani@uq.edu.au

Card Electrophysiol Clin 6 (2014) 525–534
http://dx.doi.org/10.1016/j.ccep.2014.05.003
1877-9182/14/$ – see front matter © 2014 Elsevier Inc. All rights reserved.

cardiacEP.theclinics.com

GENERAL PRINCIPLES SURROUNDING THE ECG CHARACTERISTICS OF VT

- VT presents on the surface ECG as a wide complex tachycardia (WCT) with ventriculoatrial (VA) dissociation or QRS morphology features of a ventricular origin (see later discussion). If the sinus rhythm ECG shows a wide QRS complex, a narrower QRS during tachycardia is diagnostic of VT.
- Left ventricular (LV) free wall sites of origin give rise to right bundle branch block (RBBB) configurations (net positive QRS complex in V1).
- Left bundle branch block (LBBB) configurations (negative QRS complex in V1) are seen with septal and right ventricular (RV) sites of origin.
- Septal sites of VT origin give rise to narrower QRS complexes as a result of simultaneous rather than sequential LV and RV activation.
- The QRS axis varies most closely with the craniocaudal direction of net ventricular activation (eg, left bundle left superior axis VT exiting from basal septal side of an inferior infarct scar).
- Positive QRS concordance is seen with basal VT origins activating the ventricles toward the anteroapical region, in the direction of the precordial ECG electrodes. This process may also be seen with preexcited tachycardia with antegrade conduction over a bypass tract that inserts into the basal annular region of the ventricle.
- Negative QRS concordance is seen with apical VT sites of origin, in which the net activation vector proceeds away from the precordial leads.

ECG CHARACTERISTICS OF VT IN CORONARY ARTERY DISEASE

An initial analysis of the sinus rhythm ECG may help in ECG interpretation during VT.

- The absence of pathologic Q waves during sinus rhythm is unusual in patients with postinfarct VT because of the presence of large, often aneurismal, scars. However, on many occasions, Q waves are better appreciated during VT than during sinus rhythm.
- Anteroseptal Q waves or a poor precordial R wave progression suggest previous anterior or septal infarction. Similarly, inferior or lateral Q waves suggest an inferolateral infarct scar.
- Baseline bundle branch blocks in patients with coronary artery disease (CAD) are usually RBBB. The presence of LBBB is unusual after infarct and should raise suspicion of a

nonischemic dilated cardiomyopathy (NICM). Such patients may have coexisting CAD, but their VT substrate and electrophysiologic characteristics are typical for NICM.[11]
- Atrial, RV, or biventricular pacing may also be seen, given that many of these patients have implantable cardioverter-defibrillators (ICDs).

In the setting of previous infarction, the RV is rarely involved in VT circuits. Thus the following rules apply:

- RBBB configuration VTs exit the infarct scar on the LV free wall.[9]
- LBBB configuration implies a VT exit on or adjacent to the septum.[9]

Further interpretation of VT QRS morphology is assisted by knowledge of the infarct location. Because of the typically smaller scar mass, ECG localization of VT exit site is more accurate with previous inferior infarction.

Previous Inferior Infarction

- Most VTs in these patients have a basal exit and consequent preserved precordial R waves. However, more extensive infarction can result in apical exits.
- RBBB morphology VT typically exits from the basal lateral aspect of the inferior scar, usually with right superior axis. More superior exits along the lateral wall lead to an increasingly more inferior frontal plane axis (**Fig. 1**).
- LBBB morphology VT (especially with a left superior axis) in this context characteristically exits on the inferobasal septum (see **Fig. 1**).
- Some VTs having these configurations in patients with inferior infarct have the mitral annulus as 1 boundary of their diastolic corridor (so-called mitral isthmus VTs) and may exit this slow zone on either the septal or the lateral aspect of the annulus (see **Fig. 1**).[12]

Previous Anterior Infarction

- LBBB morphology VTs with left superior axis usually exit from the apical septum (**Fig. 2**). However, large anteroseptal infarcts may result in negative precordial concordance with these VTs, with additional Q waves in I and aVL.
- RBBB morphology VTs with right or left superior axis are the most difficult to localize and can arise from multiple regions around the apex. More posterolateral exits distinguish themselves with a greater R wave in aVR than aVL.
- LBBB VT with right inferior axis generally exits from the superior midseptal aspect of the

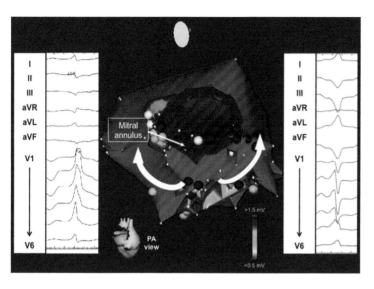

Fig. 1. Posteroanterior (PA) view of an electroanatomic voltage map depicting an inferior myocardial infarct scar underneath the mitral annulus. Two VTs were induced in this patient, 1 of right bundle, left superior axis morphology (*left*) and the other of left bundle, left superior axis morphology (*right*). These are examples of paired mitral isthmus VTs.

anterior scar, although it can also exit just off the septum (see **Fig. 2**).

- RBBB VT with right inferior axis can exit from the superolateral regions of the scar but also superiorly on the septum. The QS ratio in aVR and aVL may help distinguish these entities.
- Negative QS complexes in V4-V6 reflect apical origins, but the ECG alone cannot distinguish apicoseptal and apical free-wall exits (**Fig. 3**).

Papillary Muscle Infarction

- Papillary muscle involvement in an infarct scar is more common with inferior infarction and can result in reentrant VT circuit formation.[13]
- These infarctions are generally of RBBB morphology with a right or left superior axis with posteromedial papillary muscle origin and a right inferior axis with anterolateral papillary muscle exit.
- The mechanism of VT that arises from the papillary muscle may be focal, even in the presence of myocardial infarction that involves the papillary muscle (**Fig. 4**).

Epicardial VT

- Epicardial VT exits are uncommon in postinfarct VT, because of the subendocardial nature of the underlying substrate (**Fig. 5**).
- Interval criteria reflect the remoteness of an epicardial exit from the endocardial His-Purkinje network and include pseudo-δ wave of greater than 34 milliseconds, intrinsicoid deflection of greater than 85 milliseconds in V2 and shortest precordial RS duration of

greater than 121 milliseconds, but these have not been specifically validated in an ischemic cardiomyopathy context.[14] Morphology criteria cannot be applied in the presence of previous infarction.

Bundle Branch Reentry VT

- More commonly seen in NICM, bundle branch reentry VT should be considered a possibility in any rapid LBBB morphology VT, even in patients with ischemic cardiomyopathy.

The algorithms described by Miller and colleagues and Segal and colleagues[15] both apply these principles to VT localization, although Segal and colleagues' algorithm was validated independent of knowledge regarding the infarct location.

DIFFERENTIAL DIAGNOSIS

Patients with WCT may have any of the following diagnostic possibilities:

1. VT
2. Supraventricular tachycardia (SVT) with fixed or rate-related (aberrant) bundle branch block
3. Preexcited tachycardias
4. Paced tachycardias
5. Artifact

The last 2 can usually be rapidly excluded in the absence of a pacemaker or an ECG recording problem. Preexcited tachycardias are rare and unlikely without baseline preexcitation. In most cases, the practical distinction that needs to be made is between VT and aberrantly conducted SVT. Special consideration should be given to

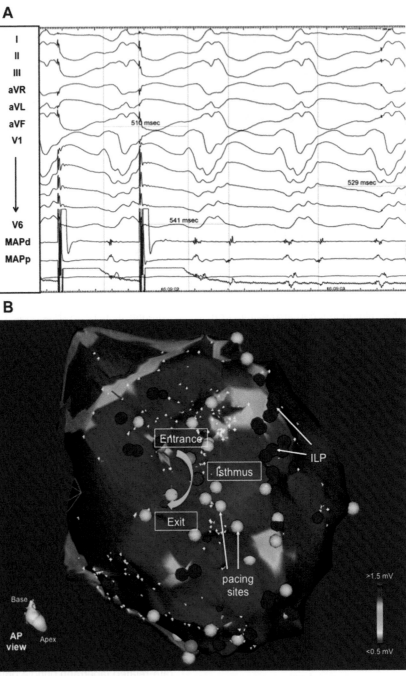

Fig. 2. On the right side of (*A*), the surface VT morphology of a patient with previous anteroseptal myocardial infarction is shown, depicting a left bundle inferior axis configuration with cycle length 529 milliseconds (msec). Intracardiac recordings from an ablation catheter placed on the septal scar are shown with a middiastolic potential seen at the end of the QRS. On the left side of (*A*), overdrive pacing entrains the tachycardia at 510 milliseconds with a long stimulus-QRS interval. The surface ECG shows concealed fusion with a notch-perfect QRS morphology during pacing compared with spontaneous VT. The postpacing interval of 541 milliseconds approximates the VT cycle length, proving this site to be in the central diastolic isthmus of this VT. (*B*) The various VT circuit components characterized by entrainment shown on the electroanatomic voltage map, with confluent anteroseptal scar shown in red. Ablation in the diastolic corridor resulted in early VT termination. AP, anteroposterior; ILP, isolated late potential.

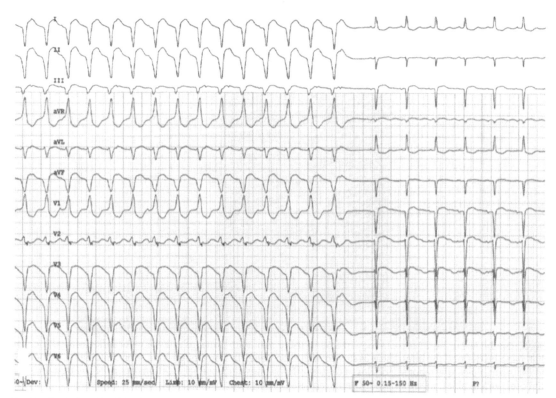

Fig. 3. The right side of this figure shows the sinus rhythm ECG characteristics of a 72-year-old man with ischemic cardiomyopathy and previous anterior and inferior infarcts. During VT, RBBB morphology with northwest axis, VA dissociation, and extensive inferoapicoseptal Q waves were seen. This VT was ablated in the apicolateral LV free wall.

A

B

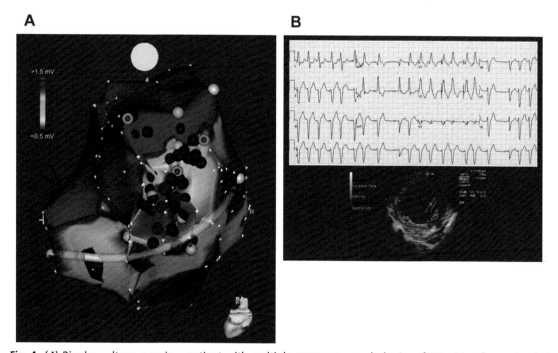

Fig. 4. (*A*) Bipolar voltage map in a patient with multiple reentrant morphologies of VT arising from a healed inferior infarction. (*B*) A relatively slow right bundle superior tachycardia with start/stop behavior (suggesting a nonreentrant mechanism); using intracardiac echocardiography, this VT was localized to the posterior medial papillary muscle, which was not involved in the field of infarction.

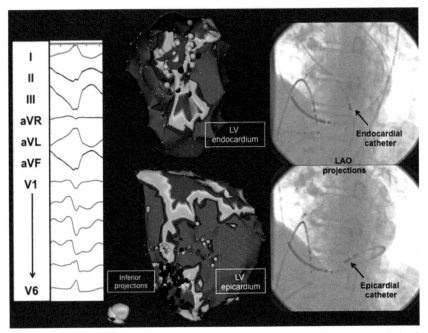

Fig. 5. On the *left* is the VT morphology of a 69-year-old man with previous inferior myocardial infarct. Endocardial mapping defined the infarct scar as shown in the *top panel*, but only outer loop sites could be found here on entrainment. Epicardial mapping disclosed central isthmus sites at epicardial locations opposite the best endocardial sites, where ablation terminated VT and rendered it noninducible. LAO, left anterior oblique.

excluding atrial flutter with 1:1 conduction. When the WCT rate is near 300 bpm, this diagnosis is readily apparent (**Fig. 6**). However, the atrial flutter cycle length may be slowed by atrial scar, atrial dilatation, or conduction-slowing agents such as flecainide, and this may facilitate 1:1 conduction, with resulting ventricular rates as slow as 200 bpm. In the presence of a previous infarct

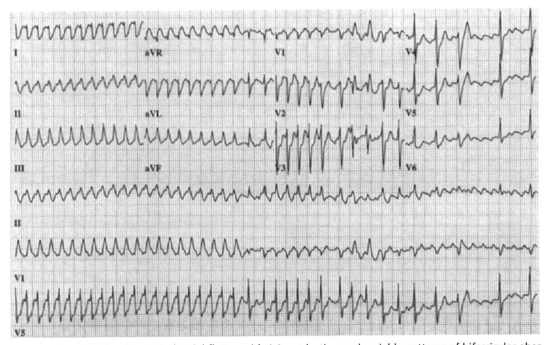

Fig. 6. Surface ECG showing typical atrial flutter with 1:1 conduction and variable patterns of bifascicular aberrance, resolving to narrow complex conduction when AV nodal conduction slows.

scar, there is a greater than 95% probability of VT being the correct diagnosis. The following ECG features are essentially diagnostic of VT:

1. VA dissociation
2. Negative precordial concordance reflecting a VT origin from the anteroapical LV (positive concordance may be seen with preexcited tachycardias)
3. Capture beats and fusion beats
4. Narrower QRS during VT than during sinus rhythm
5. Absence of RS complexes in all precordial leads[16]
6. RS interval duration greater than 100 milliseconds in any precordial lead[16]
7. An initial R in lead aVR[17]

In the absence of these features, the diagnosis of aberrant SVT may be entertained if specific morphology criteria for typical LBBB and RBBB configurations are satisfied. VT is highly likely with atypical LBBB and RBBB patterns (eg, qR or Rs RBBB morphology) in V1 (**Fig. 7**).

MANAGEMENT

Acute management of the patient presenting with postinfarct VT is centered on the prompt termination of tachycardia. Tachycardia should be terminated with electrical cardioversion if there is any suggestion of hemodynamic compromise. Pharmacologic cardioversion with intravenous procainamide, sotalol, or amiodarone may be considered for stable patients. A 12-lead ECG should be recorded whenever possible before and after cardioversion.

Most patients with monomorphic VT in this context present many years or even decades after their index myocardial infarction. After tachycardia termination, an extensive cardiac evaluation is required, including determination of scar size, location, and LV ejection fraction, as well as excluding significant CAD requiring revascularization. However, acute coronary syndromes and myocardial infarction do not typically present with monomorphic VT. Many patients are diagnosed with advanced ischemic cardiomyopathy during this process and require medical management of heart failure.

After initial evaluation, in the absence of significant competing comorbidity, most patients are offered an ICD. Contrary to popular belief, this procedure is not to treat the presenting VT morphology but rather to mitigate against the high sudden death risk that these patients have during follow-up. ICDs are not a treatment of VT, and ICD shocks are painful and associated with increased morbidity and mortality. After ICD insertion, to treat and prevent recurrences of the clinical VT, patients are offered pharmacologic therapy with antiarrhythmic drugs (commonly amiodarone), catheter ablation, or both.

ELECTROPHYSIOLOGY STUDY AND CATHETER ABLATION

The primary indication for electrophysiology study (EPS) and catheter ablation of postinfarct VT remains frequent ICD shocks, although some

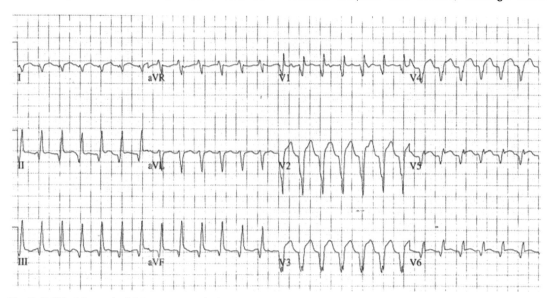

Fig. 7. WCT with atypical QR RBBB morphology and VA dissociation. This VT shows deep, broad anteroseptal Q waves and right inferior axis and was ablated at the superior lateral border of this patient's anterior LV endocardial scar.

patients are ablated before ICD insertion. At EPS, VT is induced by programmed stimulation, and the diagnosis confirmed by recording the HV interval during tachycardia (shorter than in sinus rhythm and usually negative) or by pacing maneuvers to confirm VA dissociation. Typically, several morphologies are inducible in patients with ischemic cardiomyopathy. If sustained and hemodynamically tolerated, the critical constrained diastolic isthmus of the VT circuit can be mapped with entrainment techniques, in which the responses to overdrive pacing are used to define the circuit components within the scar. The analysis of the surface 12-lead ECG is critical in entrainment mapping, because overdrive pacing within the constrained diastolic isthmus during VT results in a perfectly identical QRS match to the VT morphology. This process is known as entrainment with concealed fusion. Application of radiofrequency (RF) energy at critical isthmus sites may terminate the tachycardia, and further linear ablation is performed to completely abolish VT inducibility.[3]

VT that is not sustained or tolerated cannot be mapped by entrainment, and this represents the most frequent scenario in postinfarct VT ablation.[18] Substrate mapping techniques have been developed to deal with this problem.[19] The essential principle behind them is to define the footprints of VT circuit sites in sinus rhythm and the surface 12-lead ECG is again essential for this. The key components of this process are as follows:

- Definition of the scar extent and geometry using electrogram sampling and recording with a three-dimensional electroanatomic recording system. Scar regions are defined by bipolar electrogram voltage less than 1.5 mV, with dense infarct core less than 0.5 mV.[19] Within the dense core, areas of relatively preserved voltage compared with surrounding regions are defined, because they may form conduction channels during VT.[7]
- Sites of slow conduction are identified within the scar by pacing and recording a long duration from the pacing stimulus to the QRS onset.
- Sites of good match between the paced QRS morphology and the VT morphology are identified, particularly those with slow conduction.
- Sites where pacing produces multiple QRS morphologies or induces VT after cessation of pacing.
- Sites where electrograms contain isolated late potentials after the QRS complex, representing delayed activation into surviving myocyte bundles within dense scar.[8,20]

Once these targets have been defined, extensive RF ablation lesions are delivered to these sites in an effort to homogenize the scar and prevent VT inducibility.

OUTCOMES OF CATHETER ABLATION

For tolerated VTs, medium-term success rates for entrainment mapping and ablation are reasonable overall, ranging from 67% to 86% of patients free of VT recurrence over 2-year to 3-year follow-up.[21–23] The results of substrate ablation are comparable, with 2 recent randomized trials[24,25] examining these techniques with the use of modern mapping systems and irrigated ablation catheters. These trials showed a 13% to 21% absolute risk reduction in VT and appropriate ICD therapies over a mean follow-up of around 2 years. When patients present with further VT after ablation, the development of new VT morphologies not seen or targeted at the initial procedure represents the biggest cause for recurrence. Yokokawa and colleagues[26] found that nearly 80% of the 34% of patients who had recurrence over a 35-month follow-up after ablation had developed a new VT. Many of these patients have very advanced structural heart disease, and despite good arrhythmia control with catheter ablation, 12% to 30% succumb to progressive cardiac failure during medium-term follow-up.[21,22]

COMPLICATIONS

The advanced nature of the cardiac disease as well as the commonly attendant comorbidities in these patients makes ablation a potentially hazardous procedure. Possible complications include death, myocardial infarction, stroke, perforation and tamponade, cardiogenic shock, valve trauma, heart block, coronary artery injury, and access site misadventures. Major complications occur in around 6% of patients.[27] These risks are higher (up to 14%) if epicardial mapping and ablation are required.[28] To reduce these risks, meticulous preprocedural planning is vital, as is the vigilant management of anticoagulation and hemodynamic balance during the case.

SUMMARY

The diagnosis, definition, localization, and management of postinfarct VT in the patient with CAD depends critically on the surface 12-lead ECG. A systematic analysis of both the sinus rhythm and tachycardia ECGs provides much information that is critical for further decision making. The 12-lead ECG is used to exclude the other differential diagnostic possibilities, outline the substrate for postinfarct VT, and define the likely region of VT exit from the scar border, as well as allow for detailed intracardiac analysis using entrainment and pace mapping during catheter ablation procedures.

REFERENCES

1. de Bakker JM, van Capelle FJ, Janse MJ, et al. Reentry as a cause of ventricular tachycardia in patients with chronic ischemic heart disease: electrophysiologic and anatomic correlation. Circulation 1988;77:589–606.

2. Fenoglio JJ, Pham TD, Harken AH, et al. Recurrent sustained ventricular tachycardia: structure and ultrastructure of subendocardial regions in which tachycardia originates. Circulation 1983;68:518–33.

3. Stevenson WG, Khan H, Sager P, et al. Identification of reentry circuit sites during catheter mapping and radiofrequency ablation of ventricular tachycardia late after myocardial infarction. Circulation 1993;88:1647–70.

4. de Chillou C, Lacroix D, Klug D, et al. Isthmus characteristics of reentrant ventricular tachycardia after myocardial infarction. Circulation 2002;105:726–31.

5. de Bakker JM, van Capelle FJ, Janse MJ, et al. Slow conduction in the infarcted human heart. 'Zigzag' course of activation. Circulation 1993;88:915–26.

6. Perez-David E, Arenal A, Rubio-Guivernau JL, et al. Noninvasive identification of ventricular tachycardia-related conducting channels using contrast-enhanced magnetic resonance imaging in patients with chronic myocardial infarction: comparison of signal intensity scar mapping and endocardial voltage mapping. J Am Coll Cardiol 2011;57:184–94.

7. Arenal A, del Castillo S, Gonzalez-Torrecilla E, et al. Tachycardia-related channel in the scar tissue in patients with sustained monomorphic ventricular tachycardias: influence of the voltage scar definition. Circulation 2004;110:2568–74.

8. Bogun F, Good E, Reich S, et al. Isolated potentials during sinus rhythm and pace-mapping within scars as guides for ablation of post-infarction ventricular tachycardia. J Am Coll Cardiol 2006;47:2013–9.

9. Miller JM, Marchlinski FE, Buxton AE, et al. Relationship between the 12-lead electrocardiogram during ventricular tachycardia and endocardial site of origin in patients with coronary artery disease. Circulation 1988;77:759–66.

10. Osswald S, Wilber DJ, Lin JL, et al. Mechanisms underlying different surface ECG morphologies of recurrent monomorphic ventricular tachycardia and their modification by procainamide. J Cardiovasc Electrophysiol 1997;8:11–23.

11. Aldhoon B, Tzou WS, Riley MP, et al. Nonischemic cardiomyopathy substrate and ventricular tachycardia in the setting of coronary artery disease. Heart Rhythm 2013;10:1622–7.

12. Wilber DJ, Kopp DE, Glascock DN, et al. Catheter ablation of the mitral isthmus for ventricular tachycardia associated with inferior infarction. Circulation 1995;92:3481–9.

13. Bogun F, Desjardins B, Crawford T, et al. Post-infarction ventricular arrhythmias originating in papillary muscles. J Am Coll Cardiol 2008;51:1794–802.

14. Berruezo A, Mont L, Nava S, et al. Electrocardiographic recognition of the epicardial origin of ventricular tachycardias. Circulation 2004;109:1842–7.

15. Segal OR, Chow AW, Wong T, et al. A novel algorithm for determining endocardial VT exit site from 12-lead surface ECG characteristics in human, infarct-related ventricular tachycardia. J Cardiovasc Electrophysiol 2007;18:161–8.

16. Brugada P, Brugada J, Mont L, et al. A new approach to the differential diagnosis of a regular tachycardia with a wide QRS complex. Circulation 1991;83:1649–59.

17. Vereckei A, Duray G, Szenasi G, et al. New algorithm using only lead aVR for differential diagnosis of wide QRS complex tachycardia. Heart Rhythm 2008;5:89–98.

18. Stevenson WG, Wilber DJ, Natale A, et al. Irrigated radiofrequency catheter ablation guided by electroanatomic mapping for recurrent ventricular tachycardia after myocardial infarction: the multicenter thermocool ventricular tachycardia ablation trial. Circulation 2008;118:2773–82.

19. Marchlinski FE, Callans DJ, Gottlieb CD, et al. Linear ablation lesions for control of unmappable ventricular tachycardia in patients with ischemic and nonischemic cardiomyopathy. Circulation 2000;101:1288–96.

20. Arenal A, Glez-Torrecilla E, Ortiz M, et al. Ablation of electrograms with an isolated, delayed component as treatment of unmappable monomorphic ventricular tachycardias in patients with structural heart disease. J Am Coll Cardiol 2003;41:81–92.

21. Stevenson WG, Friedman PL, Kocovic D, et al. Radiofrequency catheter ablation of ventricular tachycardia after myocardial infarction. Circulation 1998;98:308–14.

22. Della Bella P, De Ponti R, Uriarte JA, et al. Catheter ablation and antiarrhythmic drugs for haemodynamically tolerated post-infarction ventricular tachycardia: long-term outcome in relation to acute electrophysiological findings. Eur Heart J 2002;23:414–24.

23. Rothman SA, Hsia HH, Cossu SF, et al. Radiofrequency catheter ablation of postinfarction ventricular tachycardia: long-term success and the significance of inducible nonclinical arrhythmias. Circulation 1997;96:3499–508.

24. Reddy VY, Reynolds MR, Neuzil P, et al. Prophylactic catheter ablation for the prevention of defibrillator therapy. N Engl J Med 2007;357:2657–65.

25. Kuck KH, Schaumann A, Eckardt L, et al. Catheter ablation of stable ventricular tachycardia before defibrillator implantation in patients with coronary heart disease (VTACH): a multicentre randomised controlled trial. Lancet 2010;375:31–40.

26. Yokokawa M, Desjardins B, Crawford T, et al. Reasons for recurrent ventricular tachycardia after catheter ablation of post-infarction ventricular tachycardia. J Am Coll Cardiol 2013;61:66–73.

27. Bohnen M, Stevenson WG, Tedrow UB, et al. Incidence and predictors of major complications from contemporary catheter ablation to treat cardiac arrhythmias. Heart Rhythm 2011;8:1661–6.

28. Sarkozy A, Tokuda M, Tedrow UB, et al. Epicardial ablation of ventricular tachycardia in ischemic heart disease. Circ Arrhythm Electrophysiol 2013; 6:1115–22.

Ventricular Tachycardia in Nonischemic Dilated Cardiomyopathy
Electrocardiographic and Intracardiac Electrogram Correlation

Karin K.M. Chia, MBBS, PhD, FRACP, FCSANZ[a],
Henry H. Hsia, MD, FHRS[b],*

KEYWORDS

- Nonischemic cardiomyopathy • Ventricular tachycardia • Catheter ablation
- Electroanatomic mapping • Epicardial

KEY POINTS

- The substrate for ventricular tachycardia (VT) in nonischemic cardiomyopathy (NICMP) is frequently basal scar that is epicardial and midmyocardial.
- VTs with an epicardial exit take longer to engage the His-Purkinje system, with greater initial slurring of the QRS and time to maximal deflection seen on electrocardiography.
- Anisotropic conduction through scar in NICMP results in late potentials and local abnormal ventricular activity that can be targeted for ablation.
- Unipolar electrograms with a wider field of view are useful for identifying epicardial and intramural substrate endocardially.

INTRODUCTION

Ventricular tachycardia (VT) is part of the clinical sequelae of nonischemic cardiomyopathy (NICMP) with dysfunction of the left ventricle (LV) in the absence of occlusive coronary artery disease or congenital heart disease. The prevalence of NICMP, also commonly referred to as idiopathic cardiomyopathy and dilated cardiomyopathy, is difficult to estimate, because of the heterogeneity in definitions and diagnostic criteria, selection bias, and geographic variation. In addition, there are clear differences in population characteristics between community-based studies versus analyses of populations from referral centers.[1] The estimated prevalence of NICMP is 36 to 40/100,000.[2] Its incidence discovered at autopsy is estimated to be 4.5 cases per 100,000 population per year, whereas the clinical incidence is 2.45 cases per 100,000 population per year.[3]

There is an estimated annual mortality of 7%, despite optimal medical therapy in patients with NICMP.[4] Sudden unexplained death accounts for 50%, and although primary bradyarrhythmias and asystole are contributory, VT/ventricular fibrillation accounts for many of these sudden cardiac deaths.[5] Consistent with this finding, a meta-analysis of implantable cardioverter-defibrillator

The authors have nothing to disclose.
[a] Department of Cardiology, James Mayne Building Level 3, Royal Brisbane and Women's Hospital-(University of Queensland), Herston, Queensland 4029, Australia; [b] Electrophysiology Service, VA-San Francisco, University of California, San Francisco, Building 203, Room 2A-52A, 4150 Clement Street, San Francisco, CA 94121, USA
* Corresponding author.
E-mail address: Henry.hsia@ucsf.edu

(ICD) trials in patients with NICMP showed a 26% mortality reduction with ICD therapy,[6] which indicates that a significant proportion of deaths in patients with NICMP is tachyarrhythmia related. Accordingly, there has been an increase in the proportion of patients with NICMP and VT compared with ischemic cardiomyopathy (ICMP) in recent years, which may reflect: (1) more aggressive reperfusion strategies for acute myocardial infarction, reducing the number of patients with ICMP who need VT ablation, (2) more patients with NICMP with VT surviving to require ablation as a result of advanced medical therapy, and (3) greater use of ICDs or changes in referral patterns.[7]

The acute success of catheter ablation in NICMP has varied from 21% to 79% and is generally lower than for ICMP.[8–11] Unlike ICMP, endocardial mapping and ablation alone are often insufficient to achieve noninducibility in NICMP, because circuits are frequently intramural or epicardial.[12,13] This situation partially accounts for the lower success rates of initial series of VT ablation in NICMP, before the more routine access of the epicardial space.

Recognizing the electrocardiographic (ECG) characteristics that localize the exit or focus of the VT and intracardiac electrogram (EGM) features that delineate the substrate of the arrhythmia that can be targeted for ablation is essential to the development of a successful ablation strategy. These ECG and EGM characteristics are also useful to predict success and durability of the procedure, which influences the management approach for the patient's arrhythmia. This article focuses on these ECG and EGM characteristics of VT in NICMP.

PATHOLOGY

The most common arrhythmia mechanisms in patients with NICMP include (1) scar-based reentry, (2) abnormal automaticity, and (3) Purkinje system–related arrhythmias.[9,14] Autopsy series of explanted hearts in patients with NICMP have shown interstitial and replacement fibrosis. A necropsy study of 152 patients with idiopathic dilated cardiomyopathy reported a high incidence of myocardial fibrosis (57%), despite a relative paucity of visible scar (14%). The ventricular myocardium is histologically characterized by variable degrees of myocyte hypertrophy and atrophy, with replacement by fibrosis, leading to multiple patchy areas of fibrosis and myofiber disarray.[15–18] Unlike in ICMP, these changes are not limited to the endocardium but also have a predilection to the midmyocardial and epicardial layers of the basilar and perivalvular regions of the LV.[19,20] In addition to the presence of fibrosis and scar, the electric conduction properties of the myocardium are also altered. The altered cellular processes and abnormal membrane potentials associated with myocyte hypertrophy may be arrhythmogenic. Altered automaticity from delayed after-depolarizations or early after-depolarizations resulting in focal VT has been reported in patients and animal models of dilated cardiomyopathy.[21–23]

Similar to ICMP, the most common mechanism for monomorphic VT in NICMP is reentry.[10,14] The electrophysiologic mapping and histologic examination of hearts from transplant recipients with dilated cardiomyopathy have shown areas of fibrosis that form the substrate for VT by creating conduction barriers with fractionated EGMs and heterogeneous patterns of epicardial and endocardial activations with marked conduction disturbances that are the nidus for reentry.[22,24] The amount of fibrosis and myofiber disarray correlated with higher levels of nonuniform anisotropy and generation of reentrant wave fronts. The patients with greater degrees of electric abnormality were noted to have a greater burden of nonsustained ventricular arrhythmia on Holter monitoring.[24]

The conduction slowing in NICMP may occur within the specialized His-Purkinje system. Conduction delay in the His-Purkinje system can provide the requisite substrate for monomorphic ventricular arrhythmias from bundle branch reentry (BBR) or fascicular reentry; the average HV interval in patients with BBR VT is approximately 80 milliseconds.[25] BBR has been reported as the arrhythmia mechanism in 30% to 40% of patients with NICMP presenting with monomorphic VT.[19,26] The macro reentrant circuit of BBR typically initiates with a premature ventricular beat, which conducts slowly up the left bundle with retrograde block in the right bundle. The delay in left bundle conduction provides sufficient time for recovery of the right bundle and hence, subsequent antegrade conduction down the right bundle followed by transeptal intramyocardial conduction (Fig. 1). Less commonly, the reentrant circuit can be depolarized in the opposite direction, generating a QRS morphology with a right bundle branch block (RBBB) configuration. The same mechanism with difference in conduction velocity and refractory periods between the left fascicles can result in an interfascicular VT.[27]

ECG CHARACTERISTICS

For VT resulting from myocardial reentry in patients with NICMP, there are ECG characteristics

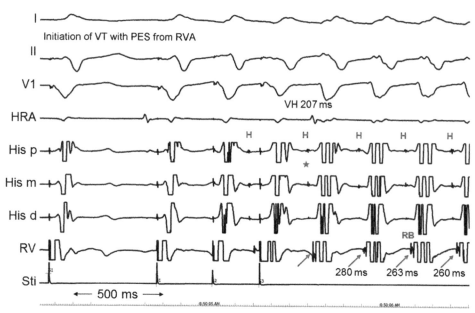

Fig. 1. BBR VT in a patient with nonischemic dilated cardiomyopathy. VT is induced by programmed stimulation (PES) from the right ventricular apex (RVA). Initiation of VT is associated with a sudden prolongation of VH interval to 207 milliseconds (*star*). BBR VT has a typical left bundle branch block pattern, suggesting anterograde conduction down the right bundle (RB). His (H) activation during VT precedes RB activation during tachycardia. Spontaneous cycle length oscillation is observed, with changes in H-H intervals preceding changes in V-V intervals. HRA, high right atrium. (*Adapted from* Hsia HH, Marchlinski FE. Electrophysiology studies in patients with dilated cardiomyopathies. Card Electrophysiol Rev 2002;6(4):478; with permission.)

that are useful in defining the location and the substrate, both during sinus rhythm (SR) and during arrhythmia.

ECG in SR

Electroanatomic mapping and magnetic resonance imaging (MRI) studies have found that patients with VT and NICMP affecting the LV typically have basal lateral scar (**Fig. 2**).[9,10,19,28,29] A recent study by Tzou and colleagues[30] developed criteria in the SR 12-lead ECG to predict the presence of such scar as defined by bipolar low voltage on electroanatomic mapping. Comparing the 12-lead SR ECG of patients with NICMP, VT and basal lateral scar with that of patients with NICMP but no VT or scar, R wave in lead V1 of 0.15 mV or greater and S wave in lead V6 of 0.15 mV or greater predicted the presence of low-voltage areas at the basal lateral LV. This finding may be useful in predicting the presence of LV scar and the risk of VT in patients with NICMP.

Furthermore, ECG criteria have been developed to distinguish ischemic versus nonischemic scar (which frequently may not involve the endocardium) in the same anatomic distribution. In patients whose ECG is without bundle branch block or ventricular paced rhythms, there are features

that help characterize the anticipated substrate in patients with VT that can aid the development of an ablative strategy, such as the need for epicardial mapping.[31] Betensky and colleagues compared the ECGs of patients undergoing VT ablation with endocardial/epicardial basal inferolateral nonischemic scar with that of patients with inferior/inferolateral myocardial infarction. After multivariate analysis of various parameters, (1) lateral lead QRS fragmentation (as defined by complex notching with various multiphasic RSR patterns or ≥ 2 R' or the presence of numerous high-frequency deflections), (2) lack of inferior q waves and (3) lead V_6 S/R ratio were the only independent predictors of NICMP. An algorithm with a stepwise assessment of these 3 parameters was developed (**Fig. 3**); when tested in a prospective cohort, it was found to have a sensitivity of 93%, negative predictive value of 87%, specificity of 57% and positive predictive value of 72%.

ECG During Ventricular Arrhythmia

Careful analysis of the surface ECG during ventricular arrhythmia is also essential for mapping strategy and procedural planning. Berruezo and colleagues[32] described the QRS morphologic characteristics of epicardial versus endocardial origins of ventricular activation. Derived from 3

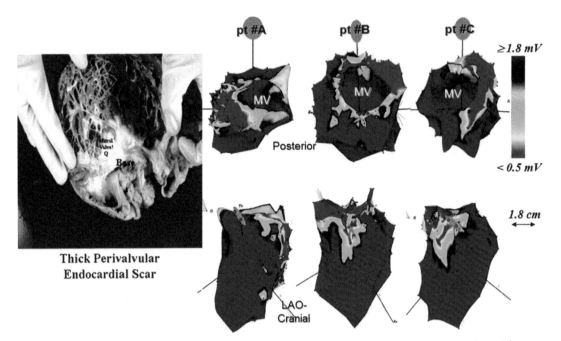

Fig. 2. Endocardial three-dimensional electroanatomic mapping in patients with NICMP presenting with mono-morphic VT. Purple areas represent normal endocardium (amplitude ≥1.8 mV) with dense scar depicted as red (amplitude <0.5 mV). The border zone (amplitude 0.5–1.8 mV) is defined as areas with the color gradient be-tween red and purple. The voltage maps typically show modest-sized low-voltage endocardial EGM abnormalities or scar, located near the ventricular base in the perivalvular region. (*Left*) A pathologic specimen that shows peri-valvular scarring at the ventricular base and corresponds to the observed low-voltage areas on the voltage maps. LAO, left anterior oblique; MV, mitral valve. (*Adapted from* Wang P, Hsia HH, Al-Ahmad A, et al, editors. Ventric-ular arrhythmias and sudden cardiac death: mechanism, ablation and defibrillation. New York: Wiley-Blackwell; 2008; with permission.)

groups of patients who were successfully ablated from the endocardium, epicardium, or unsuccess-fully from the endocardium, the parameters that favored an epicardial VT were (1) a pseudo-δ wave (the earliest ventricular activation to the earliest fast deflection in any precordial lead) of 34 milliseconds or greater; (2) an intrinsicoid deflection time (the interval measured from the earliest ventricular activation [to the peak of the R wave]) in lead V2 of 85 milliseconds or greater, the shortest RS complex duration (the interval measured from the earliest ventricular activation to the nadir of the first S wave in any precordial lead) of 121 milliseconds or greater, and a longer QRS duration (**Fig. 4**A). These parameters in the surface ECG reflect the slow myocardial propaga-tion time associated with epicardial activation, with a delayed endocardial access to the rapid conducting specialized Purkinje network, resulting in greater slurring and delay in the initial upstroke of the QRS.

This finding was further supported by a novel metric to measure the initial precordial QRS acti-vation: the maximal deflection index (MDI). MDI was described to predict an epicardial exit site for idiopathic VT, arising remotely from the sinus of Valsalva in patients with structurally normal hearts.[33] The MDI is defined by the shortest time to maximal deflection in the precordial leads, divided by the total QRS duration (see **Fig. 4**B). A delayed MDI of 0.55 or greater identified epicardial VT with a sensitivity of 100% and a specificity of 98.7% relative to all other sites of origin.

Furthermore, site-specific ECG features have recently been described that distinguish epicardial LV VT in patients without previous myocardial infarctions.[34] A q wave in lead I was more commonly seen in epicardial origin compared with the corresponding endocardial sites from basal superior, apical superior LV. A q wave in the inferior leads during VT with a superior axis identified epicardial basal inferior and apical infe-rior sites, whereas the absence of q wave in the inferior leads in a VT with an inferior axis sug-gested epicardial basal superior origin (**Fig. 5**). These criteria identified 16 of 19 spontaneous epicardial VTs, and the presence of a q wave in lead I and the absence of a q wave in the inferior leads were observed for almost all VTs arising from the epicardial basal superior LV.

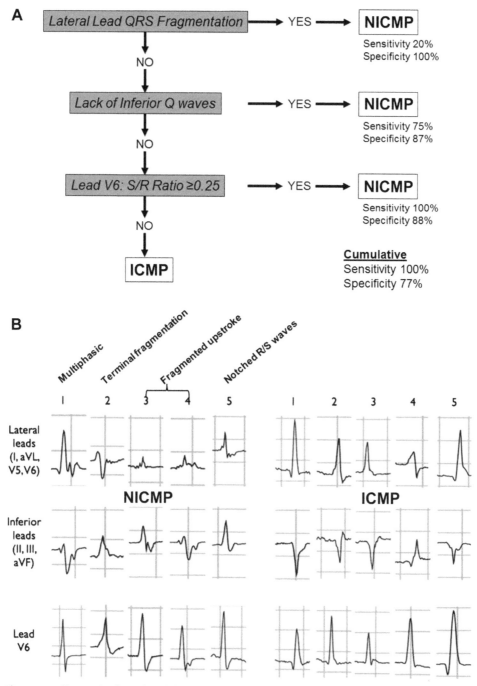

Fig. 3. Three-step diagnostic algorithm. (*A*) Stepwise assessment of lateral lead QRS fragmentation, lack of inferior q waves, and V6 S/R ratio for discriminating between ICMP and NICMP VT substrates. (*B*) Examples of ECGs in NICMP versus ICMP are represented. (*Left*) ECGs from 5 patients with NICMP showing variations of lateral lead QRS fragmentation, lack of inferior q waves, and V6 S/R ratios greater than 0.25. Various types of QRS fragmentation are described (1–5). (*Right*) ECGs from 5 patients with previous infarction showing inferior q waves, small V6 S/R ratios, and lack of lateral lead QRS fragmentation. (*Adapted from* Betensky BP, Deyell MW, Tzou WS, et al. Sinus rhythm electrocardiogram identification of basal lateral ischemic versus nonischemic substrate in patients with ventricular tachycardia. J Interv Card Electrophysiol 2012;35:311–21; with permission.)

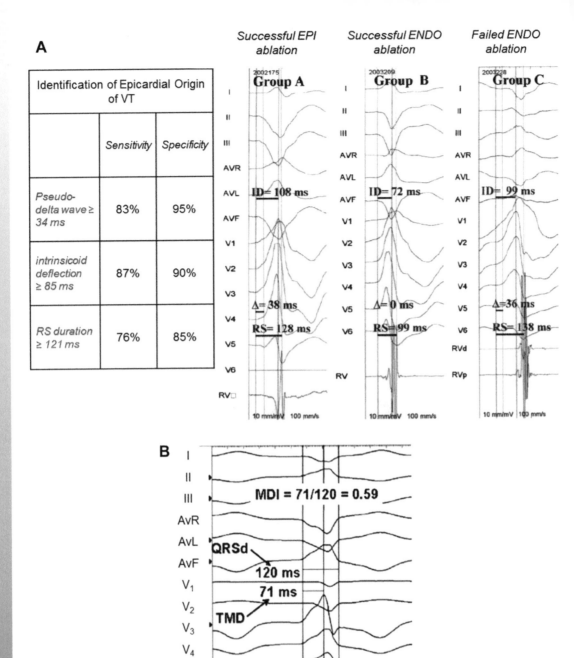

Fig. 4. Epicardial (EPI) versus endocardial (ENDO) VTs: QRS morphologic features. (*A*) Group A patients had a successful epicardial ablation, group B patients had VTs successfully ablated from the endocardium, and group C patients were unsuccessfully ablated from the endocardium. Overall, epicardial VTs (groups A and C) showed a significantly longer pseudo-δ wave (Δ), intrinsicoid deflection (ID), and RS complex duration (RS) compared with VT with endocardial origin (group B). The sensitivity and specificity of ECG parameters for identifying epicardial origin of VT were compared. (*B*) Time to maximum deflection (TMD) was measured from the onset of the QRS complex to the maximum deflection in each precordial lead; the maximum deflection was defined as the largest amplitude deflection either above or below the isoelectric line. The maximal deflection index (MDI) is defined by the shortest time to maximal deflection in the precordial leads, divided by the total QRS duration. (*Adapted from* [*A*] Berruezo A, Mont L, Nava S, et al. Electrocardiographic recognition of the epicardial origin of ventricular tachycardias. Circulation 2004;109:1842–7, with permission; and [*B*] Daniels DV, Lu YY, Morton JB, et al. Idiopathic epicardial LV tachycardia originating remote from the sinus of Valsalva: electrophysiological characteristics, catheter ablation, and identification from the 12-lead electrocardiogram. Circulation 2006;113:1659–66, with permission.)

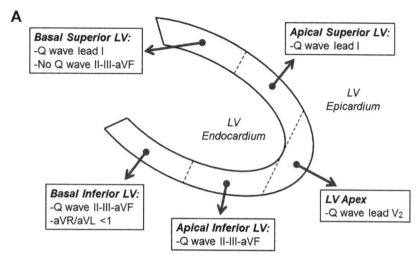

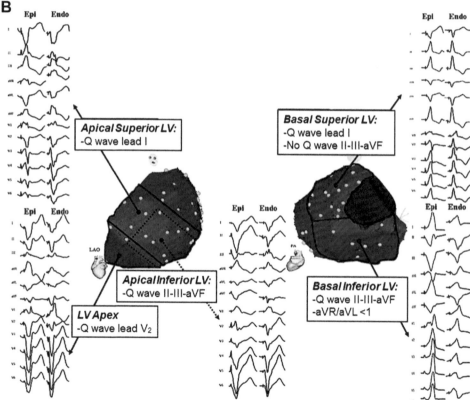

Fig. 5. Site-specific ECG features for identifying an epicardial origin. (*A*) The LV regions and their corresponding ECG patterns that suggest an epicardial origin are represented. (*B*) ECG morphologic characteristics between endocardial (Endo) and epicardial (Epi) activations at specific regions. (*Adapted from* Bazan V, Gerstenfeld EP, Garcia FC, et al. Site-specific twelve-lead ECG features to identify an epicardial origin for LV tachycardia in the absence of myocardial infarction. Heart Rhythm 2007;4:1403–10; with permission.)

ECG features to identify an epicardial exit for VTs arising from the right ventricle (RV) have also been described.[35] For VTs with an inferior exit, a q wave in lead II, III and aVF identified an epicardial exit, whereas a q wave in lead I and a QS in lead V2 identified an epicardial exit in anterior RV sites.

A more updated ECG criterion to identify epicardial VT in NICMP was proposed by Valles and colleagues.[36] These investigators identified 4 criteria: (1) q waves in inferior leads, (2) pseudo-δ wave 75 milliseconds or greater, (3) maximum deflection index 0.59 or greater, and (4) a q wave in lead I having 95% specificity or greater and 20% sensitivity or greater in identifying epicardial/endocardial origin for VT. In addition, a 4-step algorithm for identifying epicardial origin of ventricular arrhythmia from basal superior and lateral LV in the setting of NICMP was developed (**Fig. 6**), achieving a sensitivity of 96% and a specificity of 93%.

The various ECG criteria for identifying an epicardial exit are summarized in **Table 1**. The findings were consistent and indicate that an epicardial exit results in a longer time to engagement of the His-Purkinje system, with a greater initial slurring of the QRS and greater time to maximal deflection. These findings may have been influenced by antiarrhythmic drug, geometry and orientation of the heart, and the cycle length of the VTs. Although they predict the exit site being potentially epicardial, the critical isthmus of the reentrant circuit may be located and hence, ablated endocardially. Nonetheless, recognizing the

ECG parameters that indicate the potential need for epicardial mapping is crucial in planning VT ablation in patients with NICMP.

INTRACARDIAC EGM CHARACTERISTICS

Identification of the electroanatomic substrate for ventricular arrhythmia in NICMP relies on similar intracardiac EGM features to that seen in ICMP, namely low amplitude, long duration, fractionated signals, and late potentials (LPs).[37] Anisotropic and slow conduction via surviving myocardial bundles through patchy fibrosis and myocyte disarray results in long duration, fractionated, or late EGM recordings.[19,38] Unlike ICMP, in which the location of these abnormal EGMs is related to the location of previous myocardial infarction that extends from the subendocardium, the location of scar and hence abnormal EGMs in NICMP do not follow any vascular distribution.[39]

Differences in Substrate Between ICMP and NICMP

The relationship of LP recordings or local abnormal ventricular activities (LAVA) to the critical isthmus of VTs has been examined and a potential-based ablation strategy has been shown to be effective in controlling VT recurrence.[40–43]

Using ultrahigh-density mapping, Nakahara and colleagues[44] characterized the arrhythmogenic substrate in patients with NICMP. Endocardial scar area was twice the epicardial scar area in patients with ICMP, whereas patients with NICMP had equal extent of scar on the endocardium and epicardium. Significantly lower numbers of LPs and very late potentials (vLPs), with less slow conduction, were noted in patient with NICMP on both endocardium and epicardium (**Fig. 7**). Although an LP-targeted ablation strategy was effective in patients with ICMP, patients with NICMP had less favorable outcomes.[44] These findings were consistent with the findings of Kuhne and colleagues,[42] who assessed the prevalence of LPs in patients with NICMP undergoing VT ablation.

Basal Perivalvular Location

Hsia and colleagues[10] studied 19 patients with NICMP and monomorphic VT and found the predominant distribution of abnormal endocardial EGM recordings (with low voltage defined as <1.8 mV) to be located at the LV base, frequently involving the perivalvular regions (see **Fig. 2**). The VT in these patients also typically originated from the basal regions of the LV, corresponding to anatomic location of the endocardial substrate. This basal perivalvular predilection of the

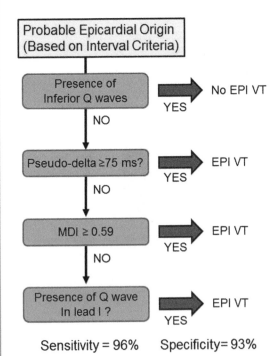

Fig. 6. Four-step algorithm for identifying epicardial (EPI) activation origin from basal superior and lateral LV in the setting of NICMP. A probable epicardial activation origin was initially suspected based on interval criteria. The 3 top steps have a high specificity, and the last step is the most accurate. The total sensitivity and specificity of the algorithm in the study population for localization reach 96% and 93%, respectively. MDI, maximal deflection index. (*Adapted from* Vallès E, Bazan V, Marchlinski FE. ECG criteria to identify epicardial ventricular tachycardia in nonischemic cardiomyopathy. Circ Arrhythm Electrophysiol 2010;3:63–71; with permission.)

Table 1
ECG criteria predictive of an epicardial exit for a VT

Author, Year	Ventricular Region	ECG Criteria Predictive of Epicardial Exit	Sensitivity (%)	Specificity (%)
Berruezo et al,[32] 2004	LV	Precordial pseudo-δ wave ≥34 ms	83	95
		Intrinsicoid deflection time in V2 ≥85 ms	87	90
		Shortest precordial RS duration ≥121 ms	76	85
Bazan et al,[35] 2006	Inferior RV Anterior exit	q waves in inferior leads	71	74
		q wave in lead I	52	94
		QS complex in V2	67	61
Bazan et al,[34] 2007	Basal superior LV	q wave in lead I	86	81
	Apical superior LV	q wave in lead I	84	74
	Basal inferior LV	q waves in inferior leads	74	51
	Apical inferior LV	q waves in inferior leads	94	61
Valles et al,[36] 2010	Basal superior and lateral LV	Algorithm with the parameters of a. Absence of q waves in inferior leads b. Precordial pseudo-δ wave ≥75 ms c. Precordial MDI ≥0.59 d. q wave in lead I	96 (pace map) 88 (VT)	93 (pace map) 88 (VT)

Abbreviations: MDI, maximal deflection index; RV, right ventricular.

abnormal substrate was also confirmed by others, both with catheter mapping[9] and with noninvasive imaging.[8,45]

Nonendocardial Substrate

Based on delayed enhancement MRI and electroanatomic mapping in patients with NICMP with monomorphic VT or premature ventricular complexes (PVCs), the distribution of scar is often noted to be epicardial or intramural, or endocardial with extension into the former.[9,28,39,46,47] The epicardial substrate has been found to be greater in volume than the endocardial substrate in patients for whom endocardial ablation has failed or in whom VT is of epicardial origin (**Table 2**).[9,28]

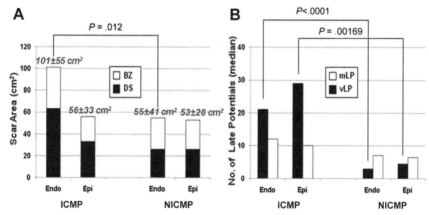

Fig. 7. Differences in scar area and LPs between ischemic and NICMP substrate. (*A*) Endocardial (Endo) scar area (101 ± 55 cm²) was twice the epicardial (Epi) scar area (56 ± 33 cm²) in patients with ICMP, whereas patients with NICMP had equal extent of scar on the endocardium and epicardium (55 ± 41 cm² vs 53 ± 28 cm²). Less dense scar (DS) (*solid bars*) was observed in patients with NICMP. Open bars indicate border zone (BZ). (*B*) Patients with NICMP had significantly less slow conduction, with fewer LP recordings, than patients with ICMP, particularly the vLP. (*Adapted from* Nakahara S, Tung R, Ramirez RJ, et al. Characterization of the arrhythmogenic substrate in ischemic and nonischemic cardiomyopathy: implications for catheter ablation of hemodynamically unstable ventricular tachycardia. J Am Coll Cardiol 2010;55:2355–65; with permission.)

Table 2
Substrate in sustained monomorphic VT

Total Area of Scar	Epicardium	Endocardium	P
NICMP			
Area of abnormal EGM (cm^2)	37.5 ± 10.4	16.5 ± 8.1	<.05
ICMP			
Area of abnormal EGM (cm^2)	15.0 ± 1.5	42.2 ± 1.1	<.01

Data from Soejima K, Stevenson WG, Sapp JL, et al. Endocardial and epicardial radiofrequency ablation of ventricular tachycardia associated with dilated cardiomyopathy: the importance of low-voltage scars. J Am Coll Cardiol 2004;43(10):1834–42; and Cesario DA, Vaseghi M, Boyle NG, et al. Value of high-density endocardial and epicardial mapping for catheter ablation of hemodynamically unstable ventricular tachycardia. Heart Rhythm 2006;3(1):1–10.

The epicardial EGM recordings have been characterized to define scar and to differentiate scar from epicardial fat. Based on detailed endocardial and epicardial mapping in patients with structurally normal hearts and idiopathic VT, excluding regions of large coronary vessels and the atrioventricular (AV) groove ± epicardial fat, Cano and colleagues[28] defined normal epicardial signal amplitude to be greater than 1.0 mV, because more than 95% of all bipolar epicardial signals in these normal controls were higher than 0.94 mV. On this basis, 22 patients with suspected epicardial VT who were studied were found to have epicardial scar in 82%, with 77% having greater epicardial scar than endocardial scar. These epicardial low-voltage areas also had abnormal EGMs, which were wide (>80 ms), split (having ≥2 distinct components), or late (with a distinct onset after the QRS).

The importance of taking into account EGM characteristics in distinguishing between

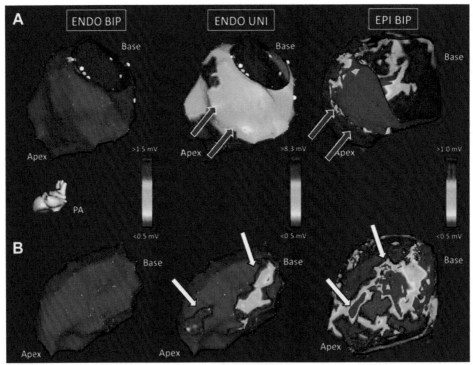

Fig. 8. Endocardial unipolar voltage mapping to detect epicardial VT substrate in nonischemic LV cardiomyopathy. Voltage maps taken from 2 patients with nonischemic LV cardiomyopathy. The LV endocardial bipolar (ENDO BIP) voltage maps (*left*) are normal in both patients. (*A*) Patient has extensive LV endocardial unipolar (ENDO UNI) low voltage involving the entire lateral and inferior LV walls (*red arrows*). There is a large region of corresponding LV epicardial bipolar (EPI BIP) low-voltage scar, corresponding spatially with the ENDO UNI abnormality. (*B*) Patient has 2 confluent low ENDO UNI voltage regions at the basal midlateral and apical LV segments (*white arrows*). The corresponding LV EPI BIP map shows 2 corresponding low-voltage areas. (*Adapted from* Hutchinson MD, Gerstenfeld EP, Desjardins B, et al. Endocardial unipolar voltage mapping to detect epicardial ventricular tachycardia substrate in patients with nonischemic left ventricular cardiomyopathy. Circ Arrhythm Electrophysiol 2011;4:49–55; with permission.)

epicardial fat and scar was shown in an analysis of EGMs from high-density epicardial mapping in a porcine infarct model, which was correlated with gross and histopathologic examination of the 7 hearts. The mean epicardial bipolar EGM voltage was not useful in differentiating epicardial fat (0.77 ± 0.34 mV) from an epicardial scar (0.75 ± 0.38 mV; P = not significant). The distinguishing differences lay in epicardial scar having EGMs that were longer in duration (68.8 ± 18.9 vs 50.1 ± 11.6 ms; P<.0001), more fractioned recordings (8.5 ± 3.1 vs 4.7 ± 1.8 deflections; P<.0001) and contained LPs that was 99% specific for scar.[48]

With a larger field of view compared with bipolar recordings, endocardial unipolar recordings may be useful in identifying epicardial and intramural substrate. Hutchinson and colleagues[49] defined the reference value for normal endocardial

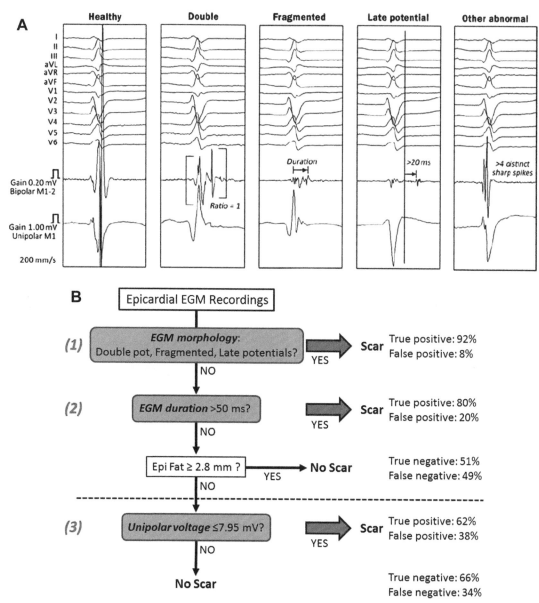

Fig. 9. (*A*) EGM morphology categories recorded on the epicardial surface. (*B*) Three-step algorithm for differentiation between epicardial (Epi) scar and viable myocardium areas. (*Adapted from* Piers SR, van Huls van Taxis CF, Tao Q, et al. Epicardial substrate mapping for ventricular tachycardia ablation in patients with non-ischaemic cardiomyopathy: a new algorithm to differentiate between scar and viable myocardium developed by simultaneous integration of computed tomography and contrast-enhanced magnetic resonance imaging. Eur Heart J 2013;34:586–96; with permission.)

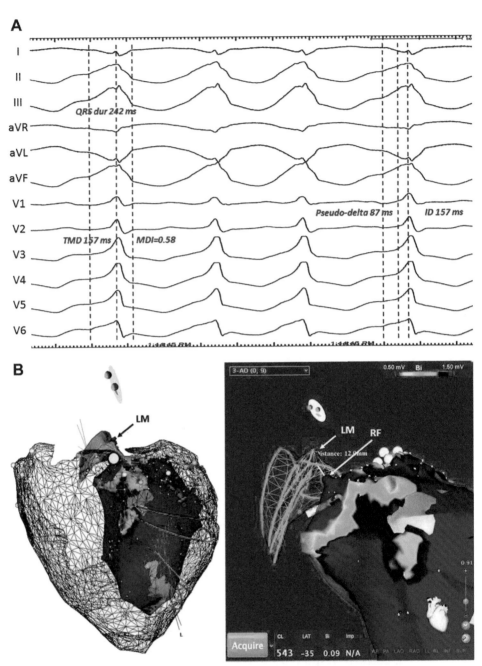

Fig. 10. An example of VT originating from the aortic sinus cusp in a patient with familial NICMP. (*A*) A 12-lead ECG of the inducible VT with an RBBB, right inferior QRS axis with slurred upstroke. Notice a pseudo-δ interval of 87 (>34) milliseconds, intrinsicoid deflection of 157 (>85) milliseconds, and an R/S ratio of greater than 121 milliseconds. The MDI was 0.58 (>0.55). These findings along with the presence of q wave in lead I suggest an epicardial (or nonendocardial) site of origin. (*B*) Electroanatomic mapping with the epicardial mesh superimposed on the endocardial shell. The color gradient was the same as that in **Fig. 2**. Minimal endocardial and epicardial low-voltage area was noted, except for a dense scar just underneath the aortic cusp. The successful ablation site (*yellow dot*, RF) was inside the left aortic cusp, 12.0 mm from the left main coronary ostium (LM). (*C*) Mapping from the left aortic cusp showed a presystolic (-92 ms before the onset of QRS) potential (*arrows*) with a good unipolar recordings during VT. ID, intrinsicoid deflection; TMD, time to maximum deflection.

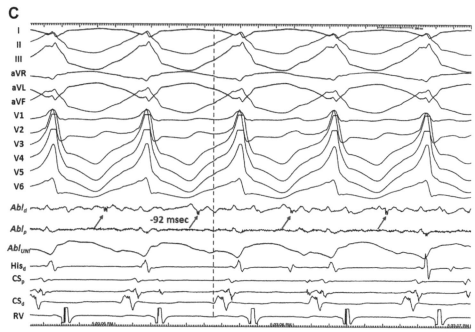

Fig. 10. (*continued*)

unipolar voltages from patients without structural heart disease as greater than 8.27 mV in the LV. Using this value (82%), patients who had low bipolar voltage regions on epicardium were found to have corresponding low-voltage unipolar recordings from the endocardial surface (**Fig. 8**). For the RV epicardium in patients with arrhythmogenic RV dysplasia, an endocardial unipolar voltage of less than 5.5 mV was found to indicate epicardial scar.[50]

The difficulty in distinguishing epicardial fibrosis and epicardial fat in patients with NICMP was addressed by Piers and colleagues[47] using computed tomography–derived epicardial fat measurement and contrast-enhanced MRI-derived scar integrated with electroanatomic mapping. At epicardial sites covered with less than 2.8 mm of fat, a bipolar voltage less than 1.81 mV and a unipolar voltage less than 7.95 mV and an EGM duration of greater than 50 milliseconds distinguished epicardial scar from myocardium.[47] The lower bipolar voltage cutoff reported by Cano and colleagues[28] (<1.0 mV) may be related to fat being arbitrarily defined around coronary vessels and the AV groove.[47] These voltage and EGM duration criteria were not useful when there was ≥2.8 mm of fat. However, EGM morphologic characteristics such as double potentials, fragmented potentials (amplitude/duration ratio ≤0.05 mV/ms), or LPs (inscribing after QRS and separated by an isoelectric segment >20 ms) could still help to identify epicardial scar in areas covered by ≥2.8 mm of fat during electroanatomical mapping (**Fig. 9**).

Intramural and Periaortic Substrate

Although many studies have noted a basal lateral LV scar in patients with NICMP and VT, other regions of abnormal substrate have been described. In a series of 33 patients with NICMP described by Yokokawa and colleagues,[51] the arrhythmogenic substrate extended from the basolateral LV into the aortic cusp in patients with aortic cusp VT (**Fig. 10**). EGM parameters for the presence of intramural scar as defined on delayed enhancement (DE) MRI were further characterized by Desjardins and colleagues.[12] A unipolar EGM voltage cutoff value of 6.78 mV and a bipolar voltage cutoff value of 1.55 mV best separated endocardial recordings overlying scar from that not overlying scar. In contrast, with epicardial voltage mapping, Piers and colleagues[47] found that in the absence of fat, a unipolar voltage less than 7.95 mV could detect intramural scar, whereas bipolar voltages were not affected (**Table 3**). Isolated septal substrate was also found in 11.6% (31/266) of consecutive patients with NICMP undergoing VT ablation, defined by bipolar EGMs less than 1.5 mV or unipolar EGMs less than 8.3 mV.[52] In 8 patients, there was no LV endocardial scar seen as defined by bipolar EGMs; however, unipolar EGMs were abnormal, indicating the possibility of exclusively intramural substrate deep in the interventricular septum (**Fig. 11**). These patients with intramural/septal scar often present with multiple VTs with variable axis and early breakthrough in the

Table 3
Summary of voltage criteria for identifying scar

Scar Location	Endocardial Mapping (mV)	Epicardial Mapping (mV)
LV endocardial scar	BV <1.5[56]	—
LV epicardial scar	UV <8.25[49]	BV <1.0[28]
RV endocardial scar	BV <1.5[56]	—
RV epicardial scar	UV <5.5[50]	BV <1.0
Intramural scar	BV <1.55 UV <6.78[12]	UV <7.95[47]

Abbreviations: BV, bipolar voltage; UV, unipolar voltage.

periseptal region and represent a challenge in VT ablation/management.

The presence of intramural septal scar can also be suggested by abnormal LV transeptal activation during RV septal pacing.[53] In patients with evidence of septal scar, as defined by DE-MRI and low septal unipolar (<8.3 mV) and bipolar (<1.5 mV) voltages, the LV transeptal activation time was significantly prolonged (55.3 ± 33.0 vs 25.7 ± 8.8 milliseconds; $P = .003$) compared with those without septal scar. A delayed transeptal activation time of greater than 40 milliseconds and EGM duration of greater than 95 milliseconds identified intramural VT substrate. Furthermore, some patients with NICMP with extensive scar had disrupted transeptal activation patterns, because activation propagated around the scar rather than directly transmural, with the earliest LV activation displaced to the apical region (**Fig. 12**).

Unipolar EGM and Irreversibility of NICMP

The unipolar EGM recordings may also be useful to identify potential reversible myocardial dysfunction in the absence of macroscopic scar on MRI.[54] When the endocardial unipolar LV voltage maps of patients with NICMP and no evidence of macroscopic scar were compared, those with irreversible cardiomyopathy had a lower median voltage

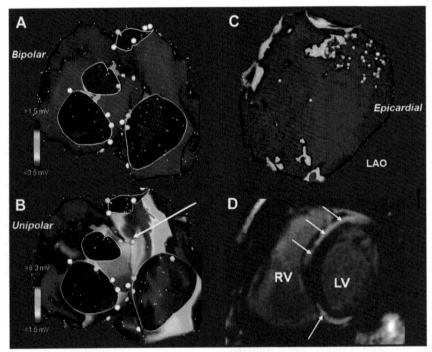

Fig. 11. Intramural septal scar in patients with NICMP. (*A*) Normal LV and RV endocardial bipolar voltage in the posteroanterior view. (*B*) Unipolar endocardial voltage maps showing septal low voltage (<8.3 mV) area (*arrows*), raising suspicion of the deeper intramural scar. (*C*) Epicardial map was unremarkable, with no abnormal EGMs and preserved bipolar voltages. (*D*) This was confirmed by cardiac MRI, which showed extensive midmyocardial and intramural septal delayed gadolinium enhancement (*arrows*). LAO, left anterior oblique. (*Adapted from* [*A, B*] Haqqani HM, Tschabrunn CM, Tzou WS, et al. Isolated septal substrate for ventricular tachycardia in non-ischemic dilated cardiomyopathy: incidence, characterization, and implications. Heart Rhythm 2011;8(8):1169–76, with permission; and [*C, D*] Hutchinson MD, Marchlinski FE. Epicardial ablation of VT in patients with nonischemic LV cardiomyopathy. Card Electrophysiol Clin 2010;2:93–103.)

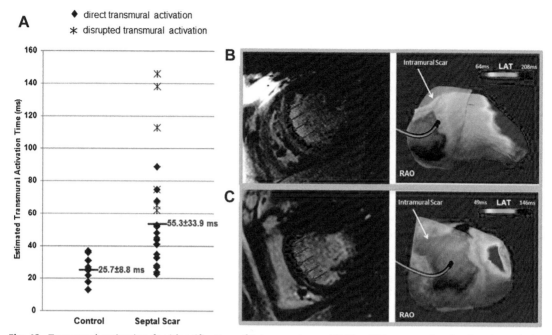

Fig. 12. Transeptal activation for identification of intramural scar. (*A*) The LV transmural activation times during right opposite septal pacing was prolonged in group 2 (with septal scar) compared with group 1 (without evidence of septal scar) (55.3 ± 33.9 milliseconds vs 25.7 ± 8.8 milliseconds, *P* = .003). All group 1 patients had rapid direct transmural activation (*black diamonds*), whereas some of the group 2 patients had disrupted transmural activation (*asterisks*) with displaced LV early activation site. Two patients (*B, C*) who showed disrupted transeptal activation are shown with earliest LV activation at the apical region. (*Left*) Short-axis MRIs showing intramural midwall delayed enhancement of the interventricular septum (*red arrows*). (*Right*) MRI three-dimensional septal scar reconstruction defined intramural scar and registration with corresponding CARTO (Biosense Webster, Diamond Bar, CA, USA) activation maps during basal RV septal pacing. LAT, local activation time; RAO, right anterior oblique. (*Adapted from* Betensky BP, Kapa S, Desjardins B, et al. Characterization of trans-septal activation during septal pacing: criteria for identification of intramural ventricular tachycardia substrate in nonischemic cardiomyopathy. Circ Arrhythm Electrophysiol 2013;6:1123–30; with permission.)

(7.6 mV) then those with reversible PVC-mediated cardiomyopathy (13.6 mV), which was lower than those with structurally normal hearts (16.3 mV). This finding is in keeping with the finding of an inverse relation between the amplitude of unipolar endocardial recording and the burden of myocardial fibrosis described in an experimental model of NICMP.[55] Areas of unipolar abnormality represented a larger proportion of the total LV surface in those in whom the cardiomyopathy did not reverse compared with those in whom it did. A unipolar abnormality area cutoff of 32% was 96% sensitive and 100% specific in identifying irreversible cardiomyopathy in patients with LV dysfunction. Unipolar electroanatomic mapping may have prognostic value in clinical decision making in patients with NICMP.

SUMMARY

VT in NICMP most commonly results from scar-based reentry arising from basal scar, which is frequently epicardial and midmyocardial and can be identified by ECG features in SR. The ECG in VT also has characteristic features to identify non-endocardial substrate, a result of longer time to engagement of the His-Purkinje system, with a greater initial slurring of the QRS and greater time to maximal deflection. Anisotropic slow conduction, which occurs through scar in NICMP, similarly results in LP and LAVA EGMs, which have been shown to be good targets in a potential-based ablation strategy. Aside from bipolar EGMs, unipolar EGMs with a wider field of view are useful for identifying epicardial and intramural substrate and for identifying potentially reversible myocardial dysfunction. These ECG and EGM characteristics, when taken into account, allow for better planning and outcomes in ablation of VT in NICMP.

REFERENCES

1. Wu AH. Management of patients with non-ischaemic cardiomyopathy. Heart 2007;93(3):403–8.

2. Dec GW, Fuster V. Idiopathic dilated cardiomyopathy. N Engl J Med 1994;331(23):1564–75.

3. Rakar S, Sinagra G, Di Lenarda A, et al. Epidemiology of dilated cardiomyopathy. A prospective post-mortem study of 5252 necropsies. The Heart Muscle Disease Study Group. Eur Heart J 1997; 18(1):117–23.

4. Effect of metoprolol CR/XL in chronic heart failure: Metoprolol CR/XL Randomised Intervention Trial in Congestive Heart Failure (MERIT-HF). Lancet 1999;353(9169):2001–7.

5. Grimm W, Maisch B. Sudden cardiac death in dilated cardiomyopathy–therapeutic options. Herz 2002;27(8):750–9.

6. Theuns DA, Smith T, Hunink MG, et al. Effectiveness of prophylactic implantation of cardioverter-defibrillators without cardiac resynchronization therapy in patients with ischaemic or non-ischaemic heart disease: a systematic review and meta-analysis. Europace 2010;12(11):1564–70.

7. Sacher F, Tedrow UB, Field ME, et al. Ventricular tachycardia ablation: evolution of patients and procedures over 8 years. Circ Arrhythm Electrophysiol 2008;1(3):153–61.

8. Piers SRD, Leong DP, van Taxis CFBvH, et al. Outcome of ventricular tachycardia ablation in patients with nonischemic cardiomyopathy: the impact of noninducibility. Circ Arrhythm Electrophysiol 2013;6(3):513–21.

9. Soejima K, Stevenson WG, Sapp JL, et al. Endocardial and epicardial radiofrequency ablation of ventricular tachycardia associated with dilated cardiomyopathy: the importance of low-voltage scars. J Am Coll Cardiol 2004;43(10):1834–42.

10. Hsia HH, Callans DJ, Marchlinski FE. Characterization of endocardial electrophysiological substrate in patients with nonischemic cardiomyopathy and monomorphic ventricular tachycardia. Circulation 2003;108(6):704–10.

11. Vergara P, Trevisi N, Ricco A, et al. Late potentials abolition as an additional technique for reduction of arrhythmia recurrence in scar related ventricular tachycardia ablation. J Cardiovasc Electrophysiol 2012;23(6):621–7.

12. Desjardins B, Yokokawa M, Good E, et al. Characteristics of intramural scar in patients with nonischemic cardiomyopathy and relation to intramural ventricular arrhythmias. Circ Arrhythm Electrophysiol 2013;6(5):891–7.

13. Tokuda M, Tedrow UB, Kojodjojo P, et al. Catheter ablation of ventricular tachycardia in nonischemic heart disease. Circ Arrhythm Electrophysiol 2012; 5(5):992–1000.

14. Hsia HH, Marchlinski FE. Electrophysiology studies in patients with dilated cardiomyopathies. Card Electrophysiol Rev 2002;6(4):472–81.

15. Roberts WC, Siegel RJ, McManus BM. Idiopathic dilated cardiomyopathy: analysis of 152 necropsy patients. Am J Cardiol 1987;60(16):1340–55.

16. Unverferth DV, Baker PB, Swift SE, et al. Extent of myocardial fibrosis and cellular hypertrophy in dilated cardiomyopathy. Am J Cardiol 1986; 57(10):816–20.

17. Nakayama Y, Shimizu G, Hirota Y, et al. Functional and histopathologic correlation in patients with dilated cardiomyopathy: an integrated evaluation by multivariate analysis. J Am Coll Cardiol 1987; 10(1):186–92.

18. de Leeuw N, Ruiter DJ, Balk AHMM, et al. Histopathologic findings in explanted heart tissue from patients with end-stage idiopathic dilated cardiomyopathy. Transpl Int 2001;14(5):299–306.

19. Hsia HH, Marchlinski FE. Characterization of the electroanatomic substrate for monomorphic ventricular tachycardia in patients with nonischemic cardiomyopathy. Pacing Clin Electrophysiol 2002; 25(7):1114–27.

20. Marchlinski FE. Perivalvular fibrosis and monomorphic ventricular tachycardia: toward a unifying hypothesis in nonischemic cardiomyopathy. Circulation 2007;116(18):1998–2001.

21. Pogwizd SM. Nonreentrant mechanisms underlying spontaneous ventricular arrhythmias in a model of nonischemic heart failure in rabbits. Circulation 1995;92(4):1034–48.

22. Pogwizd SM, McKenzie JP, Cain ME. Mechanisms underlying spontaneous and induced ventricular arrhythmias in patients with idiopathic dilated cardiomyopathy. Circulation 1998;98(22):2404–14.

23. Delacretaz E, Stevenson WG, Ellison KE, et al. Mapping and radiofrequency catheter ablation of the three types of sustained monomorphic ventricular tachycardia in nonischemic heart disease. J Cardiovasc Electrophysiol 2000;11(1):11–7.

24. Anderson KP, Walker R, Urie P, et al. Myocardial electrical propagation in patients with idiopathic dilated cardiomyopathy. J Clin Invest 1993;92(1): 122–40.

25. Blanck Z, Dhala A, Deshpande S, et al. Bundle branch reentrant ventricular tachycardia: cumulative experience in 48 patients. J Cardiovasc Electrophysiol 1993;4(3):253–62.

26. Blanck Z, Sra J, Dhala A, et al. Bundle branch reentry: mechanism, diagnosis, and treatment. In: Jalife J, Zipes DP, editors. Cardiac electrophysiology: from cell to bedside. Philadelphia: Saunders; 1995. p. 878–85.

27. Nogami A. Purkinje-related arrhythmias part I: monomorphic ventricular tachycardias. Pacing Clin Electrophysiol 2011;34(5):624–50.

28. Cano O, Dhala A, Deshpande S, et al. Electroanatomic substrate and ablation outcome for suspected

epicardial ventricular tachycardia in left ventricular nonischemic cardiomyopathy. J Am Coll Cardiol 2009;54(9):799–808.

29. Giesbrandt KJ, Bolan CW, Shapiro BP, et al. Diffuse diseases of the myocardium: MRI-pathologic review of cardiomyopathies with dilatation. Am J Roentgenol 2013;200(3):W274–82.

30. Tzou WS, Zado ES, Lin D, et al. Sinus rhythm ECG criteria associated with basal-lateral ventricular tachycardia substrate in patients with nonischemic cardiomyopathy. J Cardiovasc Electrophysiol 2011; 22(12):1351–8.

31. Betensky BP, Deyell MW, Tzou WS, et al. Sinus rhythm electrocardiogram identification of basal-lateral ischemic versus nonischemic substrate in patients with ventricular tachycardia. J Interv Card Electrophysiol 2012;35(3):311–21 [discussion: 321].

32. Berruezo A, Mont L, Nava S, et al. Electrocardiographic recognition of the epicardial origin of ventricular tachycardias. Circulation 2004;109(15): 1842–7.

33. Daniels DV, Lu YY, Morton JB, et al. Idiopathic epicardial left ventricular tachycardia originating remote from the sinus of Valsalva: electrophysiological characteristics, catheter ablation, and identification from the 12-lead electrocardiogram. Circulation 2006;113(13):1659–66.

34. Bazan V, Gerstenfeld EP, Garcia FC, et al. Site-specific twelve-lead ECG features to identify an epicardial origin for left ventricular tachycardia in the absence of myocardial infarction. Heart Rhythm 2007;4(11):1403–10.

35. Bazan V, Bala R, Garcia FC, et al. Site-specific twelve-lead ECG features to identify an epicardial origin for left ventricular tachycardia in the absence of myocardial infarction. Heart Rhythm 2006;3(10): 1132–9.

36. Vallès E, Bazan V, Marchlinski FE. ECG criteria to identify epicardial ventricular tachycardia in nonischemic cardiomyopathy. Circ Arrhythm Electrophysiol 2010;3(1):63–71.

37. Cassidy DM, Vassallo JA, Miller JM, et al. Endocardial catheter mapping in patients in sinus rhythm: relationship to underlying heart disease and ventricular arrhythmias. Circulation 1986;73(4):645–52.

38. Mathuria N, Tung R, Shivkumar K. Advances in ablation of ventricular tachycardia in nonischemic cardiomyopathy. Curr Cardiol Rep 2012;14(5): 577–83.

39. Cesario DA, Vaseghi M, Boyle NG, et al. Value of high-density endocardial and epicardial mapping for catheter ablation of hemodynamically unstable ventricular tachycardia. Heart Rhythm 2006;3(1): 1–10.

40. Hsia H, Lin D, Sauer W, et al. Relationship of late potentials to the ventricular tachycardia circuit defined by entrainment. J Interv Card Electrophysiol 2009;26(1):21–9.

41. Ouyang F, Antz M, Deger FT, et al. An underrecognized subepicardial reentrant ventricular tachycardia attributable to left ventricular aneurysm in patients with normal coronary arteriograms. Circulation 2003;107(21):2702–9.

42. Kuhne M, Abrams G, Sarrazin JF, et al. Isolated potentials and pace-mapping as guides for ablation of ventricular tachycardia in various types of nonischemic cardiomyopathy. J Cardiovasc Electrophysiol 2010;21(9):1017–23.

43. Jais P, Maury P, Khairy P, et al. Elimination of local abnormal ventricular activities: a new end point for substrate modification in patients with scar-related ventricular tachycardia. Circulation 2012;125(18):2184–96.

44. Nakahara S, Tung R, Ramirez RJ, et al. Characterization of the arrhythmogenic substrate in ischemic and nonischemic cardiomyopathy: implications for catheter ablation of hemodynamically unstable ventricular tachycardia. J Am Coll Cardiol 2010; 55(21):2355–65.

45. Nazarian S, Bluemke DA, Lardo AC, et al. Magnetic resonance assessment of the substrate for inducible ventricular tachycardia in nonischemic cardiomyopathy. Circulation 2005;112(18):2821–5.

46. Bogun FM, Desjardins B, Good E, et al. Delayed-enhanced magnetic resonance imaging in nonischemic cardiomyopathy: utility for identifying the ventricular arrhythmia substrate. J Am Coll Cardiol 2009;53(13):1138–45.

47. Piers SRD, van Huls van Taxis CFB, Tao Q, et al. Epicardial substrate mapping for ventricular tachycardia ablation in patients with non-ischaemic cardiomyopathy: a new algorithm to differentiate between scar and viable myocardium developed by simultaneous integration of computed tomography and contrast-enhanced magnetic resonance imaging. Eur Heart J 2013;34(8):586–96.

48. Tung R, Nakahara S, Ramirez R, et al. Distinguishing epicardial fat from scar: analysis of electrograms using high-density electroanatomic mapping in a novel porcine infarct model. Heart Rhythm 2010; 7(3):389–95.

49. Hutchinson MD, Gerstenfeld EP, Desjardins B, et al. Endocardial unipolar voltage mapping to detect epicardial ventricular tachycardia substrate in patients with nonischemic left ventricular cardiomyopathy. Circ Arrhythm Electrophysiol 2011;4(1): 49–55.

50. Polin GM, Haqqani H, Tzou W, et al. Endocardial unipolar voltage mapping to identify epicardial substrate in arrhythmogenic right ventricular cardiomyopathy/dysplasia. Heart Rhythm 2011;8(1): 76–83.

51. Yokokawa M, Good E, Crawford T, et al. Ventricular tachycardia originating from the aortic sinus cusp in patients with idiopathic dilated cardiomyopathy. Heart Rhythm 2011;8(3):357–60.

52. Haqqani HM, Tschabrunn CM, Tzou WS, et al. Isolated septal substrate for ventricular tachycardia in nonischemic dilated cardiomyopathy: incidence, characterization, and implications. Heart Rhythm 2011;8(8):1169–76.

53. Betensky BP, Kapa S, Desjardins B, et al. Characterization of trans-septal activation during septal pacing: criteria for identification of intramural ventricular tachycardia substrate in nonischemic cardiomyopathy. Circ Arrhythm Electrophysiol 2013;6(6):1123–30.

54. Campos B, Jauregui ME, Park KM, et al. New unipolar electrogram criteria to identify irreversibility of nonischemic left ventricular cardiomyopathy. J Am Coll Cardiol 2012;60(21):2194–204.

55. Psaltis PJ, Carbone A, Leong DP, et al. Assessment of myocardial fibrosis by endoventricular electromechanical mapping in experimental nonischemic cardiomyopathy. Int J Cardiovasc Imaging 2011; 27(1):25–37.

56. Marchlinski FE, Callans DJ, Gottlieb CD, et al. Linear ablation lesions for control of unmappable ventricular tachycardia in patients with ischemic and nonischemic cardiomyopathy. Circulation 2000;101(11):1288–96.

Electrocardiogram Characteristics of Outflow Tract Ventricular Tachycardia

Amit Mehrotra, MD, MBA, Sanjay Dixit, MD*

KEYWORDS

- Outflow tract • Electrocardiogram • Ventricular tachycardia • Idiopathic ventricular tachycardia
- Intracardiac electrogram

KEY POINTS

- The mechanism underlying outflow tract ventricular tachycardia (VT) is delayed after depolarization-mediated triggered activity.
- Outflow tract VT arises from a focal site, and these patients generally lack structural heart disease. Thus, pace mapping can be used to mimic the clinical VT.
- Outflow tract VTs most commonly arise from the superior right ventricular (RV) outflow tract, aortic cusp region, basal left ventricle and the great cardiac/anterior interventricular vein.
- At the site of origin, local activation precedes QRS complexes by 15 to 30 milliseconds, and pace mapping from this location matches the clinical arrhythmia.
- Electroanatomic mapping facilitates accurate catheter localization in the outflow tract region.

INTRODUCTION
Pathophysiology

Ventricular tachycardias (VTs) are usually observed in the setting of structural heart disease. However, in 10% of patients presenting with VT, routine diagnostic modalities demonstrate no myocardial damage. These arrhythmias have been called idiopathic ventricular tachycardias (IVTs).[1]

Outflow tract tachycardias comprise a subgroup of IVTs that are predominantly localized in and around the right and left ventricular outflow tracts (RVOT and LVOT, respectively). Lerman and colleagues[2] demonstrated that the mechanism underlying this group of arrhythmias appears to be triggered activity caused by delayed after depolarizations that are determined by intracellular calcium release (load). The release of calcium is negatively affected by adenosine, which is why these arrhythmias are considered adenosine sensitive.[3]

Clinical Presentation

In general, outflow tract tachycardias can manifest at any age and equally in both sexes.[4] The typical presentation of these arrhythmias consists of salvos of paroxysmal ventricular ectopic beats and nonsustained VT; sustained tachycardia is uncommon. Most patients (48%–80%) experience palpitations. Presyncope and lightheadedness may

Pertinent Disclosures: None.
Cardiovascular Division, Hospital of the University of Pennsylvania, 3400 Spruce Street, Philadelphia, PA 19104, USA
* Corresponding author. Hospital of the University of Pennsylvania, 9 Founders Pavilion, 3400 Spruce Street, Philadelphia, PA 19104.
E-mail address: Sanjay.Dixit@uphs.upenn.edu

cardiacEP.theclinics.com

also be observed (28%–50%). True syncope is infrequently seen (overall incidence, <10%), and these rhythm disorders are rarely life threatening.[5–7] Outflow tract tachycardias are typically provoked by exercise in most patients.[5,8] Other triggers for inducing or enhancing the arrhythmia include stress, anxiety, and stimulants such as caffeine. In women, outflow tachycardias are more often observed during premenstrual or perimenopausal periods and with gestation, suggesting the role of hormonal influences.

Distribution

In the earlier experience at the authors' center (January 1999 and December 2003) of 122 patients undergoing ablation for IVT, the site of origin (SOO) was localized to the RVOT region in 88 patients (72%). More recently (2004–2008), however, the authors have noted a preponderance of the SOO from the cusp region.[1,9]

This article describes the unique electrocardiogram (ECG) morphologies of outflow tract VT by means of their SOO. It also briefly outlines strategies that the authors have used for successfully ablating these arrhythmias.

ECG CHARACTERISTICS OF OUTFLOW TRACT VT
RVOT Versus LVOT

Outflow tract tachycardias typically manifest an inferior axis (positive deflections in the inferior leads) and a left or right bundle branch block pattern (LBBB and RBBB, respectively), based on QRS morphology in lead V1. These arrhythmias can manifest diverse axes and different precordial transition patterns (early, late, or none) (**Fig. 1**). A predominantly or exclusively positive deflection in lead V1 is considered RBBB morphology, which suggests origin from the LVOT, whereas a predominantly negative deflection in lead V1 is considered LBBB morphology; tachycardias manifesting this morphology can arise from either the RVOT or septal LVOT. The precordial transition is helpful in predicting whether VT manifesting LBBB is arising from the RVOT or septal LVOT or the cusp region. Typically, if the precordial transition of the VT is later than that of the QRS complexes in sinus rhythm, then the SOO is likely in the RVOT. If the precordial transition is at V3 or earlier and occurs before the transition in sinus rhythm, the QRS complex in lead V2 should be further analyzed to distinguish between an RVOT

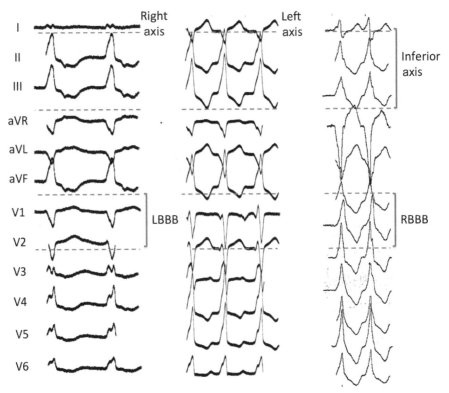

Fig. 1. Examples of variable 12-lead ECG characteristics encountered in outflow tract VT. They manifest inferior axis with either RBBB or LBBB patterns, and either a right or left axis.

versus LVOT SOO. A comparison of the R/R+S ratio of the VT in lead V2 with that in sinus allows one to distinguish between an RVOT or cusp site of origin. A ratio above or below 0.6 has been established to predict origin from cusp or RVOT, respectively (**Fig. 2**).[10]

In order to define ECGs characteristic from specific anatomic locations in the outflow tract region, the authors have developed algorithms using pace mapping with electroanatomic guidance for accurate catheter localization.

Localization of Outflow Tract Tachycardia Arising from Superior RVOT

The RVOT region is defined superiorly by the pulmonic valve and inferiorly by the superior margin of the RV inflow tract (tricuspid valve). The interventricular septum and the RV free wall constitute its medial and lateral aspects, respectively. Because of the predilection for clinical arrhythmias from the superior RVOT, the authors attempted to further characterize the ECG features of pace maps from this region. To accomplish this, the superior-most sites in a posterior-to-anterior distribution were assigned numbers 1, 2, and 3 on both the septal and free wall aspects of the

superior RVOT (**Fig. 3**). The mapping catheter was positioned serially at each of these sites, and the location was paced at the diastolic threshold for 10 to 20 beats, during which a 12-lead ECG was acquired. The ECG was specifically analyzed for (1) QRS amplitude and duration in all limb leads; (2) presence of notching of R waves in the inferior leads II and III, and/or aVF; (3) QRS transition pattern in the precordial leads (from QS/rS pattern to RS/Rs pattern) with a change at or beyond lead V4 defined as being late transition; and (4) QRS morphology in limb lead I.[11] **Fig. 4** shows clinical examples of VT/premature ventricular contractions (PVCs) arising from different locations in the superior RVOT, and **Table 1** summarizes the findings that are unique to each location in this region. In the authors' series, pace maps from superior RVOT septal sites manifested monophasic R waves in the inferior leads, which were taller and narrower when compared with those seen in the counterpart free wall locations. Likewise, the duration of the R wave in lead II at septal sites was narrower than that of the R wave at free wall sites. The contour of the R wave in the inferior leads was also helpful in differentiating septal and free wall locations in the superior RVOT. Typically, R waves from free wall sites

$$[R/R+S]_{PVC} / [R/R+S]_{SINUS} = [0.4mV/1.6mV] / [0.3mV/0.6mV] =$$

$$0.5 < 0.6 \rightarrow \text{Consistent with RVOT SOO}$$

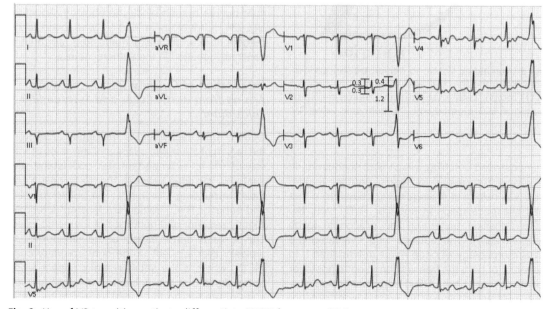

Fig. 2. Use of V2 transition ratio to differentiate RVOT from cusp SOO.

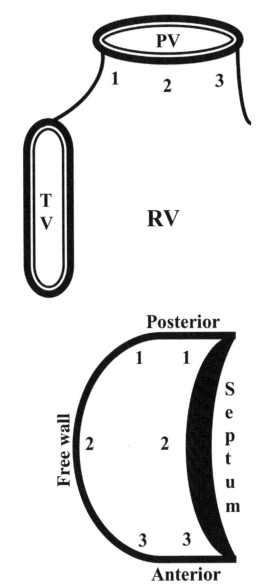

Fig. 3. Numbering system to demarcate various locations along the free wall and septum in the superior RVOT region. Each location in this region manifests a unique ECG morphology. PV, pulmonic valve; TV, tricuspid valve.

demonstrated notching, which was uncommon in R waves from septal locations. Another feature that was helpful in distinguishing septal from free wall site pace maps in superior RVOT was the QRS transition pattern in the precordial leads (late vs early). The authors also evaluated the QRS morphology of pace maps in limb lead I. In general, for both the free wall and septal posterior locations (site 1), the QRS in lead I manifested positive polarity (r waves). In comparison, anterior sites (site 3) along the septum and the free wall

demonstrated predominantly negative polarity (rs or qs). Sites midway between the anterior and posterior locations (site 2) along the septum and the free wall demonstrated either a biphasic or a multiphasic QRS morphology (qr/rs pattern), or an isoelectric segment preceding the q or r wave.[11] Using these criteria, a blinded reviewer was accurately able to predict the site of origin of clinical tachycardias arising from the superior RVOT region.[11]

Localization of Outflow Tract Tachycardia Arising from the Basal Left Ventricle

The basal left ventricle constitutes ventricular myocardium bordering the mitral valve and encompasses a wide area, including septum and anterior, lateral, and inferior walls.[4,12] The aortic valve typically sits at the superior and medial aspect of this region, distorting its otherwise circular shape. To develop ECG criteria for localizing basal LV VT, the authors performed pace mapping in a series of patients from 4 or more locations in this region, including the parahisian region, the aortomitral continuity and superior, superolateral, and lateral locations along the mitral annulus (**Fig. 5**, **Table 2**). In general, most medial basal LV sites demonstrated the narrowest QRS complexes, which were predominantly positive in lead I, whereas superolateral mitral annulus locations demonstrated the widest complexes, which were predominantly negative in lead I. With the exception of parahisian sites, which consistently demonstrate left bundle branch block morphology and early precordial transition patterns, pace maps from all other sites in this region manifested right bundle branch block morphology. Additionally, qR morphology in lead V_1 was found to be pathognomonic for pace maps from aortomitral continuity location in the authors' series.

Localization of Outflow Tract Tachycardia Arising from Aortic Cusps and Surrounding Epicardium

Outflow tract tachycardias frequently arise from the region of the aortic cusps and the sinus of Valsalva.[13,14] It is important to understand the anatomic relations between the aortic cusps and their surrounding structures. The pulmonic valve and superior RVOT region are located anteriorly, slightly superior and rightward of the aortic valve. The posterior septal aspect of the superior RVOT typically lies adjacent to the right coronary cusp (RCC), whereas the anterior septal aspect tends to be situated at the junction of the right and left cusp or anterior to the septal aspect of the latter (**Fig. 6**).[15] In some instances, a catheter in the

Localization of SOO for Superior RVOT

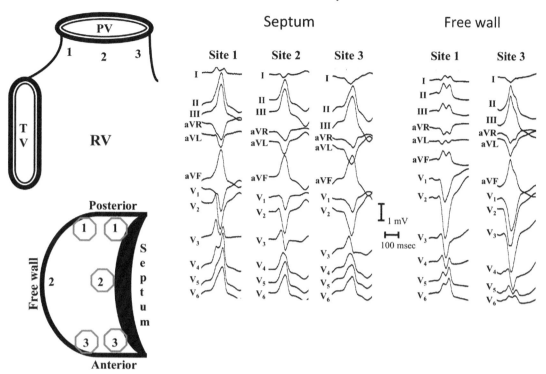

Fig. 4. 12-lead ECG morphology of clinical tachycardia that was successfully ablated from different locations in the superior RVOT region. PV, pulmonic valve; TV, tricuspid valve.

anterior–superior septal RVOT can extend far leftward almost to the left coronary cusp (LCC) location (**Fig. 7**).

To determine unique ECG characteristics of arrhythmias arising from this region, the authors performed pace mapping of the right, left, and noncoronary cusps in 20 patients with structurally normal hearts. They found lead V1 most useful in distinguishing the pace maps from various sites in the cusp region. LCC pace maps consistently produced a multiphasic component, resembling an M- or W-shaped QRS complex. RCC pacing demonstrated a QS or QR type pattern with a predominantly negative vector in V1 (**Fig. 8**). Pacing the noncoronary cusp resulted universally in capture of the atrium. Additional analysis of precordial QRS transition demonstrated that, for pace maps from the LCC, precordial transition occurred in V2 or earlier, whereas for RCC pace maps, the precordial transition was most commonly after V2. Recently, in a series of patients at the authors' center who underwent successful ablation

Table 1
Superior RV outflow tract VT location

	Septal Site 1	Septal Site 2	Septal Site 3	Free Wall Site 1	Free Wall Site 3
Inferior Lead Morphology	Monophasic	Monophasic	Monophasic	Notched	Notched
Inferior Lead Amplitude and Duration	Tall and narrow	Tall and narrow	Tall and narrow	Short and wide	Short and wide
Lead I	Positive	Biphasic	Negative	Positive	Negative
Precordial Transition	Early	Early	Early	Late	Late

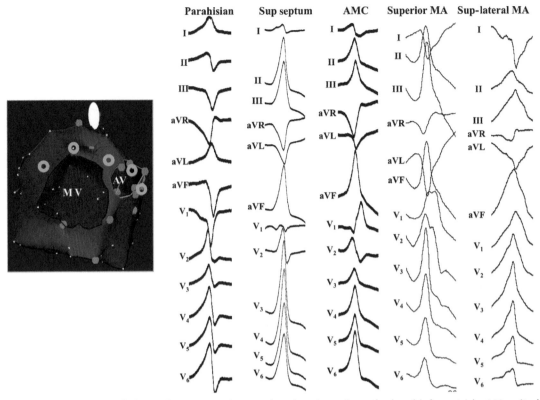

Fig. 5. 12-lead ECG morphology of pace maps from various locations along the basal left ventricle. MA, mitral annulus.

of PVC/VT from the aortic cusp region, the site of origin of the tachycardia was localized to the commissure between the LCC and RCC. Unique features of tachycardias originating from this location included QS morphology in lead V1 with notching on the downward deflection. When mapping for these arrhythmias in the cusp region, a late potential was observed during sinus rhythm at the site of earliest activation that reversed during the arrhythmia (**Fig. 9**).[16]

LOCALIZATION ALGORITHM

Several algorithms for the localization of outflow tract VT by surface ECG have been published.[17–19] Presented here is a simple algorithm that can be

used along with the figures and table in this article to help localize idiopathic VT SOO (**Fig. 10**).

LIMITATIONS AND ADDITIONAL CONSIDERATIONS

Although ECG manifestations of outflow tract tachycardias are extremely helpful in predicting their site of origin, there remain some limitations. These include lead placement and VT originating from the body of the right ventricle.

Lead Placement

Displacement of certain limb or precordial lead electrodes can change the ECG morphology of

Table 2					
Basal left ventricle VT localization					
	S-P	**AMC**	**Superior MA**	**Supero-Lateral MA**	**Lateral MA**
Lead I	R or Rs	Rs or rs	rs or rS	rS or QS	rS or rs
Lead V$_1$	QS or Qr	qR	R or Rs	R or Rs	R or Rs
Precordial Transition	Early	None	None	None	None or late S wave
Ratio of QRS in Leads II and III	>1	≤1	≤1	≤1	>1

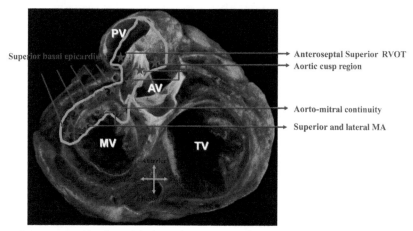

Fig. 6. Heart model transected in the axial plane demonstrates the proximity of common sites of origin of idiopathic VT: the superior RVOT, aortic cusp region, basal left ventricle and the mitral annulus. PV, pulmonic valve; TV, tricuspid valve. (*Courtesy of* Samuel Asirvatham, MD, Rochester, MN.)

the clinical arrhythmia and/or pace maps, and can adversely impact the accurate localization of the SOO. The authors examined the impact of changes in precordial leads V1 and V2 in a cohort of 18 patients as well as the influence of changes in upper limb electrode locations on QRS morphology in lead I in a separate cohort of 16 patients with outflow tract tachycardias. They found that superior displacement of leads V1 and V2 reduced the R-wave amplitude and led to a decreased R/S ratio, while inferior displacement of leads V1 and V2 resulted in increased R-wave amplitude and led to an increased R/S ratio. These changes adversely impacted the authors' ability to accurately differentiate RVOT from cusp location of the clinical arrhythmias. Similarly, anterior displacement of the arm leads from shoulders to chest resulted in a reduction in the R-wave amplitude in lead I, which limited the authors' ability to accurately differentiate between anterior and posterior locations in the superior RVOT region (**Fig. 11**).[20]

VT Originating from the Body of the Right Ventricle

Although most IVT's arise from the outflow tracts or the basal left ventricle, a small number can also arise from the body of the right ventricle. Among 278 consecutive patients who underwent radiofrequency ablation for idiopathic VT at the authors' institution between January 1999 and

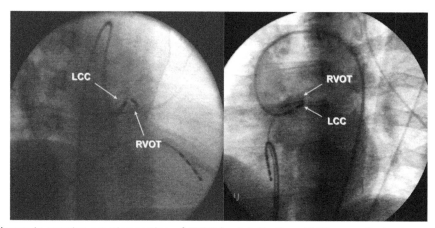

Fig. 7. Catheters in anterior–superior portion of RVOT (septal site 3) and LCC, respectively, demonstrating the proximity of these anatomic regions.

RCC

LCC

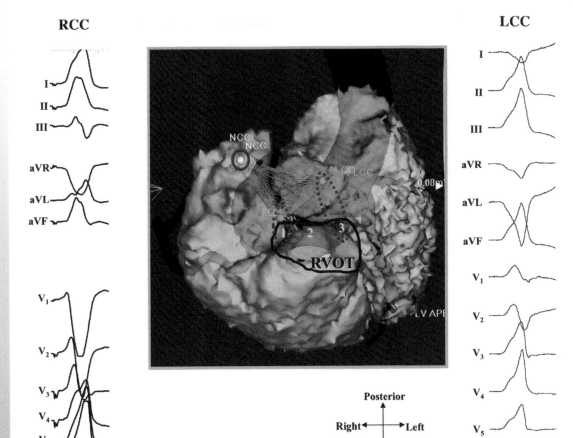

Fig. 8. 12-lead ECG morphology of right versus left coronary cusp site of origin (LCC SOO). NCC, non-coronary cusp.

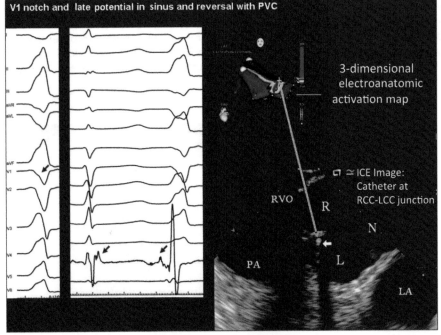

Fig. 9. 12-lead ECG morphology of VT originating from RCC–LCC junction. Late potential present in sinus rhythm that reverses with PVC. *Arrow* points to site of successful ablation. ICE, intracardiac echocardiography..

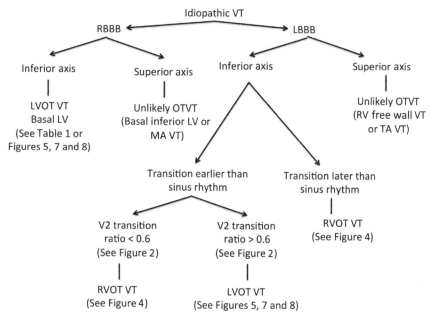

Fig. 10. Localization algorithm for IVT SOO. MA, mitral annulus.

December 2009, 29 patients were found to have VT originating from the body of the right ventricle.[21] Of these 29 patients, for 14, the SOO was within 2 cm of the tricuspid valve annulus (TVA); for 8 patients the SOO was from the basal RV, and for 7 patients, the SOO was from the apical RV segments. Among VTs from the TVA, the SOO for 8 patients was the free wall, and for 6 patients, the SOO was the septum. All but 1 RV basal or apical VT originated from the free wall. All had a left bundle branch block pattern. When the SOO was the free wall, the QRS duration was longer, and the S wave in lead V2 and V3 was deeper than in cases in which the SOO was from the septum. When the SOO was apical, the precordial R-wave transition was V6, or there was no transition; additionally, there was a smaller R wave in lead II and S wave in lead aVR compared with VT from basal RV.

MAPPING AND ABLATION

Localization of the SOO of the clinical tachycardia is accomplished by intracardiac activation and pace mapping. Careful analysis of the 12-lead ECG during tachycardia is very useful and can guide catheter localization to within 0.5 to 1 cm of the site of successful ablation.[11,12,22–24]

Although biplane fluoroscopy permits reasonable catheter localization, use of electroanatomic mapping and intracardiac echocardiography allows further refinement.

Activation and electroanatomic mapping can be used together to localize VT SOO (**Fig. 12**).[23–26] Typically, at the site of successful ablation, the local bipolar electrogram precedes QRS onset by 20 to 30 milliseconds or more.[26] Pace mapping is also performed to help confirm VT SOO. The mapping catheter is advanced to the area of interest (based on 12-lead ECG), and pacing is performed at a rate similar to the tachycardia cycle length. The goal is to achieve an identical match (all 12 leads) between the clinical arrhythmia and the pace map, paying particular attention to subtle features such as notches in the QRS complexes in various leads. Usually the site of earliest activation is also the site of the best pace map of the clinical arrhythmia.[27] The use of both localization techniques is helpful (**Fig. 13**).

Radiofrequency ablation, if done carefully (with attention to energy settings and the coronary anatomy), is a safe and highly effective (overall success rate >90%) treatment option (**Fig. 14**). For this reason, in the authors' opinion, catheter ablation may be considered first-line therapy for these arrhythmias.

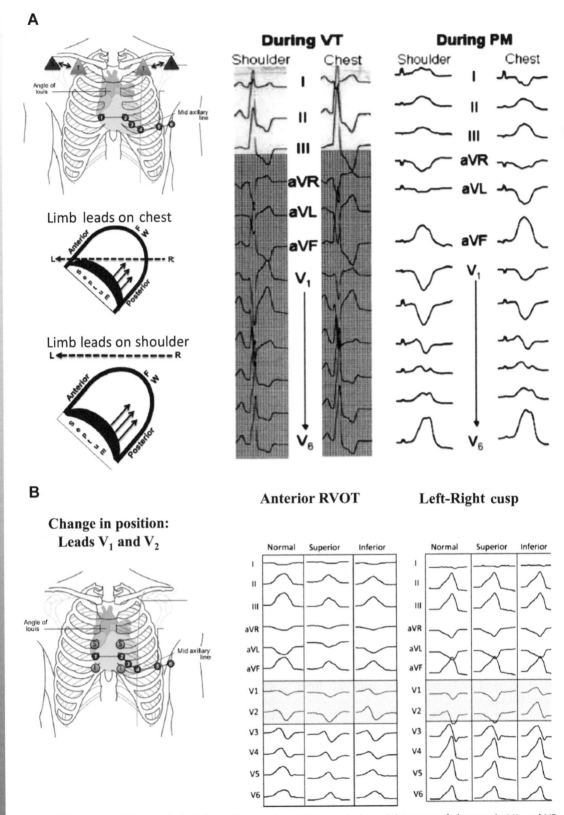

Fig. 11. (*A*) Impact of changes in limb lead placement on ECG morphology. (*B*) Impact of changes in V1 and V2 lead placement on ECG morphology.

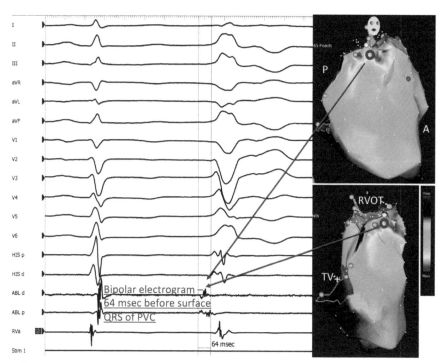

Fig. 12. Use of electroanatomic and activation mapping to facilitate localization of PVC site of origin. (*Right*) Activation mapping using local bipolar electrogram at suspected site of ventricular tachycardia origin demonstrates a signal 64 milliseconds earlier than the onset of the QRS on the 12-lead surface ECG. (*Left*) Use of 3-dimensional electroanatomic mapping to demonstrate anatomy and site of earliest activation. Color coding used to record activation timing of specific anatomic areas based on multiple points taken during tachycardia. TV, tricuspid valve.

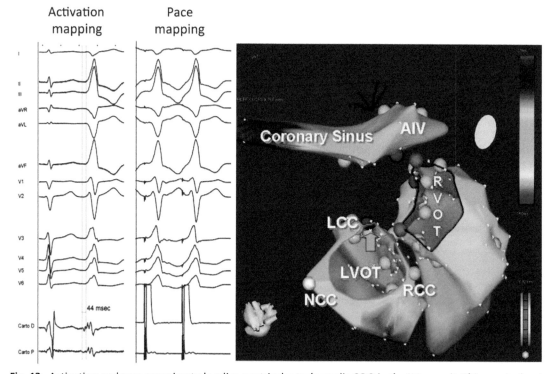

Fig. 13. Activation and pace mapping to localize ventricular tachycardia SOO in the LV summit. This area is closely abutted by the superior RVOT, aortic cusp region, junction of the great cardiac/interventricular vein, and the basal LV endocardium. Accurate localization of the SOO in this area is facilitated by electroanatomic and pace mapping. *Arrow* points to site of successful ablation. AIV, anterior interventricular vein; NCC, non-coronary cusp.

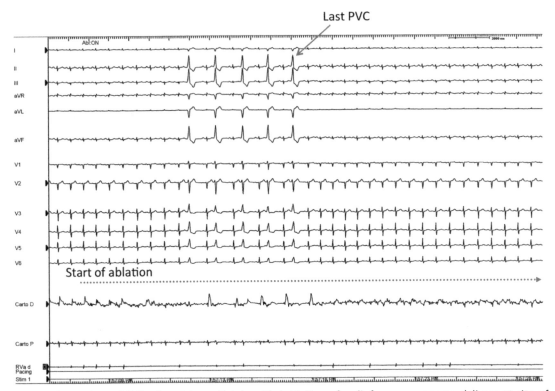

Fig. 14. Elimination of PVCs almost immediately with initiation of radiofrequency energy delivery at site of earliest activation and best pace map.

SUMMARY

Outflow tract tachycardias are thought to result from triggered activity. The 12-lead ECG during these arrhythmias manifests site-specific characteristics that can facilitate accurate localization. These arrhythmias, in general, are not life threatening and therefore can initially be managed conservatively. However, radiofrequency ablation can be curative in more than 90% of cases with a low risk (~1%) of serious complications.

REFERENCES

1. Zipes DP, Jalife J. Cardiac electrophysiology: from cell to bedside. Philadelphia: Elsevier Health Sciences; 2013.

2. Lerman BB, Belardinelli L, West GA, et al. Adenosine-sensitive ventricular tachycardia: evidence suggesting cyclic AMP-mediated triggered activity. Circulation 1986;74(2):270–80.

3. Lerman BB. Response of non reentrant catecholamine-mediated ventricular tachycardia to endogenous adenosine and acetylcholine. Evidence for myocardial receptor-mediated effects. Circulation 1993;87(2):382–90.

4. Lerman BB, Stein KM, Markowitz SM. Idiopathic right ventricular outflow tract tachycardia: a clinical

approach. Pacing Clin Electrophysiol 1996; 19(12 Pt 1):2120–37.

5. Buxton AE, Waxman HL, Marchlinski FE, et al. Right ventricular tachycardia: clinical and electrophysiologic characteristics. Circulation 1983;68(5): 917–27.

6. Proclemer A, Ciani R, Feruglio GA. Right ventricular tachycardia with left bundle branch block and inferior axis morphology: clinical and arrhythmological characteristics in 15 patients. Pacing Clin Electrophysiol 1989;12(6):977–89.

7. Lemery R, Brugada P, Bella PD, et al. Nonischemic ventricular tachycardia. Clinical course and long-term follow-up in patients without clinically overt heart disease. Circulation 1989;79(5):990–9.

8. Mont L, Seixas T, Brugada P, et al. Clinical and electrophysiologic characteristics of exercise-related idiopathic ventricular tachycardia. Am J Cardiol 1991;68(9):897–900.

9. Lerman BB, Stein KM, Markowitz SM. Mechanisms of idiopathic left ventricular tachycardia. J Cardiovasc Electrophysiol 1997;8(5):571–83. http://dx.doi.org/10.1111/j.1540-8167.1997.tb00826.x.

10. Betensky BP, Park RE, Marchlinski FE, et al. The V2 transition ratio: a new electrocardiographic criterion for distinguishing left from right ventricular outflow tract tachycardia origin. J Am Coll Cardiol 2011;

57(22):2255–62. http://dx.doi.org/10.1016/j.jacc.2011.01.035.

11. Dixit S, Gerstenfeld EP, Callans DJ, et al. Electrocardiographic patterns of superior right ventricular outflow tract tachycardias: distinguishing septal and free-wall sites of origin. J Cardiovasc Electrophysiol 2003;14(1):1–7. http://dx.doi.org/10.1046/j.1540-8167.2003.02404.x.

12. Callans DJ, Menz V, Schwartzman D, et al. Repetitive monomorphic tachycardia from the left ventricular outflow tract: electrocardiographic patterns consistent with a left ventricular site of origin. J Am Coll Cardiol 1997;29(5):1023–7.

13. Kanagaratnam L, Tomassoni G, Schweikert R, et al. Ventricular tachycardias arising from the aortic sinus of Valsalva: an under-recognized variant of left outflow tract ventricular tachycardia. J Am Coll Cardiol 2001;37(5):1408–14.

14. Ouyang F, Fotuhi P, Ho SY, et al. Repetitive monomorphic ventricular tachycardia originating from the aortic sinus cusp: electrocardiographic characterization for guiding catheter ablation. J Am Coll Cardiol 2002;39(3):500–8.

15. Lin D, Ilkhanoff L, Gerstenfeld E, et al. Twelve-lead electrocardiographic characteristics of the aortic cusp region guided by intracardiac echocardiography and electroanatomic mapping. Heart Rhythm 2008;5(5):663–9. http://dx.doi.org/10.1016/j.hrthm.2008.02.009.

16. Bala R, Garcia FC, Hutchinson MD, et al. Electrocardiographic and electrophysiologic features of ventricular arrhythmias originating from the right/left coronary cusp commissure. Heart Rhythm 2010;7(3):312–22. http://dx.doi.org/10.1016/j.hrthm.2009.11.017.

17. Cole CR, Marrouche NF, Natale A. Evaluation and management of ventricular outflow tract tachycardias. Card Electrophysiol Rev 2002;6(4):442–7.

18. Ito S, Tada H, Naito S, et al. Development and validation of an ECG algorithm for identifying the optimal ablation site for idiopathic ventricular outflow tract tachycardia. J Cardiovasc Electrophysiol 2003;14(12):1280–6.

19. Zhang F, Chen M, Yang B, et al. Electrocardiographic algorithm to identify the optimal target ablation site for idiopathic right ventricular outflow tract ventricular premature contraction. Europace 2009;11(9):1214–20.

20. Anter E, Frankel DS, Marchlinski FE, et al. Effect of electrocardiographic lead placement on localization of outflow tract tachycardias. Heart Rhythm 2012;9(5):697–703. http://dx.doi.org/10.1016/j.hrthm.2011.12.007.

21. Van Herendael H, Garcia F, Lin D, et al. Idiopathic right ventricular arrhythmias not arising from the outflow tract: prevalence, electrocardiographic characteristics, and outcome of catheter ablation. Heart Rhythm 2011;8(4):511–8. http://dx.doi.org/10.1016/j.hrthm.2010.11.044.

22. Dixit S, Gerstenfeld EP, Lin D, et al. Identification of distinct electrocardiographic patterns from the basal left ventricle: distinguishing medial and lateral sites of origin in patients with idiopathic ventricular tachycardia. Heart Rhythm 2005;2(5):485–91. http://dx.doi.org/10.1016/j.hrthm.2005.01.023.

23. Jadonath RL, Schwartzman DS, Preminger MW, et al. Utility of the 12-lead electrocardiogram in localizing the origin of right ventricular outflow tract tachycardia. Am Heart J 1995;130(5):1107–13.

24. Movsowitz C, Schwartzman D, Callans DJ, et al. Idiopathic right ventricular outflow tract tachycardia: narrowing the anatomic location for successful ablation. Am Heart J 1996;131(5):930–6.

25. Gepstein L, Hayam G, Ben-Haim SA. A novel method for nonfluoroscopic catheter-based electroanatomical mapping of the heart: in vitro and in vivo accuracy results. Circulation 1997;95(6):1611–22. http://dx.doi.org/10.1161/01.CIR.95.6.1611.

26. Marchlinski FE, Lin D, Dixit S, et al. Ventricular tachycardia from the aortic cusps: localization and ablation. In: Antonio R, editor. Cardiac arrhythmias. Milano (Italy): Springer Milan; 2004. p. 357–70. http://dx.doi.org/10.1007/978-88-470-2137-2_47.

27. Coggins DL, Lee RJ, Sweeney J, et al. Radiofrequency catheter ablation as a cure for idiopathic tachycardia of both left and right ventricular origin. J Am Coll Cardiol 1994;23(6):1333–41.

Fascicular Tachycardia

Rakesh Latchamsetty, MD*, Frank Bogun, MD

KEYWORDS

- Fascicular tachycardia • Ventricular tachycardia • Catheter ablation • Calcium channel blockers

KEY POINTS

- Fascicular ventricular tachycardia (VT) has characteristic ECG findings with a relatively narrow QRS complex, right bundle branch block (RBBB), and most commonly left axis deviation.
- Fascicular tachycardia is slightly more prevalent in men, usually presents in young adults without structural heart disease, and has a favorable long-term prognosis.
- The most frequently described tachycardia mechanism is a macroreentrant circuit involving the left posterior fascicle with an adjacent slowly conducting zone.
- Fascicular tachycardia is usually responsive both acutely and chronically to calcium channel blockers and resistant to adenosine.
- Catheter ablation offers high success rates for tachycardia elimination with low complication rates. Ablation can be performed during tachycardia or sinus rhythm.
- The Purkinje fiber system can also be involved in different ventricular arrhythmias in patients with structural heart disease.

VT emanating from the left fascicular system has been described as early as 1972[1] and has frequently been referred to as *verapamil-sensitive tachycardia* or *idiopathic left VT*. This reentrant intrafascicular tachycardia, however, is often but not universally responsive to verapamil,[2] and other forms of idiopathic left ventricular tachycardia exist (eg, left ventricular outflow tract tachycardia).

Idiopathic fascicular tachycardia is usually seen in patients between 15 and 40 years of age without structural heart disease and has a male predominance (60%–80%).[3] The most common presentation is exercise-induced palpitations but patients can also present with tachycardia at rest. Occasionally, incessant fascicular tachycardia can result in development of a tachycardia-induced cardiomyopathy and patients can present with symptoms of heart failure.[4] Sudden cardiac death is infrequent in patients with fascicular tachycardia.

Diagnosis of fascicular tachycardia is suggested by a correlation of symptoms to characteristic findings on ECG and verified through an electrophysiology study mapping the tachycardia to the left fascicular conduction system.

ECG CHARACTERISTICS OF FASCICULAR ARRHYTHMIAS

There are 3 recognized morphologies of fascicular VT classified by their regional involvement of the left fascicular system and characterized by distinct ECG patterns.[5] The most common form involves the left posterior fascicle and on ECG presents with a characteristic RBBB with left axis deviation (**Fig. 1**). Occasionally, the left anterior fascicle is involved and the subsequent ECG pattern displays an RBBB with a right axis pattern (**Fig. 2**). Rarely, an upper septal fascicular VT with a narrow QRS complex and normal or right axis deviation has also been described. The distribution of these 3 morphologies of fascicular VT are approximately 90%, 10%, and less than 1%, respectively.[5,6]

Left fascicular arrhythmias should be differentiated from those of papillary muscle origin, which

---

The authors have nothing to disclose.
Department of Internal Medicine, University of Michigan Hospital, 1500 East Medical Center Drive, Ann Arbor, MI 48109-5853, USA
* Corresponding author. CVC, SPC 5853, 1500 East Medical Center Drive, Ann Arbor, MI 48109-5853.
E-mail address: rakeshl@umich.edu

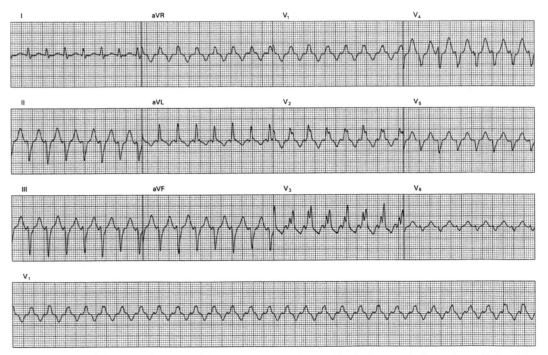

Fig. 1. Twelve-lead electrocardiogram of the most common form of fascicular ventricular tachycardia involving the left posterior fascicle. Note the characteristic right bundle branch block and left axis deviation.

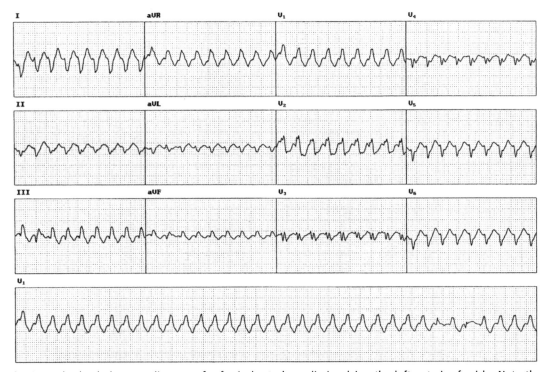

Fig. 2. Twelve-lead electrocardiogram of a fascicular tachycardia involving the left anterior fascicle. Note the right bundle branch block and rightward axis.

can have a similar axis (**Fig. 3**). A key distinguishing ECG characteristic between these 2 origins includes a narrower QRS (127 ± 11 vs 150 ± 15 milliseconds) in fascicular arrhythmias due to rapid activation via the specialized conduction system.[7] Another key feature of fascicular arrhythmias is the rsR pattern in V_1 indicating that the initial activation is in the direction of V_1 (ie, left to right) due to the left septal origin. Alternatively, arrhythmias originating from the papillary muscles often have a qR pattern in V_1. Fascicular arrhythmias more often have small Q waves in leads I and aVL, indicating early activation of the septum from left to right as opposed to a papillary muscle origin, which is further away from the septum. Arrhythmias originating from the distal Purkinje fiber system may be mapped to the papillary muscles close to the Purkinje-myocardial interface.[7,8]

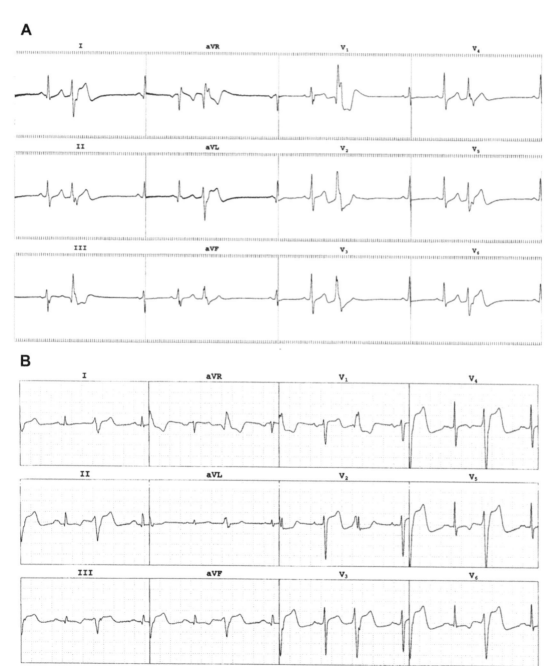

Fig. 3. Premature ventricular contractions from the left ventricular anterolateral (*A*) and posteromedial (*B*) papillary muscles. See text for discussion.

Both a myocardial origin and an origin from the Purkinje fiber system have been described for papillary muscle arrhythmias (**Fig. 4**).

The use of intracardiac ultrasound has been particularly helpful in mapping arrhythmias from the papillary muscles (**Fig. 5**). Some prior reports in patients with fascicular tachycardia have demonstrated the presence of a muscular strand, or false tendon, in the left ventricle between the septum and a papillary muscle.[9] Excision of this tendon has been reported to eliminate the tachycardia,[10] implicating the false tendon as a potential critical limb in the reentrant circuit. This finding, however, has not been universally seen.

In addition to the idiopathic fascicular tachycardias described, several other tachycardias involving the left fascicular system exist. Bundle branch reentry tachycardia forms a reentrant circuit using the His-Purkinje system with involvement of both the left and right bundles and is usually seen in patients with structural heart disease. This tachycardia more commonly presents with antegrade conduction through the right bundle branch manifesting as a left bundle branch block morphology on ECG but can also travel in the reverse direction (**Fig. 6**) and produce an RBBB morphology.

Patients postinfarction can also present with VT with a relatively narrow QRS complex (**Fig. 7**), where the tachycardia exit site involves the Purkinje network (**Fig. 8**). These VTs may be difficult to distinguish from idiopathic fascicular tachycardia by ECG alone but are also amenable to catheter ablation.[11] Q waves in the inferior leads are absent in patients with fascicular tachycardia without structural heart disease; in patients with prior inferior wall myocardial infarction, however, Q waves during VT indicate the presence of a prior myocardial infarction (see **Fig. 7**). Interfascicular reentry VT is another distinct ventricular arrhythmia that can have similar ECG findings and is usually seen in patients with large anterior wall myocardial infarctions. In these patients, an RBBB and delayed conduction in one of the left fascicles enables a macroreentrant circuit using both left fascicles. Most often, the anterior fascicle serves as the antegrade limb and the posterior fascicle as the retrograde limb (**Fig. 9**). A hallmark of interfascicular reentry VT is the similar QRS complex during sinus rhythm compared with VT with an RBBB morphology and left fascicular hemiblock. The His is activated retrograde and the His to ventricle interval during interfascicular reentry VT is shorter than during sinus rhythm.[5,12]

Frequent premature ventricular contractions (PVCs) can also be localized to the Purkinje system and be idiopathic or seen in patients with underlying structural heart disease. PVCs from the fascicular system have been reported to trigger ventricular fibrillation (VF) and can be a cause of sudden cardiac death.[13] PVC ablation in these patients may eliminate VF triggers.

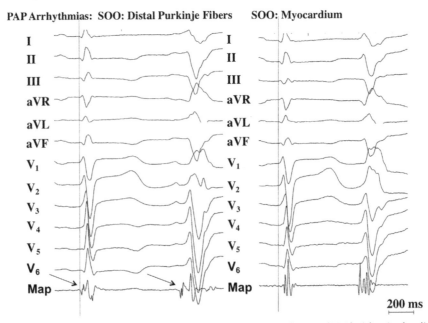

Fig. 4. Mapping of papillary (PAP) muscle arrhythmias can reveal a site of origin (SOO) either in the distal Purkinje fibers or in the ventricular myocardium. Note the sharp local Purkinje potentials (*arrows*) when the SOO is in the Purkinje fibers.

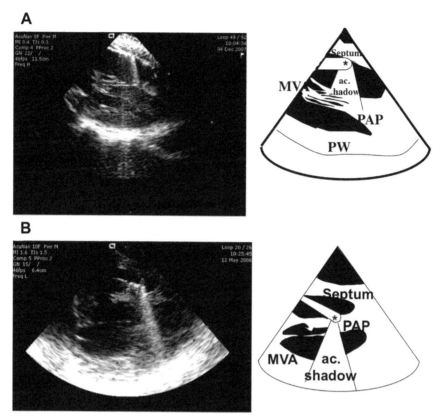

Fig. 5. Intracardiac echocardiography can offer real-time catheter visualization and facilitate navigation, particularly in relation to the papillary muscles. The image shows the catheter in contact with the left ventricular septum (*A*) and then along a papillary muscle (*B*). ac, acoustic; MVA, mitral valve annulus; PAP, papillary muscle; PW, posterior wall. (*Adapted from* Good E, Desjardins B, Jongnarangsin K, et al. Ventricular arrhythmias originating from a papillary muscle in patients without prior infarction: a comparison with fascicular arrhythmias. Heart Rhythm 2008;5:1534; with permission.)

A rare condition has also been described in patients that can present with frequent multifocal PVCs emanating from throughout the fascicular system (**Fig. 10**). Depending on the PVC burden, this may result in a PVC-induced cardiomyopathy. Given the more diffuse involvement of the Purkinje fiber system, catheter ablation in these patients can be more challenging. A mutation in the SCN5A gene has been implicated in a cohort of such patients and suggests a potential role for antiarrhythmic medications.[14]

MANAGEMENT
Medical Treatment

In a patient presenting in VT with ECG and clinical characteristics of idiopathic fascicular tachycardia, acute management focuses on restoration of sinus rhythm. Although direct current cardioversion is the preferred method in a hemodynamically unstable patient, conversion to sinus rhythm in a stable patient can often be achieved with intravenous verapamil. Although other idiopathic left VTs, such as outflow tract tachycardias, are also frequently sensitive to verapamil, fascicular tachycardia is differentiated by its resistance to treatment with adenosine.

It has been suggested that propagation through a slow conduction zone forms a requisite limb for reentrant fascicular tachycardia. Conduction through the distal portion of this zone seems primarily calcium channel dependent and may explain the sensitivity of fascicular tachycardia to verapamil.[15] Adenosine has been shown to terminate outflow tract tachycardias primarily targeting cyclic adenosine monophosphate-mediated triggered activity, and the lack of response in fascicular tachycardias lends further support to its proposed reentrant mechanism.[16]

Catheter Ablation

Chronic treatment of fascicular tachycardia can either be pharmacologic or through electrophysiology study and catheter ablation. Despite the

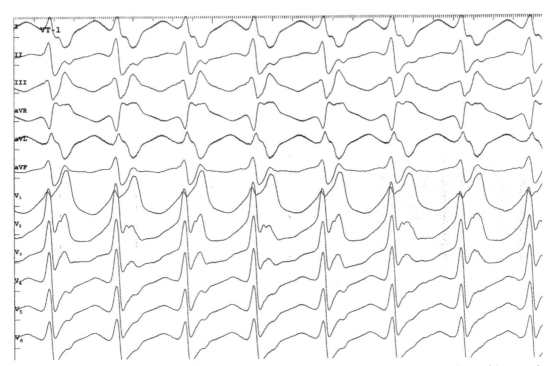

Fig. 6. Twelve-lead electrocardiogram (ECG) of a patient with bundle branch reentry tachycardia. In this example, the tachycardia propagates antegrade via the left bundle and retrograde via the right bundle, creating a right bundle branch block morphology on ECG.

effectiveness of intravenous verapamil during acute management of fascicular tachycardia, the response to oral verapamil for long-term suppression is variable.[17] In patients in whom symptoms are refractory to pharmacologic management, catheter ablation offers an effective and safe treatment option.

Description of recurrent VT sensitive to verapamil during electrophysiology study and successful catheter ablation of fascicular tachycardias has been reported as early as the 1980s.[18,19] Proposed mechanisms responsible for the tachycardia include automaticity, triggered activity, microreentry, and macroreentry.[19–21] The majority of evidence supports a macroreentrant circuit involving most commonly the left posterior fascicle with an adjacent area of slower conduction, which may also be part of the Purkinje fiber system.[21,22]

Different ablation strategies for patients with suspected fascicular tachycardia have been proposed and have resulted in successful ablation of fascicular VT. Although this discussion focuses on patients with fascicular tachycardia involving the left posterior fascicle, similar strategies are applied to the left anterior fascicle.

Mapping in patients with documented fascicular VT can be performed during sinus rhythm or during tachycardia. During sinus rhythm, Purkinje potentials are recorded along the posterior aspect of the interventricular septum, identifying the course of the posterior fascicle. Detailed mapping also reveals an adjacent area with lower-amplitude electrograms, suggesting the presence of a slow conduction zone involved in the reentrant circuit (**Fig. 11**).[22] As discussed later, in patients in whom tachycardia is not inducible, these serve as potential ablation targets.

If tachycardia is inducible and tolerated, mapping during tachycardia is preferable. Tachycardia is induced with atrial or ventricular pacing and sometimes requires administration of isoproterenol. The VT reentrant circuit proceeds antegrade over a zone of slow conduction and retrograde over the posterior fascicle (**Fig. 12**).[23] The turnaround point where the antegrade limb connects to the retrograde limb marks a site where the earliest Purkinje potentials during VT are recorded. The exit site is often more distal to this turnaround point.

Multiple approaches have been described to target different components of the reentrant circuit. One approach targets the antegrade limb of slow conduction during VT, where lower-amplitude potentials preceding the QRS complex by approximately 30 to 60 ms[22,24] are identified

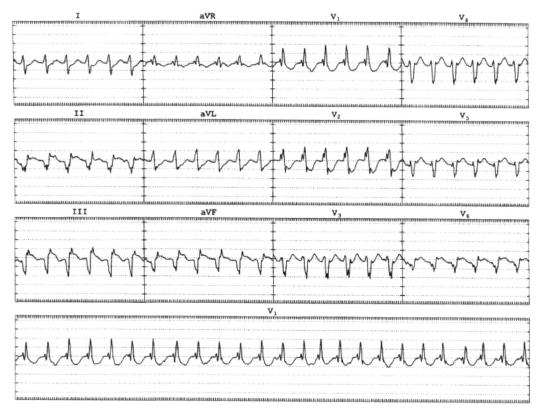

Fig. 7. Twelve-lead electrocardiogram of a postinfarction ventricular tachycardia with exit site localized to the left posterior fascicle. Note the relatively narrow QRS complex and Q waves present in the inferior leads.

during late diastole (**Fig. 13**). Often Purkinje potentials are also present at these sites, indicating retrograde activation via the posterior fascicle. The earliest Purkinje potential, which typically precedes the QRS complex by approximately 15 to 40 ms, can also be targeted.[5,22,24] The posterior fascicle itself can also be targeted and ablation at any point in its course may eliminate VT. A distal location is preferable to avoid damage to the proximal conduction system.

Mechanical trauma to the fascicles may render fascicular VTs noninducible. In these patients as well as in patients without inducible VT at baseline, ablation is performed during sinus rhythm. Pace mapping is often used when mapping is performed for reentrant VT in an attempt to identify the VT exit site. Unfortunately, in fascicular VT, pace mapping is not as reliable in identifying an optimal target site for ablation during sinus rhythm because the critical parts of the reentrant circuit

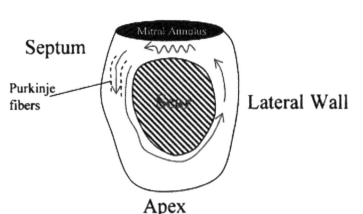

Fig. 8. Schematic illustration of a reentrant circuit around an inferoseptal scar. Surviving muscle bundles within the myocardium and in the Purkinje system are components of the reentrant circuit with the exit site at the Purkinje fibers. (*From* Bogun F, Good E, Reich S, et al. Role of purkinje fibers in post-infarction ventricular tachycardia. J Am Coll Cardiol 2006;48:2506; with permission.)

Interfascicular Reentry

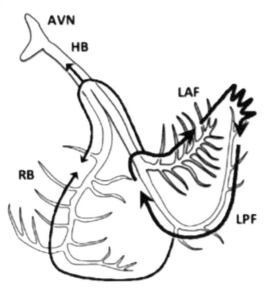

Fig. 9. Schematic illustration of an interfascicular reentrant circuit with antegrade conduction over the left anterior fascicle and retrograde conduction over the left posterior fascicle. Note the underlying right bundle branch block. AVN, atrioventricular node; HB, his bundle; LAF, left anterior fascicle; LPF, left posterior fascicle; RB, right bundle. (*From* Nogami A. Purkinje-related arrhythmias part I: monomorphic ventricular tachycardias. Pacing Clin Electrophysiol 2011;34:643; with permission.)

may be remote from the VT exit site into the ventricular myocardium.[25] Pacing at successful ablation sites often captures both local myocardial tissue and the Purkinje fiber system, generating a QRS morphology that can be very different from the QRS morphology of the clinical VT, whereas pacing at a distal location closer to the myocardial breakthrough site may provide an excellent match with the targeted VT but may not represent an effective ablation site (**Fig. 14**). Some investigators, however, have described ablation of the more distally located Purkinje-myocardial interface. Effective ablations have been described using this area as a target; however, more extensive ablation lesions are required here to render VT noninducible, most likely because of arborization of the distal Purkinje fiber system.[26] An advantage of this technique is that the conduction in the fascicular system is not impaired postablation.

Another ablation strategy during sinus rhythm targets the area of slow conduction that is adjacent to the posterior fascicle. At these sites, both low-amplitude electrograms attributable to the slow conduction zone and sharp and more prominent Purkinje potentials are present (see **Fig. 11**).[22] Conduction through the distal portion of the slow conduction zone during sinus rhythm is believed retrograde and the identification of the earliest of these retrograde signals has been

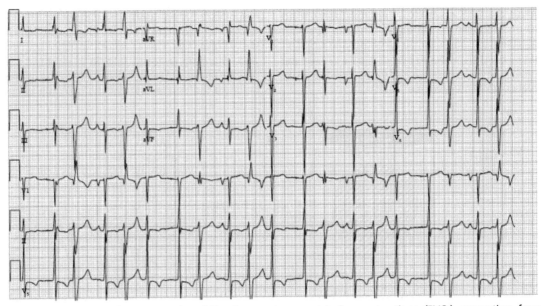

Fig. 10. Patient with frequent and multifocal premature ventricular contractions (PVCs) emanating from throughout the conduction system. Note the narrow QRS morphologies of the PVCs and varying axes.

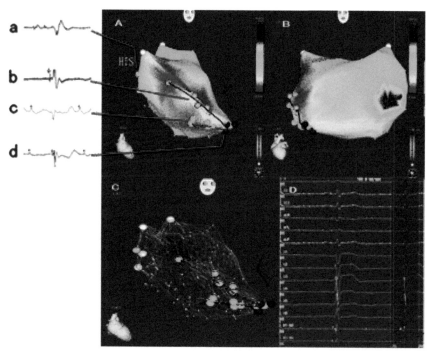

Fig. 11. Identification of the left posterior fascicle and slow conduction zone during sinus rhythm in patients with idiopathic fascicular tachycardia. Note that the slow conduction zone characterized with diastolic potentials (DPs) is located within the inferoposterior septum and marked with green tags; the area with Purkinje potentials (PP) is located within the posterior septum and marked with pink tags. The black line delineates part of the left posterior fascicle and the red line represents the slow conduction zone. From the intracardiac electrograms a–d, the arrows indicate the PP, the asterisks indicate the DP. (*A*) Right anterior oblique view. (*B*) Left anterior oblique view. (*C*) Mesh mapping at right anterior oblique view. (*D*) The electroanatomic map of the effective target site. (*From* Chu J, Sun Y, Zhao Y, et al. Identification of the slow conduction zone in a macroreentry circuit of verapamil-sensitive idiopathic left ventricular tachycardia using electroanatomic mapping. J Cardiovasc Electrophysiol 2012;23:841; with permission.)

proposed as the ideal ablation target when ablating during sinus rhythm.[21] In many patients, however, the lower-amplitude signals associated with a proposed slow conduction zone are either not identified or similar nonspecific electrograms are seen ubiquitously throughout the ventricular chamber.

Yet another ablation strategy, particularly useful in patients in whom sustained VT is not inducible, is the empiric creation of a linear lesion set perpendicular to the long axis of the ventricle at the mid- to midinferior septum. Ablation here is likely to transect the reentrant circuit and has been shown to have favorable outcomes, albeit with risk of left posterior fascicular block.[27] The long-term ramifications of such a block are not clear and creating a block has been proposed as an effective endpoint to ablation.

Targeted endpoints to the ablation can vary and can include termination of induced tachycardia, noninducibility, ablation, and possible elimination of target electrograms during sinus rhythm, or development of left posterior fascicular block. Wissner and colleagues[28] targeted ablation at the earliest retrograde Purkinje potential primarily during sinus rhythm in 24 patients and showed a 92% arrhythmia-free survival at a median of 8.9 years' follow-up with no patients suffering a left posterior fascicular block. In a recent study by Kataria and colleagues,[26] the distal posterior fascicle was targeted until block was achieved from the local myocardium to the fascicle and 100% arrhythmia-free survival was reported in 15 patients at a mean follow-up of 20.8 months. Overall, long-term success rates seem generally high and exceed 90% to 95%.[29] Although complication rates are difficult to accurately ascertain due to the limited sample sizes, most studies report no or rare complications.[29] In particular, atrioventricular block is very rare due to the distal ablation targets and left posterior fascicular block may or may not be an intended goal of ablation.

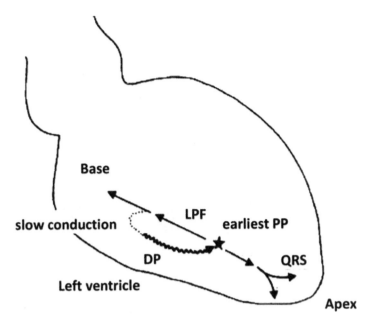

Fig. 12. Schematic illustration of the reentrant circuit of idiopathic fascicular tachycardia. During tachycardia, conduction is antegrade through a zone of slow conduction and retrograde over the left posterior fascicle (LPF). Low-amplitude signals (DP) at the terminal end of the slowly conducting limb or sharp and early Purkinje potentials (PP) are potential ablation targets during tachycardia. (*Adapted from* Aiba T, Suyama K, Aihara N, et al. The role of Purkinje and pre-Purkinje potentials in the reentrant circuit of verapamil-sensitive idiopathic LV tachycardia. Pacing Clin Electrophysiol 2001;24:342; with permission.)

Despite involvement of similar anatomic structures, ablation strategies and targets for other ventricular arrhythmias from the Purkinje system can be quite different. In patients with PVCs originating from the fascicles or the Purkinje fiber system, mapping of the earliest Purkinje potential during PVCs identifies the site of origin where radiofrequency energy can be applied (**Fig. 15**). In patients

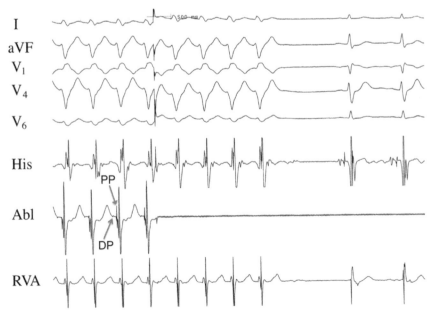

Fig. 13. Successful site of ablation terminating fascicular tachycardia. Note the presence of both a sharp Purkinje potential (PP) as well as a late and low-amplitude diastolic potential (DP) on the ablation electrogram.

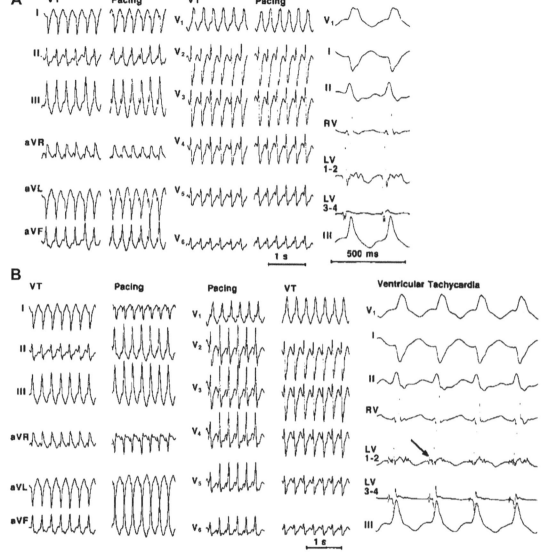

Fig. 14. (*A*) Pacemapping performed on a patient with fascicular tachycardia involving the anterior fascicle revealed an excellent match to the clinical ventricular tachycardia (VT) at the site of exit to the ventricular myocardium. Ablation here had no effect on the VT. Note the local electrogram recorded from the distal ablation catheter preceded the QRS complex by 20 ms. (*B*) Pace mapping from the site of the earliest sharp Purkinje potentials during tachycardia revealed a poor match to the clinical VT due to capture of local myocardial tissue in addition to the anterior fascicle. The local Purkinje potential during VT on the distal ablation catheter (*arrow*) preceded the QRS complex by 30 ms and ablation here resulted in termination of the VT. (*From* Bogun F, El-Atassi R, Daoud E, et al. Radiofrequency ablation of idiopathic left anterior fascicular tachycardia. J Cardiovasc Electrophysiol 1995;6:1114, 1115; with permission.)

with prior myocardial infarction and VT with an exit site involving the fascicular system, parts of the reentrant circuit (often located within the inferior wall scar when the posterior fascicle is involved in the VT exit) can be targeted or the exit site containing fascicular potentials can be targeted (see **Fig. 8**). The presence of concealed entrainment with matching stimulus-QRS and electrogram-QRS intervals helps to identify critical components of the reentry circuit.[11]

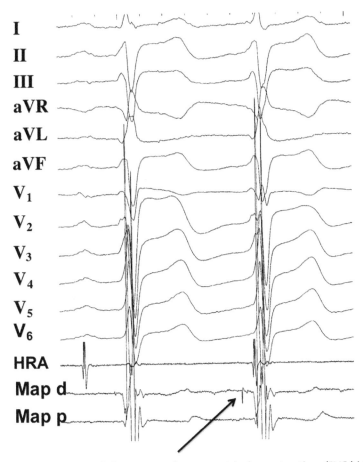

Fig. 15. Activation map in a patient with frequent premature ventricular contractions (PVCs) identified the site of origin in the left posterior fascicle. At this successful ablation site, during PVCs a sharp and early Purkinje potential (*arrow*) is seen on the distal ablation catheter (Map d) electrogram. HRA, high right atrium; Map p, proximal ablation.

SUMMARY

Fascicular VT is a reentrant tachycardia involving most commonly the left posterior fascicle with an overall favorable prognosis. Patients most commonly present with palpitations during exercise although the arrhythmia can also present at rest. Rarely, fascicular tachycardia is incessant and causes a tachycardia-mediated cardiomyopathy. Sudden cardiac death is not typically seen with this arrhythmia. Diagnosis is suggested by characteristic findings on ECG and confirmed through electrophysiology study. The rhythm is acutely susceptible to medical management most commonly with intravenous verapamil. Long-term management can be attempted with oral calcium channel blockade with varying accounts of success. Catheter ablation has a high curative rate with infrequent complications and can be considered in patients refractory to medical management or as a first-line therapy in patients who prefer to avoid long-term pharmacologic therapy or in whom medical management my be contraindicated. Ablation targets and endpoints are varied but suitable targets can be identified during tachycardia or sinus rhythm.

REFERENCES

1. Cohen HC, Gozo EG, Pick A. Ventricular tachycardia with narrow QRS complexes (left posterior fascicular tachycardia). Circulation 1972;45:1035–43.
2. Morgera T, Hrovatin E, Mazzone C, et al. Clinical spectrum of fascicular tachycardia. J Cardiovasc Med (Hagerstown) 2013;14:791–8.
3. Zipes D, Jalife J, Lerman B. Cardiac electrophysiology, from cell to bedside. Philadelphia: Saunders Elsevier; 2009.
4. Velázquez-Rodríguez E, Rodríguez-Piña H, Pacheco-Bouthillier A, et al. Cardiomyopathy induced by incessant fascicular ventricular tachycardia. Arch Cardiol Mex 2013;83:194–8.

5. Nogami A. Purkinje-related arrhythmias part I: monomorphic ventricular tachycardias. Pacing Clin Electrophysiol 2011;34:624–50.

6. Nogami A. Idiopathic left ventricular tachycardia: assessment and treatment. Card Electrophysiol Rev 2002;6:448–57.

7. Good E, Desjardins B, Jongnarangsin K, et al. Ventricular arrhythmias originating from a papillary muscle in patients without prior infarction: a comparison with fascicular arrhythmias. Heart Rhythm 2008;5: 1530–7.

8. Yokokawa M, Good E, Desjardins B, et al. Predictors of successful catheter ablation of ventricular arrhythmias arising from the papillary muscles. Heart Rhythm 2010;7(11):1654–9.

9. Thakur RK, Klein GJ, Sivaram CA, et al. Anatomic substrate for idiopathic left ventricular tachycardia. Circulation 1996;93:497–501.

10. Suwa M, Yoneda Y, Nagao H, et al. Surgical correction of idiopathic paroxysmal ventricular tachycardia possibly related to left ventricular false tendon. Am J Cardiol 1989;64:1217–20.

11. Bogun F, Good E, Reich S, et al. Role of purkinje fibers in post-infarction ventricular tachycardia. J Am Coll Cardiol 2006;48:2500–7.

12. Josephson M. Clinical cardiac electrophysiology, techniques and interpretations. Philadelphia: Lippincott Williams & Wilkins; 2008.

13. Haïssaguerre M, Shoda M, Jaïs P, et al. Mapping and ablation of idiopathic ventricular fibrillation. Circulation 2002;106:962–7.

14. Laurent G, Saal S, Amarouch MY, et al. Multifocal ectopic purkinje-related premature contractions: a new scn5a-related cardiac channelopathy. J Am Coll Cardiol 2012;60:144–56.

15. Tsuchiya T, Okumura K, Honda T, et al. Effects of verapamil and lidocaine on two components of the re-entry circuit of verapamil-sensitive idiopathic left ventricular tachycardia. J Am Coll Cardiol 2001;37:1415–21.

16. Griffith MJ, Garratt CJ, Rowland E, et al. Effects of intravenous adenosine on verapamil-sensitive "idiopathic" ventricular tachycardia. Am J Cardiol 1994; 73:759–64.

17. Chiarandà G, Di Guardo G, Gulizia M, et al. Fascicular ventricular tachycardia. Ital Heart J Suppl 2001; 2:1181–6 [in Italian].

18. Ruffy R, Kim SS, Lal R. Paroxysmal fascicular tachycardia: electrophysiologic characteristics and treatment by catheter ablation. J Am Coll Cardiol 1985; 5:1008–14.

19. Belhassen B, Rotmensch HH, Laniado S. Response of recurrent sustained ventricular tachycardia to verapamil. Br Heart J 1981;46:679–82.

20. Kottkamp H, Chen X, Hindricks G, et al. Radiofrequency catheter ablation of idiopathic left ventricular tachycardia: further evidence for microentry as the underlying mechanism. J Cardiovasc Electrophysiol 1994;5:268–73.

21. Ouyang F, Cappato R, Ernst S, et al. Electroanatomic substrate of idiopathic left ventricular tachycardia: unidirectional block and macroreentry within the purkinje network. Circulation 2002;105:462–9.

22. Chu J, Sun Y, Zhao Y, et al. Identification of the slow conduction zone in a macroreentry circuit of verapamil-sensitive idiopathic left ventricular tachycardia using electroanatomic mapping. J Cardiovasc Electrophysiol 2012;23:840–5.

23. Aiba T, Suyama K, Aihara N, et al. The role of purkinje and pre-purkinje potentials in the reentrant circuit of verapamil-sensitive idiopathic LV tachycardia. Pacing Clin Electrophysiol 2001;24:333–44.

24. Schreiber D, Kottkamp H. Ablation of idiopathic ventricular tachycardia. Curr Cardiol Rep 2010;12: 382–8.

25. Bogun F, El-Atassi R, Daoud E, et al. Radiofrequency ablation of idiopathic left anterior fascicular tachycardia. J Cardiovasc Electrophysiol 1995;6:1113–6.

26. Kataria V, Yaduvanshi A, Kumar M, et al. Demonstration of posterior fascicle to myocardial conduction block during ablation of idiopathic left ventricular tachycardia: an electrophysiological predictor of long-term success. Heart Rhythm 2013;10:638–45.

27. Lin D, Hsia HH, Gerstenfeld EP, et al. Idiopathic fascicular left ventricular tachycardia: linear ablation lesion strategy for noninducible or nonsustained tachycardia. Heart Rhythm 2005;2:934–9.

28. Wissner E, Menon SY, Metzner A, et al. Long-term outcome after catheter ablation for left posterior fascicular ventricular tachycardia without development of left posterior fascicular block. J Cardiovasc Electrophysiol 2012;23:1179–84.

29. Aliot EM, Stevenson WG, Almendral-Garrote JM, et al. EHRA/HRS expert consensus on catheter ablation of ventricular arrhythmias: developed in a partnership with the European Heart Rhythm Association (EHRA), a Registered Branch of the European Society of Cardiology (ESC), and the Heart Rhythm Society (HRS); in collaboration with the American College of Cardiology (ACC) and the American Heart Association (AHA). Heart Rhythm 2009;6: 886–933.

Ventricular Tachycardia Originating from Unusual Sites

Srikant Duggirala, MD, Edward P. Gerstenfeld, MD*

KEYWORDS

- Ventricular tachycardia • Ablation • Electrocardiography • Electrogram • Papillary muscle

KEY POINTS

- Recognition of typical electrocardiogram patterns and careful mapping are critical for localizing ventricular arrhythmia (VAs) of unusual origin.
- VAs from the right parahisian region can be differentiated from typical right ventricle outflow tract VAs by more positive R wave in lead I and flat or w pattern in lead aVL.
- Right ventricular moderator band VAs are rare and have a left bundle branch block (LBBB) pattern with late precordial transition (>V5).
- Left ventricular posterior papillary muscle premature ventricular complexes (PVCs) have a right bundle branch (RBB)/left axis that can be differentiated from posterior fascicular PVCs by a qR pattern in lead V1 and wider QRS.
- Mitral annular PVCs have a RBB pattern with positive precordial concordance.
- VAs from the great cardiac vein/anterior interventricular vein have LBBB/inferior axes with early precordial transition (by V2) and QS patterns in lead I.
- VAs from the basal cardiac crux have left bundle branch/superior axes with delayed intrinsicoid deflection.

INTRODUCTION

Ventricular arrhythmias (VAs) in the absence of structural heart disease (idiopathic) can present as premature ventricular contractions (PVCs) or sustained ventricular tachycardia (VT) and account for approximately 10% of patients with VAs. Although most of these arrhythmias originate from the right ventricular outflow tract (RVOT) or left ventricular outflow tract (LVOT), VT can also arise from other locations.[1,2] Distinct electrocardiographic and electrophysiologic features can help localize these arrhythmias. In the appropriate patients, radiofrequency (RF) catheter ablation is an effective treatment of patients with idiopathic VT.[3,4] This article discusses the electrocardiographic features of the more unusual origins of idiopathic VT. In addition, it discusses some electrophysiologic parameters and catheter-based ablation techniques used in the treatment of these arrhythmias.

RIGHT VENTRICLE
Tricuspid Annulus

The tricuspid annular region includes arrhythmias with origins from the parahisian region, midseptum, inferior tricuspid annulus, and the annular free wall. In a study of 454 consecutive patients with symptomatic VAs who underwent RF catheter

Disclosures: None.
Section of Cardiac Electrophysiology, University of California, San Francisco, 500 Parnassus Avenue, MUE 434, San Francisco, CA 94143-1354, USA
* Corresponding author. MU-East 4th Floor, 500 Parnassus Avenue, MUE 434, San Francisco, CA 94143-1354.
E-mail address: egerstenfeld@medicine.ucsf.edu

cardiacEP.theclinics.com

ablation, Tada and colleagues[5] identified 38 patients (8%) with VAs originating from the tricuspid annulus. In 74% of patients VAs arose from the septal portion of the annulus, and in 26% VAs arose from the free-wall portion of the annulus. Of those that originated from the septal portion of the annulus, nearly three-quarters originated from the anteroseptum, above the His bundle, and the remaining from the midseptum or posteroseptum. The mean QRS duration was 149 ± 20 milliseconds. All VAs originating from the tricuspid annulus showed a left bundle branch morphology (QS in V1 for anteroseptal and rS for anterior and posterolateral origins). Because the tricuspid annulus is positioned inferiorly and posteriorly to the RVOT (**Fig. 1**), the QRS axis is typically leftward and less inferiorly or superiorly directed. The precordial lead transition depends on the site of origin, with free-wall VT/PVCs all having a later transition to R>S (typically >V3); however, this was also noted in about 50% of septal VT/PVCs. In addition, VT/PVCs originating from the free wall were more likely to have QRS notching (78% vs 11%) and a longer QRS duration (167 vs 143 milliseconds). When VAs originated from the annular septum, both ventricles were activated

simultaneously, resulting in a shorter QRS duration and absence of QRS notching, whereas late activation of the left ventricular free wall accounted for the notching in free-wall VTs.

Parahisian VAs are commonly encountered and warrant special consideration. Yamauchi and colleagues[6] evaluated the electrocardiogram (ECG) characteristics of VAs originating from the His bundle in 10 patients and compared these ECG characteristics with 81 patients with RVOT VAs.

There were several ECG characteristics that could be used to differentiate VAs that originate from the His bundle from the RVOT (**Fig. 2**). Patterns that favored a His bundle origin over the RVOT included a QS pattern in lead V1 (80% vs 17%), an early precordial transition by V2/V3 (80% vs 22%), and the presence of an R wave in lead aVL (60% vs 9%). In our experience, when an RSR' (w) pattern is present in lead aVL in an inferiorly directed LBBB morphology VA, it is a valuable ECG finding suggesting a parahisian origin.[7] In addition, a significantly narrower QRS complex (113 vs 131 milliseconds) and a lower R-wave voltage ratio index (lead III/II) favored the His bundle group (65% vs 97%), meaning that lead III<II was typically present in His the bundle group. Furthermore, significantly taller R-wave amplitudes in leads V5 (2.10 vs 1.37 mV) and V6 (2.08 vs 1.36 mV) were seen the His bundle group compared with the RVOT group. The His bundle is located more inferiorly and posteriorly to the RVOT, explaining the taller, monophasic R wave in lead I, flat or w-pattern in aVL, and lower QRS amplitude in lead III. Parahisian VAs also depolarize the His-Purkinje system resulting in a shorter QRS duration and taller QRS complexes in V5 and V6.

The His bundle region is also in close proximity to the right and noncoronary aortic cusps, and thus can show similar electrocardiographic features to aortic cusp VAs.[8,9] In a study of 13 patients, Yamada and colleagues[8] identified 7 patients with ventricular arrhythmias originating from the His bundle and compared these features with those originating from the right and noncoronary cusps (6 patients). A later precordial transition (V4 vs V2) was specific for distinguishing VAs from the His bundle region from the aortic sinus cusps, but the sensitivity was low because of significant overlap among the groups. Both sites show R waves in lead I, but a QS in lead aVL was more commonly seen with VAs originating from the aortic sinus cusps.

During mapping of parahisian VAs, the presence of a QS pattern on the unipolar recording at the ablation site can be helpful to identify local activation; mapping of the aortic right and noncoronary cusps and left parahisian sites is recommended to identify the earliest site of activation.[8]

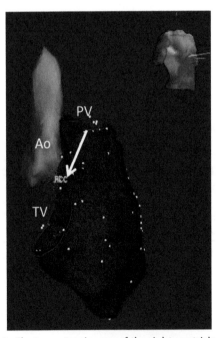

Fig. 1. Electroanatomic map of the right ventricle and aortic root in the right anterior oblique (RAO) projection. Note that the tricuspid annulus is inferior and posterior to the RVOT, which explains why PVCs/VT originating from the tricuspid annulus are less inferiorly directed and more positive in lead I compared with typical RVOT PVCs. Ao, aorta; PV, pulmonic valve; RCC, right coronary cusp; TV, tricuspid valve.

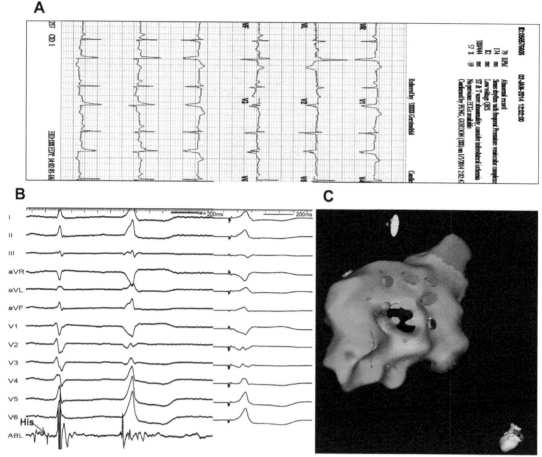

Fig. 2. Parahisian PVC. (*A*) The 12-lead ECG shows LBBB morphology (QS in V1) with left/inferior axis and precordial transition by lead V4. QRS duration is 140 milliseconds, and there is a monophasic tall R in lead I. Note smaller lead III/II ratio and positive R in aVL, which distinguishes the morphology of RV outflow tract PVCs. (*B*) The PVC and best pace map during electrophysiology study. Note the His deflection (*red arrow*) on the ablation catheter during sinus rhythm. (*C*) Electroanatomic map showing ablation site just inferior to the sites where a His bundle deflection was recorded (red tag, ablation sites; yellow tag, His bundle deflection sites).

Electrophysiologists may be less aggressive during ablation near the His bundle given the risk of injuring the atrioventricular conduction system and creating atrioventricular block; difficulty with catheter stability and adequate tissue contact can contribute to higher early recurrence rates.[10] In some cases of true parahisian origin, consideration can be given to the use of focal cryoablation to further minimize the risk to the atrioventricular conduction system and achieve more stable catheter contact. Ablation from the right coronary cusp, which is above the His bundle, is also less likely to lead to atrioventricular block than ablation from the right ventricle.

Papillary Muscles of the Right Ventricle

The anatomy of the right ventricular papillary muscles is unique compared to those of the left ventricle (**Fig. 3**). The papillary muscles make up the inlet portion of the right ventricle. The medial (or septal) papillary muscle supports the commissure between the septal and anterosuperior leaflet of the tricuspid valve. The anterosuperior leaflet is larger and is supported by a larger papillary muscle that typically arises from the moderator band. In addition, several small papillary muscles that arise from the diaphragmatic portion of the right ventricle support the posterior leaflet.[11,12]

VAs rarely originate from the right ventricular papillary muscles. Crawford and colleagues[13] described a series of 8 patients with right ventricular papillary muscle PVCs and compared this cohort with a series of patients with PVCs originating from the RVOT. Right VTs originating from the papillary muscles showed left bundle branch morphology (either rs or QS in V1). A later precordial transition (>V4) with a left/superior axis was

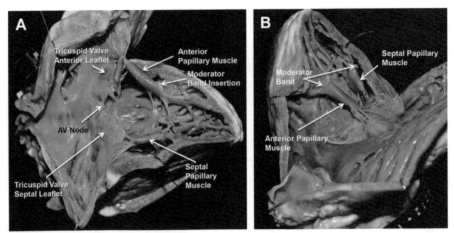

Fig. 3. Anatomy of the right ventricular papillary muscles. (*A*) A structurally normal heart identifying the papillary muscles, moderator band, and tricuspid valve leaflets in the lateral view with lateral wall exposed. (*B*) The same heart from the left superior view. The moderator band was cut during dissection; however, the insertion between the anterior papillary muscle and free wall can be seen.

seen in those originating from either the anterior or posterior papillary muscles, because these structures are located toward the apex of the right ventricle. In contrast, the septal papillary muscle is inserted toward the septal base of the right ventricle and thus an earlier precordial transition (≤V4) with a left/inferiorly directed axis is typically seen. Right ventricular papillary muscle VT/PVCs generally can be distinguished from those originating from the RVOT by a higher prevalence of notching in the precordial leads, a longer QRS duration (163 vs 141 milliseconds), a superior or less inferior axis, and typically a later precordial transition (**Fig. 4**).

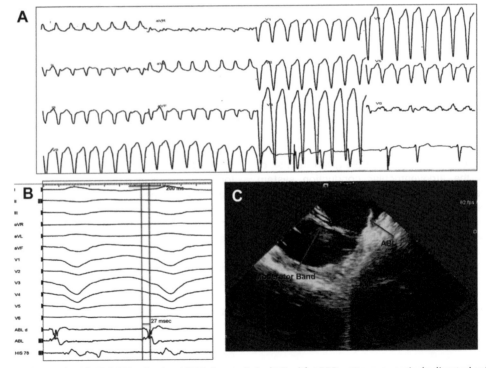

Fig. 4. Moderator band VT. (*A*) Twelve-lead ECG shows clinical VT with LBBB pattern, superiorly directed axis, and a late precordial lead transition. (*B*) Site of earliest activation before ablation with local activation 27 milliseconds before QRS onset. (*C*) Intracardiac echo image shows moderator band and ablation catheter (ABL) at the moderator band insertion site. Note echogenic area at the tip of the ablation catheter present after RF ablation.

During electrophysiologic studies, these arrhythmias were not inducible by either atrial-programmed or ventricular-programmed stimulation; induction required either burst pacing or isoproterenol infusion. Furthermore, the VT could not be entrained or terminated with overdrive pacing, suggesting automaticity rather than reentry. Two of the 8 patients also displayed a Purkinje potential at the ablation site, suggesting that the Purkinje fibers may play a role in the arrhythmia and may be similar to those described in left-sided papillary muscle VTs.[13,14] The use of real-time imaging with intracardiac echocardiography is helpful to confirm location and adequate catheter contact (see **Fig. 4**).

LEFT VENTRICLE
Mitral Annulus

In a study by Tada and colleagues,[15] the incidence of VT or PVCs originating from the mitral annulus was approximately 5%. The prevalence of mitral annular VT (MAVT) can be further designated by its location of origin, which includes the anterolateral (58%), posterior (11%), or posteroseptal (31%) sites. All patients with MAVT had a right bundle branch pattern (precordial R-wave transition usually occurs by V1 with positive concordance, and no cases had a precordial transition beyond V2), mean QRS duration of 154 ± 20

milliseconds, and the presence of an S wave in lead V6 (**Fig. 5**). The early transition and positive R-wave concordance is seen because the origin of the tachycardia initiates at the posterior base of the left ventricle and ventricular depolarization proceeds anteriorly toward the left ventricular apex and precordial leads. In anterolateral MAVT, the QRS polarity is positive in the inferior leads and negative in leads I and aVL. In contrast, posterior/posteroseptal leaflet MAVT/PVC, the polarity is negative in the inferior leads and positive in I and aVL. All anterior and posterior leaflet MAVT originating from the left ventricular free wall showed a longer QRS duration (>140 milliseconds) compared with the posteroseptal MAVT (<140 milliseconds) and showed notching of the terminal R wave in anterior leaflet MAVT or the Q wave in posterior leaflet MAVT of the inferior leads. Overall, the longer QRS duration and notching of the late phase of the QRS complex in the inferior leads was helpful in distinguishing posterior and anterolateral MAVT from posteroseptal MAVT. Posteroseptal MAVT can be further distinguished from posterior MAVT by the presence of a negative component in the QRS in V1 (qR, qr, rS, rs, or QS) and a greater Q-wave ratio of lead III to lead II (III/II) (2.3 ± 0.6 vs 1.5 ± 0.3). Kumagai and colleagues[16] corroborated similar ECG findings of MAVT and, during electrophysiologic testing, the arrhythmia occurred spontaneously or was induced with either isoproterenol

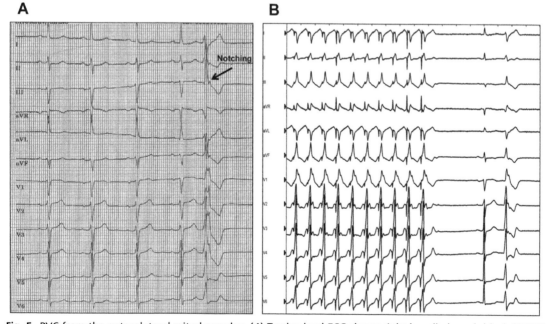

A   **B**

Fig. 5. PVC from the anterolateral mitral annulus. (A) Twelve-lead ECG shows right bundle branch block (RBBB) pattern with positive concordance in the precordial leads and inferiorly directed axis. QRS duration is 170 milliseconds with an rS in leads I and aVL. There is notching in the terminal portion of the QRS in the inferior leads (arrow). (B) Pace map from the anterolateral mitral annulus during electrophysiologic study.

or ventricular-programmed stimulation. The site of origin could easily be identified using pace mapping and successful ablation was achieved in all patients with RF energy.[15]

Papillary Muscles of the Left Ventricle

In the left ventricle there are 2 groups of papillary muscles: the posteromedial and anterolateral papillary muscles (**Fig. 6**). The posteromedial papillary muscle is located posteriorly near the junction of the posterior free wall and interventricular septum. The anterolateral papillary muscle is typically attached to the anterolateral endocardial surface. The papillary muscles are typically oriented parallel to the axis of the left ventricular cavity. During left ventricular hypertrophy the papillary muscles thicken in diameter and the orientation is typically preserved. However, in dilated cardiomyopathies, the dilatation typically affects the apical portion of the ventricle and the papillary muscles seem to move more toward the base of the heart.[17]

Anterolateral Papillary Muscle

VT/PVCs originating from the papillary muscles are rare; those that originate from the anterolateral papillary muscle (1.4%–4.4%) are less common than those from the posteromedial papillary muscle (2.4%–7.5%).[18,19] In one study of 6 patients with VT originating from the anterolateral papillary muscles, the ECG showed a right bundle branch pattern with a right/inferior axis and early precordial transition (<V1) (**Fig. 7**). The mean QRS duration was 168 ± 19 milliseconds. Lead aVR was notable for either a qR or qr pattern and an rS in lead V6.

Posteromedial Papillary Muscle

The incidence of VT/PVC originating from the posteromedial papillary muscle is approximately 2.4% to 7.5%.[19,20] In the study by Doppalapudi and colleagues,[20] the VT/PVC's demonstrated a right bundle branch block and right/superior axis in five of the seven patients and a left/superior axis in the other two patients (**Fig. 8**). The mean QRS duration was 158 milliseconds.

Given the anatomic proximity of papillary muscles to that of the mitral annulus and to the fascicles, arrhythmias that originate from these sites can show similar ECG characteristics. In the anterolateral region of the left ventricle (anterior papillary muscle, anterior fascicle, and anterolateral and lateral mitral annulus) the presence of a right bundle branch block, right/inferior axis, and precordial transition by V1 were common features. However, the presence of an rS in lead I and aVR, qR in aVL, and a qR in lead V1 was specific for distinguishing anterior papillary muscle and left anterior fascicular VTs from the MAVTs. Furthermore, an R/S ratio of less than 1 in V6 can be used to further distinguish the anterior papillary muscle from the left anterior fascicular VT (**Fig. 9**). In the posteroseptal region of the left ventricle (posterior papillary muscle, posterior fascicle, posterior and posterior-septal mitral annulus) the ECG characteristics of a right bundle branch, superior axis, and precordial transition by V1 were common. However, the presence of an Rs or rS in lead I, qR in aVL, and Q wave in V1 could be used to distinguish posterior papillary muscle and posterior fascicular VTs from the posteroseptal and posterior MAVTs. Fascicular VTs typically

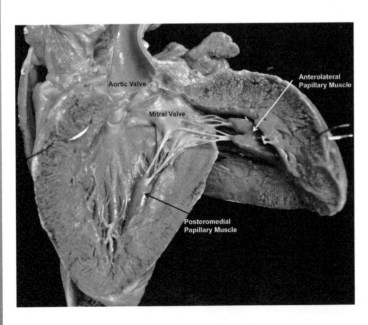

Fig. 6. Anatomy of the left ventricular papillary muscles. The left ventricle of a structurally normal heart showing the papillary muscles and mitral and aortic valvular apparatus.

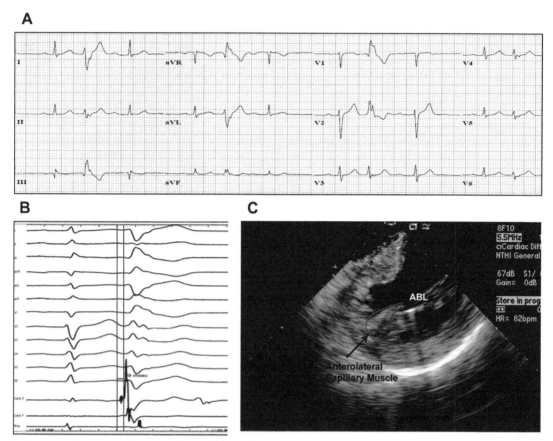

Fig. 7. Anterolateral papillary muscle PVC. (*A*) Twelve-lead ECG showing an RBBB with early precordial transition and a right/inferior axis with a qR in aVR and rS in V6. (*B*) Site of earliest activation (19 milliseconds) during electrophysiology study preceding surface ECG QRS onset. (*C*) Intracardiac echo image with ablation catheter at the base of the anterolateral papillary muscle (outlined in *red*) just before ablation.

had an rsR′ right bundle pattern in V1 that was not seen in any of the papillary muscle VTs (which usually have a qR or monophasic R in V1) and either a typical left anterior or posterior hemiblock. Although papillary muscle VTs typically had a longer mean QRS duration compared with fascicular VTs (150 ± 15 milliseconds vs 127 ± 11 milliseconds), only a QRS cutoff greater than 160 milliseconds could be used to reliably distinguish posterior papillary muscle VT/PVCs from posterior fascicular VT.[14,19]

During electrophysiology study, the presence of Purkinje potentials during sinus rhythm occurred before the QRS onset in fascicular VTs compared with occurring after QRS onset or not at all in papillary muscle VTs.[14,20] In addition, programmed ventricular or atrial stimulation did not induce VT in any of the papillary muscle VT/PVCs, but the arrhythmia was inducible with either isoproterenol or epinephrine, suggesting a nonreentrant mechanism. These arrhythmias were also more likely to present as PVCs than

sustained episodes of VT. Pace mapping of papillary muscle VTs was successful in matching the clinical arrhythmia for papillary muscle but not patients with fascicular VT. Although pace mapping can be used to localize papillary muscle arrhythmias, difficulty with catheter stability makes this less reliable and local activation mapping can be more helpful. For anterolateral papillary muscle VT/PVCs earliest activation occurred at the base or the middle portion of the anterior papillary muscle and successful ablation often required high-power irrigated tip ablation catheters to be successful. For posteromedial papillary muscle VT/PVCs earliest activation was at the base of the papillary muscle and the site of successful ablation was located at the inferior wall, lateral to the septum and approximately one-third of the distance from the left ventricle apex to the mitral annulus. Postablation echocardiography has not revealed a significant increase in mitral regurgitation after papillary muscle ablation.[18–20]

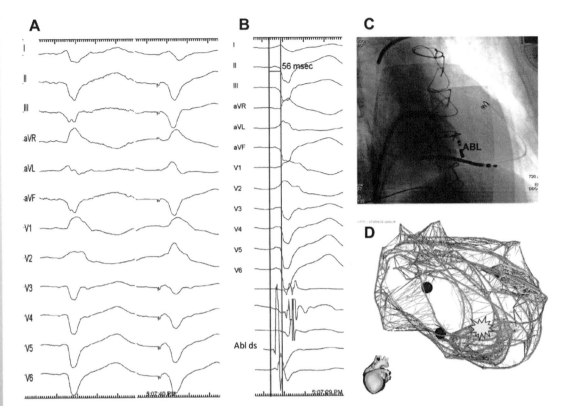

Fig. 8. Posteromedial papillary muscle. (*A*) Twelve-lead ECG shows an RBBB pattern with superior axis and monophasic R in V1. The second QRS complex shows pace map from the lateral side of the posteromedial papillary muscle. (*B*) Earliest activation occurred at the posteromedial papillary muscle and preceded the surface QRS by 56 milliseconds. (*C*) Cardiac fluoroscopy with ablation catheter at base of posteromedial papillary muscle. (*D*) Electroanatomic map using 3D intracardiac echo image depicting the anterolateral (*yellow*) and posteromedial (*blue*) papillary muscles. Ablation was performed at the base of the posteromedial papillary muscle (*yellow star*). Red dots refer to the tricuspid annulus.

CARDIAC VENOUS SYSTEM

Idiopathic VTs and PVCs have also been described arising from the epicardial side of the LVOT, and these arrhythmias can sometimes be mapped and ablated from within the coronary venous system.[21–26] Two common sites of VA origin within the cardiac veins are the anterior interventricular vein (AIV) and the cardiac crux at the inferior junction between the right and left ventricles.

The great cardiac vein (GCV) is located anteriorly in the atrioventricular groove and subsequently transitions to the AIV at the bifurcation of the left main coronary artery where it runs parallel to the left anterior descending artery.[25]

VAs originating from the junction of the GCV/AIV or AIV typically have a left bundle branch pattern and an early precordial lead transition (V1 or V2), often with slurring of the r wave in V1, inferiorly directed axis with tall R waves in the inferior leads, a Q wave in aVL, and an rS or QS in lead I (**Fig. 10**).

VT from the distal AIV typically had lower amplitude in the inferior leads compared with the septal RVOT.[25,26] Furthermore, ECG indices used to identify VT with an epicardial origin, such as the R-wave duration index (>50%), R/S amplitude index in leads V1 or V2 (>30%), and precordial maximum deflection index (MDI) greater than 0.55 can also be used to predict VTs from the AIV.[9] Using these parameters, Kaseno and colleagues[25] found that 8 of the 10 patients with AIV PVCs had an R-wave amplitude index greater than 50%, an R/S amplitude index greater than 30, and an MDI greater than 0.55.

The ECG characteristics of VAs originating from the cardiac veins also guide whether ablation can be successfully performed via an endocardial approach from the left sinus Valsalva (LSV) or an epicardial approach via the AIV. Ito and colleagues[7] developed an ECG algorithm for identifying the optimal ablation site for idiopathic ventricular outflow tract tachycardia. As part of their algorithm, they reported that a Q-wave ratio

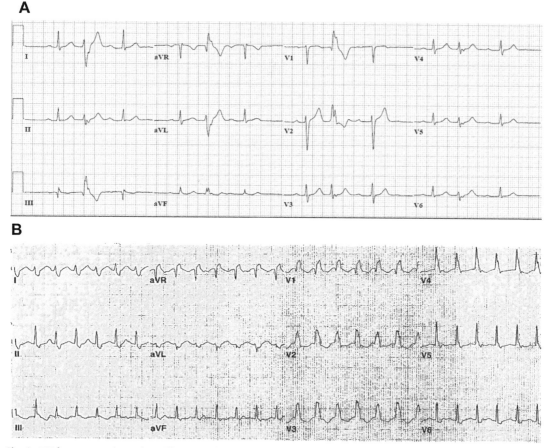

Fig. 9. VT from anterolateral papillary muscle versus left anterior fascicle. (*A*) The 12-lead ECG of PVC originating from the anterolateral papillary muscle shows RBBB (early transition) with right/inferior axis, a qR in aVR, and an rS in V6. (*B*) Twelve-lead ECG of left anterior fascicular VT shows RBBB pattern with right/inferior axis with positive concordance across the precordium. Note that the rsR' in V1, R/S greater than 1 in V6, and narrower QRS complex in this tracing favors fascicular VT.

in leads aVL/aVR greater than 1.4 or the presence of an S wave in V1 greater than 1.2 mV indicated that the VT originated from the left ventricular epicardium remote from the LSV. In contrast, if it did not fulfill both criteria, the VT was located in the region of the LSV. Similar results regarding the Q-wave ratio were seen in the study by Abularach and colleagues.[27] A Q-wave ratio of less than 1.45 in aVL/aVR, an R-wave amplitude ratio in lead III/II of less than 1.13, and a close anatomic distance of less than 13.5 mm between the LSV and the coronary veins suggested that successful ablation can be performed from the LSV. Otherwise ablation needed to be performed from within the AIV or via epicardial access.[27]

In another study by Ito and colleagues[28] using simultaneous mapping of the LSV and coronary venous system in 25 patients, it was hypothesized that analysis of the electrograms from the LSV and the transitional zone from the GCV to the AIV could

be used to successfully predict successful RF catheter ablation from within the LSV. A ventricular activation time from the transition zone of the GCV to the AIV that preceded the LSV activation by less than 10 milliseconds was useful in identifying the LSV as a successful ablation site. These findings had a high sensitivity of 88% and a specificity and positive predictive value of 100%. Mapping from both the AIV and LSV is often necessary to identify the best site for ablation.

Ablation within the coronary venous system with RF energy is often challenging and can be associated with complications such as cardiac tamponade or injury to adjacent coronary arteries. Irrigated RF is nearly always needed in order to deliver adequate power. Coronary angiography should always be performed before ablating within the AIV to determine proximity to the left anterior descending coronary artery, and ablation should be avoided if the distance is less than 5 mm.[29]

A

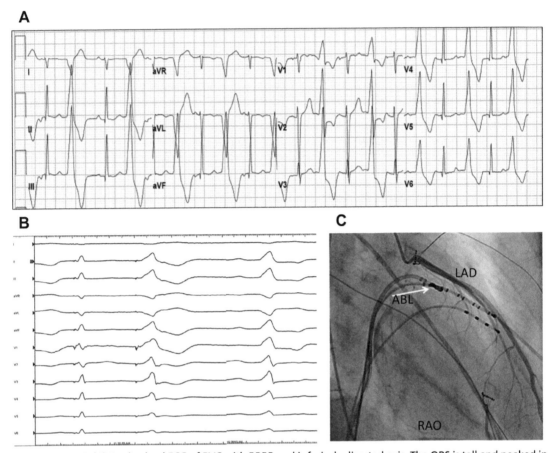

B

C

Fig. 10. AIV PVC. (*A*) Twelve-lead ECG of PVC with RBBB and inferiorly directed axis. The QRS is tall and peaked in the inferior leads with QRS amplitude greater than 15 mV. Lead I and aVL show a QS, and aVL/aVR greater than 1.4 suggests epicardial origin. (*B*) PVC and corresponding pace map from the AIV during electrophysiologic study. (*C*) Cardiac fluoroscopy showing ablation catheter in the AIV near the base of the heart. LAD, left anterior descending artery.

Lower power (15–30 W) should be used. However, experienced operators can often perform ablation safely.[9,27]

The cardiac crux is another epicardial anatomic region identified as a source of idiopathic VT that can be targeted from within the coronary venous system. The cardiac crux is located posteroseptally and occupies a 4-sided pyramidal space at the confluence of the 4 cardiac chambers at the junction of the atrioventricular groove.[30] The region of the cardiac crux can be accessed from the coronary sinus, typically at the origin of or within the middle cardiac vein. Epicardial access is also necessary in some cases. In a study of 4 patients, the ECG features during crux VT showed a left bundle branch pattern with left superior axis. An abrupt precordial transition in lead V2 was seen in 3 of the 4 patients, with the fourth patient having R waves present in all precordial leads. Because the VAs have an epicardial origin, the

QRS is typically wide, with a mean QRS duration of 158 milliseconds (150–165 milliseconds) with negative slurred QS complex in the inferior leads with pseudodelta waves. Using the epicardial VT criteria as described by Berruezo and Daniels,[26,31] all patients with crux VT had a pseudodelta wave greater than or equal to 34 milliseconds (mean, 54 milliseconds), an intrinsicoid deflection time in lead V2 greater than or equal to 85 milliseconds (mean, 97 milliseconds), and an MDI greater than or equal to 0.55.[32] Another study by Kawamura and colleagues[33] corroborates the ECG findings from Doppalapudi and colleagues, but further distinguishes the cardiac crux into a basal and apical origin. Apical crux VT showed a superior axis with either a left or right bundle pattern, whereas all basal crux VTs had a left bundle pattern (**Fig. 11**). A positive QRS complex in aVR and negative deflection in lead V6 suggested an apical crux origin. During electrophysiologic study, crux VAs

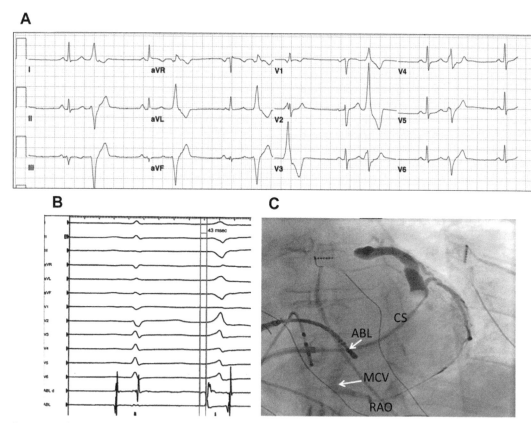

Fig. 11. Cardiac crux PVC. (*A*) The 12-lead ECG shows a PVC with right bundle branch morphology and superiorly directed axis. There is also slurring of the QRS onset in the precordial leads, a QS in lead II, and tall R wave in V2. These findings suggest an epicardial location near the basal cardiac crux. (*B*) Electrophysiologic study shows site of earliest activation at 43 milliseconds before QRS onset. (*C*) Cardiac fluoroscopy shows ablation catheter near the middle cardiac vein before ablation. CS, coronary sinus; MCV, middle cardiac vein.

were inducible with right ventricular stimulation, but failed to show entrainment, suggesting a non-reentrant mechanism. Ablation for the basal crux VAs can be achieved from within the coronary sinus at the junction with the middle cardiac vein, whereas successful apical crux VT typically required epicardial ablation. Coronary angiography should always be performed before ablation in the cardiac crux to show proximity to the posterior descending right coronary artery. Epicardial ablation at the cardiac crux can be challenging, because the site is covered by epicardial fat that may limit transmission of ablation energy. Ablation just left of the posterior descending artery was noted to be more successful because this region has less epicardial fat.[32]

SUMMARY

Unusual sites of VAs include the tricuspid and mitral annulus, right and left ventricular papillary muscles, and coronary venous system. Information garnered from the standard 12-lead ECG can be useful for identifying these sites and distinguishing them from more typical outflow origins. Mapping and ablation can often be challenging because of the limitations of delivering adequate power, maintaining catheter stability, and avoiding damage to collateral cardiac structures and arteries. Successful ablation is often possible with careful mapping, but the success rates are lower and complication rates higher than for typical RVOT VAs.

REFERENCES

1. Lerman BB, Stein KM, Markowitz SM. Mechanisms of idiopathic left ventricular tachycardia. J Cardiovasc Electrophysiol 1997;8:571–83.
2. Badhwar N, Scheinman M. Idiopathic ventricular tachycardia: diagnosis and management. Curr Probl Cardiol 2007;32:7–43.
3. Coggins DL, Lee RJ, Sweeney J, et al. Radiofrequency catheter ablation as a cure for idiopathic tachycardia of both right and eight ventricular origin. J Am Coll Cardiol 1994;23:1333–41.

4. Miller JM, Varma N, Josephson ME. Therapy of "idiopathic" ventricular tachycardia. J Cardiovasc Electrophysiol 1997;8:104–16.

5. Tada H, Tadokoro K, Ito S, et al. Idiopathic ventricular arrhythmias originating from the tricuspid annulus: prevalence, electrocardiographic characteristics, and results of radiofrequency catheter ablation. Heart Rhythm 2007;4:7–16.

6. Yamauchi Y, Aonuma K, Takahashi A, et al. Electrocardiographic characteristics of repetitive monomorphic right ventricular tachycardia originating near the His-bundle. J Cardiovasc Electrophysiol 2005; 16:1041–8.

7. Ito S, Tada H, Naito S, et al. Development and validation of an ECG algorithm for identifying the optimal ablation site for idiopathic ventricular outflow tract tachycardia. J Cardiovasc Electrophysiol 2003; 14:1280–6.

8. Yamada T, McElderry HT, Doppalapudi H, et al. Catheter ablation of ventricular arrhythmias originating in the vicinity of the His bundle: significance of mapping the aortic sinus cusp. Heart Rhythm 2008;5:37–42.

9. Ouyang F, Fotuhi P, Ho SY, et al. Repetitive monomorphic ventricular tachycardia originating from the aortic sinus cusp: electrocardiographic characterization for guiding catheter ablation. J Am Coll Cardiol 2002;39:500–8.

10. Klein LS, Shih HT, Hackett FK, et al. Radiofrequency catheter ablation of ventricular tachycardia in patients without structural heart disease. Circulation 1992;85:1666–74.

11. Ho SY, Nihoyannopoulos P. Anatomy, echocardiography, and normal right ventricular dimensions. Heart 2006;92(Suppl 1):i2–13.

12. Haddad F, Hunt SA, Rosenthal DN, et al. Right ventricular function in cardiovascular disease, Part I. Circulation 2008;117:1436–48.

13. Crawford T, Mueller G, Good E, et al. Ventricular arrhythmias originating from papillary muscles in the right ventricle. Heart Rhythm 2010;7:725–30.

14. Good E, Desjardins B, Jongnarangsin K, et al. Ventricular arrhythmias originating from a papillary muscle in patients without prior infarction: a comparison with fascicular arrhythmias. Heart Rhythm 2008;5: 1530–7.

15. Tada H, Ito S, Naito S, et al. Idiopathic ventricular arrhythmia arising from the mitral annulus: a distinct subgroup of idiopathic ventricular arrhythmias. J Am Coll Cardiol 2005;45:877–86.

16. Kumagai K, Yamauchi Y, Takahashi A, et al. Idiopathic left ventricular tachycardia originating from the mitral annulus. J Cardiovasc Electrophysiol 2005;16:1029–36.

17. Estes EH, Dalton FM, Entman ML, et al. The anatomy and blood supply of the papillary muscles of the left ventricle. Am Heart J 1966;71:356–62.

18. Yamada T, Mcelderry HT, Okada T, et al. Idiopathic focal ventricular arrhythmias originating from the anterior papillary muscle in the left ventricle. J Cardiovasc Electrophysiol 2009;20:866–72.

19. Yamada T, Doppalapudi H, McElderry HT, et al. Idiopathic ventricular arrhythmias originating from the papillary muscles in the left ventricle: prevalence, electrocardiographic and electrophysiological characteristics, and results of the radiofrequency catheter ablation. J Cardiovasc Electrophysiol 2010;21: 62–9.

20. Doppalapudi H, Yamada T, McElderry HT, et al. Ventricular tachycardia originating from the posterior papillary muscle in the left ventricle: a distinct clinical syndrome. Circ Arrhythm Electrophysiol 2008; 1:23–9.

21. de Paola A, Melo W, Távora M, et al. Angiographic and electrophysiological substrates for ventricular tachycardia mapping through the coronary veins. Heart 1998;79:59–63.

22. Hirasawa Y, Miyauchi Y, Iwasaki YK, et al. Successful radiofrequency catheter ablation of epicardial left ventricular outflow tract tachycardia from the anterior interventricular coronary vein. J Cardiovasc Electrophysiol 2005;16:1378–80.

23. Meininger GR, Berger RD. Idiopathic ventricular tachycardia originating in the great cardiac vein. Heart Rhythm 2006;3:464–6.

24. Obel OA, d'Avila A, Neuzil P, et al. Ablation of left ventricular epicardial outflow tract tachycardia from the distal great cardiac vein. J Am Coll Cardiol 2006;48:1813–7.

25. Kaseno K, Tada H, Tanaka S, et al. Successful catheter ablation of left ventricular epicardial tachycardia originating from the great cardiac vein: a case report and review of the literature. Circ J 2007;71:1983–8.

26. Daniels DV, Lu YY, Morton JB, et al. Idiopathic epicardial left ventricular tachycardia originating remote from the sinus of Valsalva: electrophysiological characteristics, catheter ablation, and identification from the 12-lead electrocardiogram. Circulation 2006;113:1659–66.

27. Abularach M, Campos B, Park KM, et al. Ablation of ventricular arrhythmias arising near the anterior epicardial veins from the left sinus of Valsalva region: ECG features, anatomic distance, and outcome. Heart Rhythm 2012;9:865–73.

28. Ito S, Tada H, Naito S, et al. Simultaneous mapping in the left sinus of Valsalva and coronary venous system predicts successful catheter ablation from the left sinus of Valsalva. Pacing Clin Electrophysiol 2005;28(Suppl 1):S150–4.

29. Giorgberidze I, Saksena S, Krol RB, et al. Efficacy and safety of radiofrequency catheter ablation of left-sided accessory pathways through the coronary sinus. Am J Cardiol 1995;76:359–65.

30. Sánchez-Quintana D, Ho SY, Cabrera JA, et al. Topographic anatomy of the inferior pyramidal space: relevance to radiofrequency catheter ablation. J Cardiovasc Electrophysiol 2001;12:210–7.

31. Berruezo A, Mont L, Nava S, et al. Electrocardiographic recognition of the epicardial origin of ventricular tachycardias. Circulation 2004;109:1842–7.

32. Doppalapudi H, Yamada T, Ramaswamy K, et al. Idiopathic focal epicardial ventricular tachycardia originating from the crux of the heart. Heart Rhythm 2009;6:44–50.

33. Kawamura M, Gerstenfeld EP, Vedantham V, et al. Idiopathic ventricular arrhythmia originating from the cardiac crux, in press.

Electrocardiographic Characteristics of Ventricular Tachycardia in Arrhythmogenic Right Ventricular Dysplasia

Kurt S. Hoffmayer, PharmD, MD[a],
Melvin M. Scheinman, MD[b],*

KEYWORDS

- Ventricular tachycardia • Electrocardiogram
- Arrhythmogenic right ventricular dysplasia/cardiomyopathy (ARVD/C)
- Idiopathic ventricular tachycardia • Genetic arrhythmia syndromes

KEY POINTS

- Ventricular arrhythmias in patients with arrhythmogenic right ventricular dysplasia/cardiomyopathy (ARVD/C) are common.
- Ventricular arrhythmias show left bundle branch block (LBBB) morphology as they arise from the right ventricle.
- Multiple forms, including LBBB/superior axis morphology, are frequently seen in ARVD/C and not idiopathic right ventricular outflow tract–ventricular tachycardia (RVOT-VT).
- Several electrocardiogram features may aid in distinguishing ARVD/C from idiopathic RVOT-VT.
- Several clinical and electrocardiographic features may aid in distinguishing ARVD/C from cardiac sarcoid.

BACKGROUND

Arrhythmogenic right ventricular dysplasia/cardiomyopathy (ARVD/C) is an inherited arrhythmia syndrome characterized by a progressive replacement of cardiac myocytes with fibrous and adipose tissue.[1] The replacement primarily affects the right ventricle but can also progress to affect the left ventricle.[1-4] The progressive replacement starts in the epicardium and eventually becomes transmural spreading to the endocardium with minimal involvement of the interventricular septum. Fibrofatty progression leads to wall thinning, aneurysms, and interference with electrical impulse conduction and is the primary cause of epsilon waves, right bundle branch block (RBBB), late potentials, and reentrant ventricular arrhythmias.[3]

Ventricular arrhythmias in ARVD/C show distinctive left bundle branch block (LBBB) QRS morphology, indicating origin from the right ventricle. They may originate from anywhere in the right ventricle with a superior axis originating from the inferior wall or apex or an inferior axis originating from the right ventricular outflow tract. Although peri-valvular origin is more common, they can originate anywhere along the base to apex (**Figs. 1–3**).[5-8]

Disclosures: Kurt Hoffmayer: None. Melvin Scheinman: He has received speakers fees from St Jude Medical, Boston Scientific, Medtronic, Biosense, and Biotronik; he has also received consultant fees from Jansen.
[a] Division of Electrophysiology, Department of Cardiology, University of Wisconsin, Madison, 600 Highland Avenue, Madison, WI 53792, USA; [b] Division of Electrophysiology, Department of Cardiology, University of California, San Francisco, 500 Parnassus Avenue, San Francisco, CA 94143, USA
* Corresponding author.
E-mail address: scheinman@medicine.ucsf.edu

Card Electrophysiol Clin 6 (2014) 595–601
http://dx.doi.org/10.1016/j.ccep.2014.05.012
1877-9182/14/$ – see front matter © 2014 Elsevier Inc. All rights reserved.

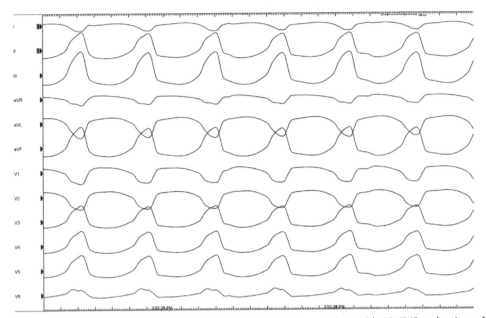

Fig. 1. Ventricular tachycardia (VT) shown on a 12-lead rhythm strip in a patient with ARVD/C at the time of catheter ablation. LBBB/inferior axis VT, mapped to the right ventricular outflow tract epicardium and successfully ablated.

CLINICAL MANIFESTATIONS AND EPIDEMIOLOGY OF VENTRICULAR ARRHYTHMIAS

Clinical manifestations of ARVD/C may present as palpitations from premature ventricular contractions (PVCs), syncope from sustained ventricular tachycardia (VT), or sudden cardiac death from ventricular fibrillation.[9] Most patients with ARVD/C come to medical attention after presenting with ventricular arrhythmias. This clinical presentation was first described in the initial series of ARVD/C cases reported by Marcus and colleagues[2] in 24 patients all presenting with ventricular arrhythmias.

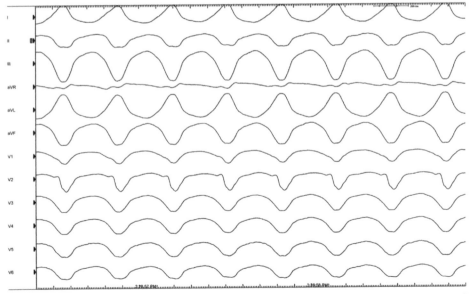

Fig. 2. Ventricular tachycardia (VT) shown on a 12-lead rhythm strip in the same patient with ARVD/C shown in **Fig. 1.** LBBB/superior axis VT, mapped to the right ventricular apical epicardium and successfully ablated.

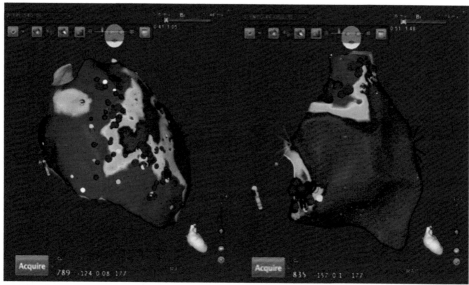

Fig. 3. CARTO voltage maps in the right anterior oblique (RAO) projection of the right ventricular epicardium (*left*) and endocardium (*right*) in the patient with ARVD/C from **Figs. 1** and **2**. Note the larger area of epicardial scar that extends beyond the limits of the endocardial abnormalities.

Although most present with ventricular arrhythmias, others do not. The North American Multidisciplinary ARVD study characterized the incidence of ventricular arrhythmias in 108 probands with suspected ARVD/C, and VT was not seen in every patient.[10] Sustained clinical VT was present in 35%; among patients undergoing electrophysiology study (75 probands), sustained VT was induced during an electrophysiology study in 49%. Among the patients with sustained VT, the morphology of LBBB/superior axis was the most common (14 out of 38, 36.8%) and then LBBB/inferior axis (10 out of 38, 26.3%), with the remaining having either LBBB/indeterminate axis (8 out of 38, 21.0%), indeterminate morphology (5 out of 38, 13.0%), and RBBB pattern (1 out of 38, 2.6%).

Because left ventricular function is usually normal in these patients, it is not unusual to see hemodynamically well-tolerated VTs with cycle lengths as fast as 240 ms.[9]

ELECTROCARDIOGRAPHIC DIFFERENTIATION BETWEEN ARVD/C AND RIGHT VENTRICULAR OUTFLOW TRACT–VT

Differentiation between idiopathic ventricular tachycardia from the right ventricular outflow tract (RVOT-VT) and ARVD/C is of utmost importance given the benign nature of the former and the need for sudden cardiac risk stratification and family screening in the latter.[8,11] Baseline sinus rhythm electrocardiography as well as electrocardiographic differences during ventricular arrhythmias (VT or PVCs) can be helpful in differentiating the 2 disease states.[8]

SINUS RHYTHM

The presence of T-wave inversion in the precordial (V1–V3 and beyond) and inferior leads during sinus rhythm may aid the diagnosis of ARVD/C. T-wave inversions in V1 to V3 may be present in only 32% of patients with ARVD/C as well as 1% to 3% of normal young patients and 4% of patients with RVOT-VT.[10,12–14] In addition, T-wave inversions V1 to V4 have been found in 12.7% of black athletes and may represent an ethnic variant of an athletic heart.[15]

Epsilon waves (the pathognomic low-amplitude signals between the end of the QRS complex to onset of the T wave in the right precordial leads [V1–V3]), if seen, are very helpful and are a major diagnostic criterium[16] but are seen in the minority of patient in most series (0% to 37%).[6–8,12,17]

The terminal portion of the QRS complex in sinus rhythm in leads V1 to V3 in patients without RBBB may also be helpful in identifying ARVC/D. The duration from the nadir to S wave back to baseline in V1 through V3 (prolonged S-wave upstroke) greater than 55 ms was the most prevalent electrocardiogram (ECG) feature, predicted disease severity and induction of VT at electrophysiology study in a cohort of 50 patients with ARVC/D.[18]

Fragmentation of the QRS complex on standard 12-lead ECG has also been recently found to be of diagnostic significance in ARVC/D and has been correlated to events, predicting fatal and nonfatal arrhythmias.[19]

VENTRICULAR ARRHYTHMIAS
Single Versus Multiple Forms

The presence of more than one form of VT should increase the pretest probability for ARVD/C as this likely reflects more diffuse disease affecting multiple sites of the right ventricle. Niroomand and colleagues[20] performed electrophysiology studies in 56 patients and found the presence of more than one type of VT in 75% of the ARVD group (n = 15) compared with 0% in the idiopathic RVOT-VT group (n = 41) (P<.0001). O'Donnell and colleagues[21] had similar findings, with more than one type of VT morphology seen in 71% of the ARVD/C group (n = 17) and 0% in the RVOT-VT group (n = 33) (P<.01).

Although this finding is of utmost importance, the predictive value is not 100% accurate. Early in the disease of ARVD/C, one may see a single form of VT. There has also been a report of multiple forms of VT seen in an idiopathic VT, but the diagnosis in these rare instances must be carefully scrutinized.

VT/PVC Morphology

The ECG morphology of the ventricular arrhythmias has been used to differentiate the 2 entities.

Multiple VT forms including LBBB/superior axis essentially excludes RVOT-VT and should shift your pretest probability toward ARVD/C.[17]

Given the anatomic substrate differences between the 2 disease states, the width of the QRS complex may be helpful. Ainsworth and colleagues[22] found that the mean QRS duration was longer in all 12 leads in patients with ARVC with a significant difference seen in leads I, III, aVL, aVF, V1, V2, and V3 (P<.05). Leads I and aVL had the largest mean difference between patients with ARVC and patients with RVOT-VT of 17.6 ± 4.7 ms and 15.8 ± 7.5 ms, respectively (P = .0001). Lead I QRS duration of 120 ms or greater had a sensitivity of 100%, specificity of 46%, positive predictive value of 61%, and negative predictive value of 100% for ARVC.

The authors' group found that several ECG criteria may aid in distinguishing ARVD/C from RVOT-VT, and they prospectively validated these criteria with an ARVD risk score.[6,7] Patients with ARVD/C had a significantly longer mean QRS duration in lead I (in agreement with Ainsworth and colleagues[22]), more often exhibited a later precordial transition, and more often had QRS notching.

The ARVD/C ECG risk score uses these principles and combines them with baseline sinus rhythm ECG (**Fig. 4, Table 1**).[6] The scoring system provides 3 points for sinus rhythm anterior T-wave inversions in leads V1 to V3 and during

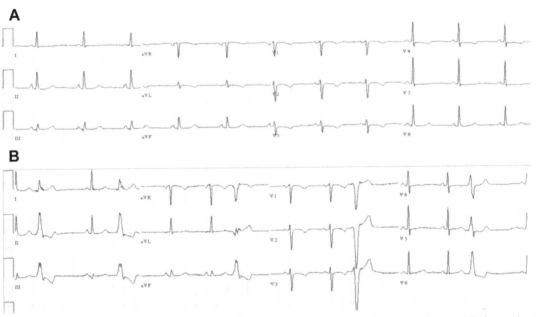

Fig. 4. Two ECGs from a patient with ARVD/C and premature ventricular contractions. The top (A) shows sinus rhythm with anterior T-wave inversions, V1 to V4. The same patient during PVCs (B) scores an 8 in the ARVD ECG risk score, as lead I QRS duration greater than 120 ms has a precordial V5 transition and has QRS notching in multiple leads (I, II, III, aVL, V4, V5) and, as noted previously, T-wave inversions V1 to V4.

Table 1
Arrhythmogenic right ventricular cardiomyopathy ECG risk score

ECG Characteristic	Points
Anterior TWI (V1–V3) in sinus rhythm	3
Lead 1 QRS ≥120 ms	2
QRS notching	2
V5 transition or later	1

Maximum score is 8 points. A score of 5 or greater was able to correctly distinguish ARVD/C from idiopathic VT 93% of the time, with a sensitivity of 84%, specificity of 100%, positive predictive value of 100%, and negative predictive value of 91%.

Abbreviation: TWI, T-wave inversions.

Adapted from Hoffmayer KS, Bhave PD, Marcus GM, et al. An electrocardiographic scoring system for distinguishing right ventricular outflow tract arrhythmias in patients with arrhythmogenic right ventricular cardiomyopathy from idiopathic ventricular tachycardia. Heart Rhythm 2013;10(4):477–82.

ventricular arrhythmia: 2 points for QRS duration in lead I of 120 ms or greater, 2 points for QRS notching, and 1 point for precordial transition at lead V5 or later. A score of 5 or greater was able to correctly distinguish ARVD/C from idiopathic VT 93% of the time, with a sensitivity of 84%, specificity of 100%, positive predictive value of 100%, and negative predictive value of 91%.

PATHOPHYSIOLOGY OF VT MORPHOLOGY

The mechanism of the differences in QRS morphology in ARVD/C compared with RVOT-VT is related to the difference in the underlying pathology in the 2 conditions. The underlying pathophysiologic mechanism in ARVD/C is the replacement of normal right ventricular myocardial tissue with fibrous and fatty tissue. This replacement may delay cell-to-cell conduction and facilitate the development of reentrant ventricular arrhythmias.[4] The fibrofatty myocyte replacement results in a greater delay from the earliest onset to local onset of the QRS complex, greater duration of the QRS complex, and irregularities of conduction manifest as notching of the QRS complex.

VT origin is another factor. Patients with ARVD/C have a greater frequency of the site of origin of the right ventricular free wall, more remote from the normal His-Purkinje conduction tissue than in those patients with RVOT-VT. These factors also explain the late precordial transition and possibly notching of the QRS. Several studies have found that the VT origin in patients with RVOT-VTs is predominately in the septum.[23,24] Therefore, differences between ECG characteristics of ventricular arrhythmias in patients with RVOT-VT versus ARVD/C are partially explained by differences in the site of origin.

DIFFERENTIATION BETWEEN ARVD/C AND CARDIAC SARCOID

Cardiac sarcoidosis is a disorder with the replacement of myocytes with noncaseating granulomas leading to scar with resultant interference in electrical impulse conduction and reentrant VT.[25] Even though the pathophysiologic process is widely different, these 2 distinct diseases may lead to very similar clinical presentations. Discrimination between the two is challenging because of common right ventricular involvement in both; often, patients with cardiac sarcoid meet the revised task force criteria for the diagnosis of ARVD/C.[9,16,26]

Recently, Dechering and colleagues[26] prospectively compared patients who presented for VT ablation with biopsy-proven cardiac sarcoid with ARVD/C. On baseline ECG, patients with cardiac sarcoid had a significantly wider QRS (0.146 ms vs 0.110 ms, $P = .004$). Programed stimulation induced an average of 3.7 different monomorphic VTs in patients with cardiac sarcoid compared with 1.8 in patients with ARVD/C ($P = .01$). VT origin more often originated in the apical region of the right ventricle in cardiac sarcoid compared with ARVD/C ($P = .001$). Ablation success was not different. In addition, they found 63% of the cardiac sarcoid fit the revised task force diagnostic criteria.

SUMMARY

Ventricular arrhythmias in patients with ARVD/C are common. The ECG can be an invaluable tool to help differentiate between ARVD/C and idiopathic RVOT-VT. Clinical and ECG features may aid in distinguishing ARVD/C from cardiac sarcoid.

REFERENCES

1. Marcus FI, Fontaine G. Arrhythmogenic right ventricular dysplasia/cardiomyopathy: a review. Pacing Clin Electrophysiol 1995;18(6):1298–314.
2. Marcus FI, Fontaine GH, Guiraudon G, et al. Right ventricular dysplasia: a report of 24 adult cases. Circulation 1982;65(2):384–98.
3. Basso C, Corrado D, Marcus FI, et al. Arrhythmogenic right ventricular cardiomyopathy. Lancet 2009; 373(9671):1289–300. http://dx.doi.org/10.1016/S0140-6736(09)60256-7. pii:S0140-6736(09)60256-7.

4. Thiene G, Nava A, Corrado D, et al. Right ventricular cardiomyopathy and sudden death in young people. N Engl J Med 1988;318(3):129–33. http://dx.doi.org/10.1056/NEJM198801213180301.

5. Marchlinski FE, Zado E, Dixit S, et al. Electroanatomic substrate and outcome of catheter ablative therapy for ventricular tachycardia in setting of right ventricular cardiomyopathy. Circulation 2004; 110(16):2293–8. http://dx.doi.org/10.1161/01.CIR.0000145154.02436.90.

6. Hoffmayer KS, Bhave PD, Marcus GM, et al. An electrocardiographic scoring system for distinguishing right ventricular outflow tract arrhythmias in patients with arrhythmogenic right ventricular cardiomyopathy from idiopathic ventricular tachycardia. Heart Rhythm 2013;10(4):477–82. http://dx.doi.org/10.1016/j.hrthm.2012.12.009.

7. Hoffmayer KS, Machado ON, Marcus GM, et al. Electrocardiographic comparison of ventricular arrhythmias in patients with arrhythmogenic right ventricular cardiomyopathy and right ventricular outflow tract tachycardia. J Am Coll Cardiol 2011;58(8): 831–8. http://dx.doi.org/10.1016/j.jacc.2011.05.017.

8. Hoffmayer KS, Scheinman MM. Electrocardiographic patterns of ventricular arrhythmias in arrhythmogenic right ventricular dysplasia/cardiomyopathy. Front Physiol 2012;3:23. http://dx.doi.org/10.3389/fphys.2012.00023.

9. Marcus FI, Abidov A. Arrhythmogenic right ventricular cardiomyopathy 2012: diagnostic challenges and treatment. J Cardiovasc Electrophysiol 2012; 23(10):1149–53. http://dx.doi.org/10.1111/j.1540-8167.2012.02412.x.

10. Marcus FI, Zareba W, Calkins H, et al. Arrhythmogenic right ventricular cardiomyopathy/dysplasia clinical presentation and diagnostic evaluation: results from the North American Multidisciplinary Study. Heart Rhythm 2009;6(7):984–92. http://dx.doi.org/10.1016/j.hrthm.2009.03.013. pii:S1547-5271(09)00288-4.

11. Calkins H. Arrhythmogenic right-ventricular dysplasia/cardiomyopathy. Curr Opin Cardiol 2006; 21(1):55–63.

12. Kazmierczak J, De Sutter J, Tavernier R, et al. Electrocardiographic and morphometric features in patients with ventricular tachycardia of right ventricular origin. Heart 1998;79(4):388–93.

13. Marcus FI. Prevalence of T-wave inversion beyond V1 in young normal individuals and usefulness for the diagnosis of arrhythmogenic right ventricular cardiomyopathy/dysplasia. Am J Cardiol 2005; 95(9):1070–1. http://dx.doi.org/10.1016/j.amjcard.2004.12.060. pii:S0002-9149(05)00185-2.

14. Morin DP, Mauer AC, Gear K, et al. Usefulness of precordial T-wave inversion to distinguish arrhythmogenic right ventricular cardiomyopathy from idiopathic ventricular tachycardia arising from the right ventricular outflow tract. Am J Cardiol 2010; 105(12):1821–4. http://dx.doi.org/10.1016/j.amjcard.2010.01.365. pii:S0002-9149(10)00524-2.

15. Papadakis M, Carre F, Kervio G, et al. The prevalence, distribution, and clinical outcomes of electrocardiographic repolarization patterns in male athletes of African/Afro-Caribbean origin. Eur Heart J 2011;32(18):2304–13. http://dx.doi.org/10.1093/eurheartj/ehr140.

16. Marcus FI, McKenna WJ, Sherrill D, et al. Diagnosis of arrhythmogenic right ventricular cardiomyopathy/dysplasia: proposed modification of the task force criteria. Circulation 2010;121(13):1533–41. http://dx.doi.org/10.1161/CIRCULATIONAHA.108.840827. pii:CIRCULATIONAHA.108.840827.

17. Arbelo E, Josephson ME. Ablation of ventricular arrhythmias in arrhythmogenic right ventricular dysplasia. J Cardiovasc Electrophysiol 2010;21(4): 473–86. http://dx.doi.org/10.1111/j.1540-8167.2009.01694.x. pii:JCE1694.

18. Nasir K, Bomma C, Tandri H, et al. Electrocardiographic features of arrhythmogenic right ventricular dysplasia/cardiomyopathy according to disease severity: a need to broaden diagnostic criteria. Circulation 2004;110(12):1527–34. http://dx.doi.org/10.1161/01.CIR.0000142293.60725.18.

19. Canpolat U, Kabakci G, Aytemir K, et al. Fragmented QRS complex predicts the arrhythmic events in patients with arrhythmogenic right ventricular cardiomyopathy/dysplasia. J Cardiovasc Electrophysiol 2013;24(11):1260–6. http://dx.doi.org/10.1111/jce.12202.

20. Niroomand F, Carbucicchio C, Tondo C, et al. Electrophysiological characteristics and outcome in patients with idiopathic right ventricular arrhythmia compared with arrhythmogenic right ventricular dysplasia. Heart 2002;87(1):41–7.

21. O'Donnell D, Cox D, Bourke J, et al. Clinical and electrophysiological differences between patients with arrhythmogenic right ventricular dysplasia and right ventricular outflow tract tachycardia. Eur Heart J 2003;24(9):801–10.

22. Ainsworth CD, Skanes AC, Klein GJ, et al. Differentiating arrhythmogenic right ventricular cardiomyopathy from right ventricular outflow tract ventricular tachycardia using multilead QRS duration and axis. Heart Rhythm 2006;3(4):416–23. http://dx.doi.org/10.1016/j.hrthm.2005.12.024. pii:S1547-5271(05)02479-3.

23. Joshi S, Wilber DJ. Ablation of idiopathic right ventricular outflow tract tachycardia: current perspectives. J Cardiovasc Electrophysiol 2005; 16(Suppl 1):S52–8. http://dx.doi.org/10.1111/j.1540-8167.2005.50163.x.

24. Dixit S, Gerstenfeld EP, Callans DJ, et al. Electrocardiographic patterns of superior right ventricular outflow tract tachycardias: distinguishing septal

and free-wall sites of origin. J Cardiovasc Electrophysiol 2003;14(1):1–7.

25. Zipse MM, Sauer WH. Electrophysiologic manifestations of cardiac sarcoidosis. Curr Opin Pulm Med 2013;19(5):485–92. http://dx.doi.org/10.1097/MCP. 0b013e3283644c6f.

26. Dechering DG, Kochhauser S, Wasmer K, et al. Electrophysiological characteristics of ventricular tachyarrhythmias in cardiac sarcoidosis versus arrhythmogenic right ventricular cardiomyopathy. Heart Rhythm 2013;10(2):158–64. http://dx.doi.org/10.1016/j.hrthm.2012.10.019.

Electrocardiographic Recognition of Epicardial Arrhythmias

Steven M. Stevens, MD[1], David Hamon, MD[1], Ricky Yu, MD,
Kalyanam Shivkumar, MD, PhD, Noel G. Boyle, MD, PhD*

KEYWORDS

- Epicardial ablation • Ventricular tachycardia • Accessory pathway

KEY POINTS

- Epicardial access for mapping and ablation has increasingly become a feasible modality for treatment of arrhythmias; therefore, the ability to recognize likely epicardial arrhythmias on electrocardiogram (ECG) is important.
- Classic criteria for identifying epicardial ventricular tachycardia (VT) are: (1) the pseudo-δ wave; (2) the intrinsicoid deflection time; and (3) the shortest RS, all of which are based on the initial QRS portion. Additional criteria include the QRS duration, maximum deflection index, and presence of Q in lead I and absence of Q wave in inferior leads for nonischemic substrates with basal lateral VT focus.
- Despite their applicability, ECG criteria for diagnosis of epicardial VT can vary widely, based on differences in underlying cardiomyopathy, ventricular site of origin, tachycardia cycle length, His-Purkinje conduction, and antiarrhythmic therapy.
- There is no single ECG criterion or unique cutoff value reliable enough to diagnose epicardial VT as a stand-alone assessment; therefore, the entire clinical picture must be considered to identify epicardial arrhythmias.
- Applying ECG criteria is one of several steps in considering an epicardial approach for ablation.

INTRODUCTION

Epicardial interventions in electrophysiology date back to the first bypass tract surgery for Wolff-Parkinson-White syndrome in 1969.[1] Nearly 30 years later, in 1996, pericardial access was moved from the operating room to the electrophysiology laboratory, when Sosa and colleagues[2] described percutaneous pericardial access from the subxiphoid space by performing a dry pericardiocentesis. Epicardial interventions are commonly performed for ablation of ventricular tachycardia (VT), reported as 17% of VT ablations at tertiary centers in a survey carried out by the Heart Rhythm Society and European Heart Rhythm Association.[3] Epicardial ventricular arrhythmias are more common in certain populations, such as those with Chagas cardiomyopathy, arrhythmogenic right ventricular cardiomyopathy, nonischemic cardiomyopathy, and ischemic cardiomyopathy with inferior scar.[3] In patients without structural heart disease, epicardial VT may originate in the outflow tracts, septum, and the crux of the heart.[4,5] With increasing feasibility of epicardial interventions, it is important that cardiac electrophysiologists are familiar with the electrocardiographic (ECG)

The authors have nothing to disclose.
UCLA Cardiac Arrhythmia Center, UCLA Health System, David Geffen School of Medicine at UCLA, Los Angeles, CA, USA
[1] The two authors contributed equally to this work.
* Corresponding author. David Geffen School of Medicine at UCLA, 100 UCLA Medical Plaza, Suite 660, Los Angeles, CA 90095-1679.
E-mail address: NBoyle@mednet.ucla.edu

Card Electrophysiol Clin 6 (2014) 603–611
http://dx.doi.org/10.1016/j.ccep.2014.05.007

recognition of tachycardias that may be most amenable to ablation therapy via an epicardial approach.

VENTRICULAR ARRHYTHMIAS

Several criteria have been published to help identify epicardial exit sites for VT. The epicardial surface has slower conduction compared with the endocardium, which contains the His-Purkinje conduction system. The transmural conduction delay from epicardium to endocardium thus leads an initial slurring or delayed upstroke of the QRS. The following 4 general measurement criteria were initially defined in 2004 by Berruezo and colleagues[6] for VTs with a right bundle branch block morphology pattern, in a series of patients with predominantly ischemic cardiomyopathy:

i. The pseudo-δ wave
ii. Intrinsicoid deflection time
iii. The shortest RS complex
iv. The QRS complex duration

These investigators analyzed the ECG patterns for 14 VTs successfully ablated from the epicardium compared with 27 VTs successfully ablated from the endocardium; a third group consisting of 28 additional VTs with unsuccessful endocardial ablation (presumed epicardial focus) were also studied. In addition, these investigators compared the ECG findings for epicardial and endocardial ventricular pacing in 9 patients undergoing cardiac resynchronization. They determined criteria for these parameters to identify epicardial VT, as described later.

Pseudo-δ Wave

The pseudo-δ wave is the interval of the earliest ventricular activation to the onset of the earliest rapid deflection of the QRS in any precordial lead. Berruezo and colleagues[6] reported that a pseudo-δ cutoff of greater than 34 milliseconds is highly suggestive of an epicardial VT focus, with a sensitivity of 83% and a 95% specificity. This parameter was validated by Bazan and colleagues[7] in a study of 19 epicardial VTs in 15 patients (9 with nonischemic cardiomyopathy), who in addition had endocardial and epicardial pace mapping performed at 5 different sites in the left ventricle (LV). These investigators found that the pseudo-δ was significantly longer from the epicardium than endocardium, and that a cutoff value of 34 milliseconds had 96% sensitivity but only 29% specificity for an epicardial focus. The pseudo-δ can be challenging to measure and may have some variability in interpretation, because onset

of the QRS and the first sharp deflection in the precordial leads may be difficult to define. In such cases, other criteria should be used.

Differences between studies may be explained by the nature and the severity of the underlying cardiomyopathy. In cases of previous myocardial infarction, transmural activation time is highly influenced in the scar region. Moreover, endocardial conduction is slower near the scar region and can mimic a pseudo-δ wave. In addition, the specific cardiac region of VT or pacing is probably a critical determinant of this heterogeneity. Bazan and colleagues showed that the pacing site location dramatically influences the ability of those criteria to predict epicardial origin. A pseudo-δ wave of 34 milliseconds or greater was present in almost 40% of patients with endocardial apical inferior pacing, and this increased to 85% when pacing was performed at an endocardial basal inferior site. The percentages were comparable for both regions in epicardial pacing, at greater than 90%. Thus, specificity decreased as the pacing site was changed from apical toward basal regions, which was reproducible with other criteria. This finding may indicate an initial slower conduction in basal rather than apical regions, reflecting the common pattern of predominantly basal fibrosis gradient in nonischemic cardiomyopathy[8] and the distance to the main stems of the His-Purkinje system. Vallès and colleagues[9] reviewed epicardial and endocardial pace maps from the basal superior lateral region in patients with nonischemic cardiomyopathy and VT and then revised the interval criteria, choosing cutoffs that were able to achieve a high specificity of 95% or greater and sensitivity of 20% or greater (**Figs. 1** and **2**).

Intrinsicoid Deflection Time

The intrinsicoid deflection time is the interval from the onset of QRS to the peak of the R wave in lead V2. Berruezo and colleagues[6] found that greater than 85 milliseconds indicates epicardial VT, with 87% sensitivity and 90% specificity. However, in the validation study by Bazan and colleagues,[7] this criterion was found to have low sensitivity (39%) and specificity (24%) values. Again, this lack of reliability may be explained by the integration of all sites of stimulation in the study, because this criterion or cutoff was not appropriate for apical sites of stimulation. In all apical sites, 20% or fewer values were 85 milliseconds or greater during epicardial pacing. Unlike in the earlier study of this group, Vallès and colleagues,[9] in their homogeneous group of patients with dilated cardiomyopathy, paced only in basal superior lateral sites. The same cutoff showed a relatively good

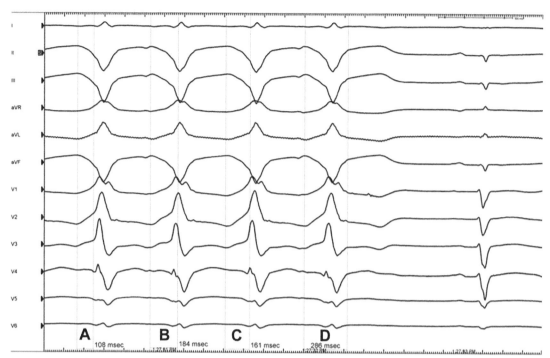

Fig. 1. Epicardial VT termination from the apical inferior septal region of the left ventricle in a patient with non-ischemic cardiomyopathy. (A) the pseudodelta is 108 ms; (B) the intrisicoid deflection time (IDT) is 184 ms; (C) and (D) the maximal deflection index (MDI) is 0.56 (161/286); all consistent with epicardial VT. The Q waves in the inferior leads are expected in epicardial VT from the inferior wall of the LV (**Fig. 4**).

sensitivity and specificity (83% and 70%, respectively). Thus, these investigators proposed an increased cutoff to 90 milliseconds which resulted in mild decrease in sensitivity and an improvement in specificity (76% and 79%, respectively).

The Shortest RS Complex

The shortest RS is measured from the earliest ventricular activation to the nadir of the first S wave in any precordial lead. A cutoff greater than 121 milliseconds was 76% sensitive and 85% specific for epicardial exit of VT in Berruezo and colleagues' study. Again, in the study by Bazan and colleagues, these values were lower, at 53% and 79%, respectively. Vallès and colleagues found that with pacing in basal superior lateral sites, the sensitivity and specificity were 74% and 57%, respectively. VT analyses in the same sites showed some differences, because those values shifted to 93% and 50%, respectively, in this population. This finding suggests longer duration of the shortest RS interval in both endocardial and epicardial VT compared with endocardial and epicardial pace mapping. Differences between cycle length of the VT and the pacing cycle length may be influenced by conduction delays, especially in the His-Purkinje system.[10] The clinical VT usually occurs at faster rates than the pacing cycle

length used for pace mapping. This situation may contribute to the differences between studies, because some used mostly VTs,[6] whereas others used mostly pace mapping to define criteria.[7,9]

QRS Complex Duration

The QRS complex duration is defined as the interval measured from the earliest ventricular activation to the offset of the QRS in precordial leads. In Berruezo and colleagues' study, epicardial terminated VTs had significantly longer QRS duration (217 ± 24 milliseconds) than endocardial terminated VTs (174 ± 37 milliseconds); however, no exact cutoff was defined.[6] In the study by Bazan and colleagues, pacing from the epicardium yielded a QRS of 213 ± 45 milliseconds compared with 191 ± 41 milliseconds from the endocardium, with significant overlap between sites.[7] Again, in this group, important differences were found in the site-specific analysis. Epicardial basal superior VT (n = 10) had greater QRS duration than apical ones (n = 2; 210 ± 34 vs 177 ± 1 milliseconds, respectively). The severity of the cardiomyopathy and myocardial remodeling may directly affect the conduction system and thus, QRS duration. In Berruezo and colleagues' study, the pacing analysis was performed in 9 patients with severe cardiomyopathy (LV ejection fraction = 24% ± 7%)

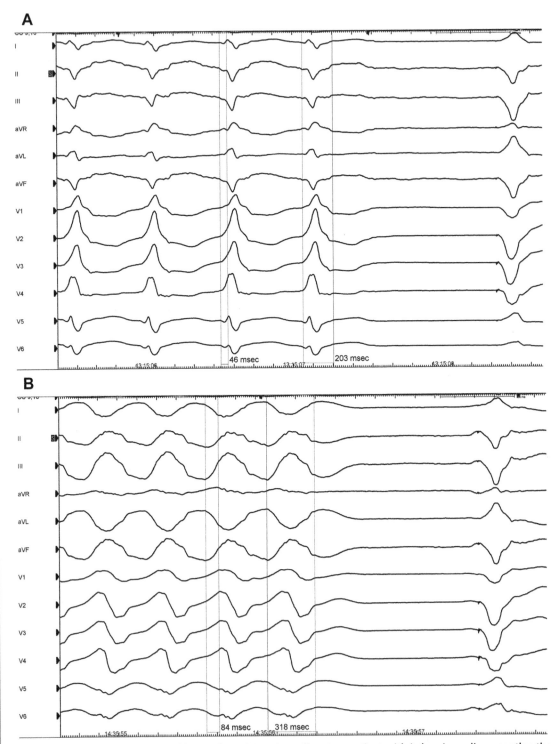

Fig. 2. (*A*) VT termination during ablation from the endocardium in a patient with ischemic cardiomyopathy; the pseudo-δ was 46 milliseconds and QRS width 203 milliseconds. (*B*) VT termination from the epicardium in the same patient; the pseudo-δ was 84 milliseconds and the QRS width 318 milliseconds.

undergoing cardiac resynchronization therapy. QRS duration during epicardial pacing with a lateral pacemaker lead and endocardial stimulation was markedly prolonged (266 ± 25 and 241 ± 39 milliseconds, respectively), as was the baseline QRS complex average duration in those patients (194 ± 19 milliseconds). Conversely, in a study of premature ventricular complexes (PVCs) with patients free from structural heart disease, Yokokawa and colleagues[11] showed short QRS duration: 159 ± 22 milliseconds and 154 ± 20 milliseconds for epicardial and endocardial PVCs, respectively. We propose that no cutoff for QRS duration should be defined and that each patient should be their own reference; thus, VT QRS duration should probably be adjusted to baseline QRS duration. Endocardial pace map QRS duration should also be compared with QRS duration of the clinical VT, because it may suggest the redirection to the epicardium.[7]

Additional criteria, including precordial maximal deflection index (MDI), precordial pattern break, and analysis of the Q wave pattern in lead I and the inferior leads, were derived in populations of patients with nonischemic cardiomyopathy.[7,9]

MDI

Maximal deflection index (MDI) is defined as the interval from the beginning of the QRS to the earliest maximal deflection (in either direction), divided by the QRS duration. A cutoff of 0.55 or greater was sensitive (100%) and specific (98.7%) for VT from the sinus of Valsalva or near the crux of the heart.[4,5]

This measure has been validated only for outflow tract morphology, because most epicardial VTs were located near the anterior interventricular vein and its junction with the great cardiac vein, with left bundle branch block morphology in 11 of 12 patients, whereas most (74%) control endocardial VTs were outflow tract VT, mainly from the right ventricle. Site-specific assessment of this criterion was not performed in Bazan and colleagues[7] study. Basal superior lateral VT and pacing site-specific evaluation of MDI was investigated in Vallès and colleagues' study,[9] in which this predictor was not reliable (sensitivity and specificity of 30% and 89%, respectively, for MDI ≥0.55). Once again, these investigators suggested a revision of the criterion, and with an MDI cutoff value of 0.45 or greater, the sensitivity increased, with a moderate decrease in specificity (76% and 75%, respectively). Nevertheless, a cutoff value of 0.59 was used in their 4-step algorithm (**Figs. 3** and **4**).[9]

Q Wave Status in Lead I and Inferior Leads

Bazan and colleagues developed this approach based on the assessment of the initial local transmural ventricular activation, representing local activation vector between the endocardium and the epicardium. The premise is that in nonischemic cardiomyopathy, VT commonly comes from the basal superior and apical superior LV. Activation from epicardium is expected to spread inferior and rightward. Thus, the presence of Q wave in lead 1 (and conversely, its absence in endocardial VT) has been found to be a reliable predictor

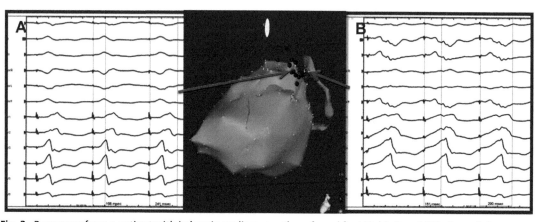

Fig. 3. Pace maps from a patient with ischemic cardiomyopathy referred for VT ablation. (*A*) Endocardial pace map from the basal anterior lateral LV endocardium with an MDI of 0.43 (108/241 milliseconds) with longer than expected QRS width (241 milliseconds) for an endocardial pace map. (*B*) Epicardial pace map from the great cardiac vein directly across from the endocardial site with an MDI of 0.51 (151/290 milliseconds) but with a slower initial upstroke, intrinsicoid deflection time 151 milliseconds and wider QRS 290 milliseconds. The center panel shows an electroanatomic Navx map (St Jude Medical, Minneapolis, MN) of the endocardial LV surface (*green*) and the epicardial surface along the coronary sinus and great cardiac vein (*gray*). The *arrows* indicate the sites of the endocardial pace map (*A*) and the pace map from great cardiac vein (*B*). The *red dots* indicate ablation sites.

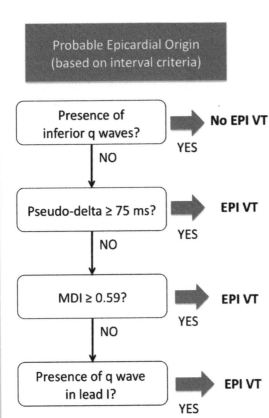

Fig. 4. Algorithm for identifying epicardial (EPI) origin of VT in nonischemic cardiomyopathy. (*From* Valles E, Bazan V, Marchlinski FE. ECG criteria to identify epicardial ventricular tachycardia in nonischemic cardiomyopathy. Circ Arrhythm Electrophysiol 2010; 3:70; with permission.)

(sensitivity and specificity of 86% and 81%, respectively) of an epicardial focus. Similarly, the absence of Q wave in inferior leads (and its presence in endocardial VT) appeared to be a sensitive but not specific finding (100% and 18%, respectively). Although most VTs were basal superior in this study, these investigators also found an expected inverse ECG pattern for this criterion in inferior LV VT. Vallès and colleagues validated those criteria in a wider subset of basal superior lateral VTs and pacing, with better predictive values, and also integrated it in their 4-step algorithm.

Because these criteria were assessed in nonischemic cardiomyopathy, they should not be used in cases of previous infarction with myocardial scar and fixed Q wave in a given region.

Precordial Pattern Break

A well-described but not overtly tested pattern is the abrupt loss of R wave in lead V2 followed by return of R wave in lead V3.[12] This is a common observation in epicardial VT coming from areas near the LV summit, such as the anterior interventricular vein.

Nonischemic Cardiomyopathy Epicardial VT Algorithm

A 4-step algorithm by Vallès and colleagues[9] was applied to 14 patients with nonischemic cardiomyopathy and basal superior lateral origin VT. It combines 2 morphology criteria and 2 modified interval criteria. The first step is that presence of Q waves in the inferior leads rules out epicardial VT, given the high sensitivity of this measurement (99% for paced QRS and 94% for VT). The second step is that a pseudo-δ of 75 milliseconds or greater favors an epicardial VT. The third step is an MDI of 0.59 or greater, and the fourth step is the presence of a Q wave in lead I, each of which indicates an epicardial VT focus. This 4-step algorithm correctly identified the origin of 109 of 115 pace maps and 21 of 24 VTs. The overall sensitivity was 96% and specificity was 93% for this algorithm (see **Fig. 4**).

Ischemic Cardiomyopathy Epicardial VT Criteria

The criteria developed in nonischemic cardiomyopathy are less accurate when applied to ischemic cardiomyopathy. Martinek and colleagues[13] could not identify features of epicardial VT that accurately identified epicardial VT in ischemic cardiomyopathy. These investigators also found that pseudo-δ wave measurement had an interobserver variability of 25%. In the study by Beruzzo and colleagues, 70% of the patients had ischemic VT, so it is reasonable to apply their 3 criteria: pseudo-δ wave greater than 34 milliseconds, intrinsicoid deflection time greater than 85 milliseconds, and shortest RS complex greater than 121 milliseconds. All endocardial VTs in this study had a QRS complex duration of less than 211 milliseconds. In a study of 444 consecutive patients undergoing ablation for ischemic VT,[14] 6% required epicardial ablation, and of these, 68% had a successful ablation site on the epicardium. In the series of 109 epicardial ablation reported by Tung and colleagues,[15] patients with ischemic VT overall did better with epicardial ablation compared with an endocardial only approach, with significantly better freedom from VT at 12 months.

Normal Sinus Rhythm Findings Suggestive of Basal Lateral Scar

Tzou and colleagues[16] compared sinus rhythm ECGs in patients with nonischemic cardiomyopathy who had VT with those without VT. Epicardial scar in the basal lateral region is commonly found in the patient population with nonischemic cardiomyopathy. An R wave greater than 0.15 mV in V1, and a V6 S wave greater than 0.15 mV, or an S/R wave ratio in V6 greater than 0.2, predicted basal lateral low voltage on electroanatomic mapping. This study did not differentiate between endocardial and epicardial scar. One limitation is that imaging was not performed routinely to confirm the scar location findings on the electroanatomic maps.

Decision Algorithm for Epicardial Mapping and Ablation in VT

ECG findings that can help the clinician determine if an epicardial approach to VT ablation is warranted are critical to recognize. The basic premise is that a slurred upstroke and widened QRS may imply that VT activation is further from the endocardial Purkinje network. An algorithm suggested by Boyle and colleagues is a 4-step approach to determine if epicardial access and ablation are required:

Step 1: determine if ECG criteria as described earlier are met to suggest epicardial VT

Step 2: if previous endocardial ablation unsuccessful, consider epicardial approach

Step 3: define if there is subepicardial or midmyocardial scar on contrast-enhanced imaging

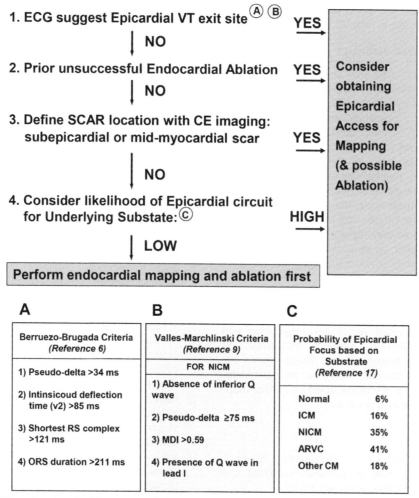

Fig. 5. Flow Chart showing decision approach for epicardial access and ablation with VT. ARVC, Arrhythmogenic Right Ventricular Cardiomyopathy; CE, contrast enhanced; CM, cardiomyopathy; ICM, ischemic cardiomyopathy; MDI, maximal deflection index; NICM, nonischemic cardiomyopathy. (*From* Boyle NG, Shivkumar K. Epicardial interventions in electrophysiology. Circulation 2012;126:1759.)

Step 4: assess if the substrate is high risk for epicardial VT (ie, arrhythmogenic right ventricular cardiomyopathy, Chagas cardiomyopathy).[17]

If some or all of the 4 criteria are met, a combined endocardial-epicardial approach to VT ablation may be warranted (**Fig. 5**).[18]

ACCESSORY PATHWAYS
Posterior Septal Pathways

The coronary sinus has musculature capable of electrical conduction and shares surfaces with both the atrium and the ventricle. This situation predisposes to epicardial accessory pathways, particularly in the case of anatomic variants, such as diverticulum in the middle cardiac vein, which is present in 30% of posterior septal pathways.[19] The most sensitive finding is an immediate negative δ wave in lead II ($\leq$87% of cases). A more specific finding is a steep positive δ in lead AVR and deep S wave in lead V6.[20]

Right Free Wall Pathways

The right atrial free wall is a common site for epicardial pathways. In a case series of 6 patients from our center,[21] a total of 7 epicardial pathways were ablated successfully, with 5 on the right atrial free wall, and 2 in the posterior septal coronary sinus (1 right and 1 left). The right atrial appendage may also touch down on the anterior wall of the right ventricle, making this a potential location of an atrioventricular connection. ECG findings of right free wall pathway (either epicardial and endocardial) include left axis with negative δ wave in V1. The decision to undertake epicardial mapping is best made after an endocardial approach does not yield an early or adequate signal for ablation.

SUMMARY

ECG criteria have been developed for the identification of epicardial ventricular arrhythmias and accessory pathways, although sensitivity and specificity are highly variable. These criteria are best used in conjunction with other clinical and imaging criteria to determine when epicardial mapping and ablation is necessary.

REFERENCES

1. Sealy WC, Hattler BG Jr, Blumenschein SD, et al. Surgical treatment of Wolff-Parkinson-White syndrome. Ann Thorac Surg 1969;8:1–11.
2. Sosa E, Scanavacca M, d'Avila A, et al. A new technique to perform epicardial mapping in the electrophysiology laboratory. J Cardiovasc Electrophysiol 1996;7:531–6.
3. Aliot EM, Stevenson WG, Almendral-Garrote JM, et al. EHRA/HRS expert consensus on catheter ablation of ventricular arrhythmias: developed in a partnership with the European Heart Rhythm Association (EHRA), a registered branch of the European Society of Cardiology (ESC), and the Heart Rhythm Society (HRS); in collaboration with the American College of Cardiology (ACC) and the American Heart Association (AHA). Heart Rhythm 2009;6(6): 886–933.
4. Daniels DV, Lu YY, Morton JB, et al. Idiopathic epicardial left ventricular tachycardia originating remote from the sinus of Valsalva: electrophysiological characteristics, catheter ablation, and identification from the 12-lead electrocardiogram. Circulation 2006;113:1659–66.
5. Doppalapudi H, Yamada T, Ramaswamy K, et al. Idiopathic focal epicardial ventricular tachycardia originating from the crux of the heart. Heart Rhythm 2009;6:44–50.
6. Berruezo A, Mont L, Nava S, et al. Electrocardiographic recognition of the epicardial origin of ventricular tachycardias. Circulation 2004;109:1842–7.
7. Bazan V, Gerstenfeld EP, Garcia FC, et al. Site-specific twelve-lead ECG features to identify an epicardial origin for left ventricular tachycardia in the absence of myocardial infarction. Heart Rhythm 2007;4:1403–10.
8. Hsia HH, Callans DJ, Marchlinski FE. Characterization of endocardial electrophysiological substrate in patients with nonischemic cardiomyopathy and monomorphic ventricular tachycardia. Circulation 2003;108:704–10.
9. Vallès E, Bazan V, Marchlinski FE. ECG criteria to identify epicardial ventricular tachycardia in nonischemic cardiomyopathy. Circ Arrhythm Electrophysiol 2010;3:63–71.
10. Goyal R, Harvey M, Daoud EG, et al. Effect of coupling interval and pacing cycle length on morphology of paced ventricular complexes implications for pace mapping. Circulation 1996;94: 2843–9.
11. Yokokawa M, Kim HM, Good E, et al. Impact of QRS duration of frequent premature ventricular complexes on the development of cardiomyopathy. Heart Rhythm 2012;9:1460–4.
12. Haqqani HM, Morton JB, Kalman JM. Using the 12-lead ECG to localize the origin of atrial and ventricular tachycardias: part 2–ventricular tachycardia. J Cardiovasc Electrophysiol 2009;20(7):825–32.
13. Martinek M, Stevenson WG, Inada K, et al. QRS characteristics fail to reliably identify ventricular tachycardias that require epicardial ablation in ischemic heart disease. J Cardiovasc Electrophysiol 2012;23(2):188–93.
14. Sarkozy A, Tokuda M, Tedrow UB, et al. Epicardial ablation of ventricular tachycardia in ischemic heart

disease. Circ Arrhythm Electrophysiol 2013;6(6): 1115–22.

15. Tung R, Michowitz Y, Yu R, et al. Epicardial ablation of ventricular tachycardia: an institutional experience of safety and efficacy. Heart Rhythm 2013;10: 490–8.

16. Tzou WS, Zado ES, Lin D, et al. Sinus rhythm ECG criteria associated with basal-lateral ventricular tachycardia substrate in patients with nonischemic cardiomyopathy. J Cardiovasc Electrophysiol 2011; 22:1351–8.

17. Sacher F, Roberts-Thomson K, Maury P, et al. Epicardial ventricular tachycardia ablation a multicenter safety study. J Am Coll Cardiol 2010;55: 2366–72.

18. Boyle NG, Shivkumar K. Epicardial interventions in electrophysiology. Circulation 2012;126:1752–69.

19. Sun Y, Arruda M, Otomo K, et al. Coronary sinus-ventricular accessory connections producing posteroseptal and left posterior accessory pathways: incidence and electrophysiological identification. Circulation 2002;106:1362–7.

20. Takahashi A, Shah DC, Jais P, et al. Specific electrocardiographic features of manifest coronary vein posteroseptal accessory pathways. J Cardiovasc Electrophysiol 1998;9:1015–25.

21. Valderrabano M, Cesario DA, Ji S, et al. Percutaneous epicardial mapping during ablation of difficult accessory pathways as an alternative to cardiac surgery. Heart Rhythm 2004;1:311–6.

Incessant Ventricular Tachycardia and Fibrillation: Electrical Storms

Amin Al-Ahmad, MD[a], Mohammad Shenasa, MD[b,c],*,
Hossein Shenasa, MD, MsC[b,c], Mona Soleimanieh, RN[b]

KEYWORDS

- Electrical storm • Ventricular tachycardia • Ventricular fibrillation

KEY POINTS

- Management of ventricular tachycardia storms is often empiric and typically depends on the identification of a cause or underlying pathophysiology that needs treatment.
- The use of the electrocardiogram (ECG) and intracardiac ECGs can be useful in deciding on a clinical strategy for treatment of electrical storm.
- Treating the underlying causes and contributing factors is often helpful in addition to the use of medical therapy and ablation.

INTRODUCTION

Electrical storm is defined as 3 or more episodes of sustained ventricular tachyarrhythmias/ventricular fibrillation (VT/VF) or appropriate implantable-cardioverter defibrillators (ICD) shocks that occur within a period of 24 hours.[1,2] Most commonly, VT storm is seen in individuals with structural heart disease and ICDs. Before ICDs, most patients with electrical storm did not survive. VT storm can also be seen in patients with a structurally normal heart, such as those with ion channel mutation.[3] The overall mortality related to electrical storm is very high.[1] Many times electrical storm occurs in the setting of end-stage cardiomyopathy or in the setting of severe medical and metabolic comorbid conditions.[4] In addition, patients who survive the storm often are treated with medications that have a high level of side effects and adverse effects, such as Amiodarone. Innovative procedures such as VT or VF ablation when done in the setting of electrical storm also have higher morbidity and mortality than when performed electively. In an extreme example, radiofrequency ablation (RFA) in the setting of VT/VF storm in patients with ventricular assist devices has been reported as high as 80% over a 6-month follow-up period.[2,5,6] Neural modulation (left stellate ganglion blockade) has recently been reported as an effective method in rare cases of VT storm.[7] Similarly, renal denervation has been used in the management of ventricular arrhythmia storm in patients with cardiomyopathy.[6]

In this communication, VT/VF storm is used interchangeably with electrical storm.

SPECIFIC CONTRIBUTING FACTORS IN ELECTRICAL STORM

Box 1 shows the common causes of VT/VF storm.

The authors have nothing to disclose.
[a] Texas Cardiac Arrhythmia Institute, 3000 N. IH 35 Suite 720, Austin, TX 78705, USA; [b] Heart & Rhythm Medical Group, 105 North Bascom Avenue, San Jose, CA 95128, USA; [c] Department of Cardiovascular Services, O'Connor Hospital, San Jose, CA, USA
* Corresponding author. Heart & Rhythm Medical Group, 105 North Bascom Avenue, Suite 204, San Jose, CA 95128.
E-mail address: mohammad.shenasa@gmail.com

Card Electrophysiol Clin 6 (2014) 613–621
http://dx.doi.org/10.1016/j.ccep.2014.05.010

> **Box 1**
> **Causes of VT/VF electrical storm**
>
> 1. Electrolyte and metabolic imbalance
> 2. Myocardial ischemia and infarction
> 3. Drug-induced proarrhythmia
> 4. VT/VF Storm in Patients with ICDs
> 5. VT storm in inherited channelopathies
> 6. Electrical storm in patients with congestive heart failure
> 7. Unknown causes

Electrolyte Imbalance

Electrolyte imbalance can often contribute to electrical storm.[4] In patients with hyperkalemia, the electrolyte imbalance can lead directly to ventricular arrhythmias, although not always as a "storm." Patients with electrical storm can often have hypokalemia. Both hyperkalemia and hypokalemia can manifest as electrocardiogram (ECG) changes before onset of ventricular arrhythmias. Correction of the electrolyte imbalance is an important step in the early management of these patients.

Myocardial Ischemia and Infarction

Acute ischemia can sometimes lead to electrical storm, usually VF. Chronic myocardial ischemia can also set the stage for reentrant arrhythmias. Patients with electrical storm should be evaluated for ischemia, and when possible, it should be reversed. In addition, treatment with β-blockers can decrease both ischemia and ventricular arrhythmias. Patients with atrial fibrillation (AF) who inherently have irregular heart rate often with short-long-short sequence in the presence of ischemia and infarction may trigger recurrent fast VT/VF, especially when antiarrhythmic medications are on board. **Fig. 1** shows an example of incessant VT in a patient after a myocardial infarction. Frequent premature ventricular complexes precede VT, and a 3-beat VT triggers sustained monomorphic VT. Urgent coronary angiography and revascularization of a subtotal left anterior descending coronary artery abolished ventricular arrhythmias.

Drug-induced Proarrhythmia

Proarrhythmia is most commonly related to prolongation of the QT interval. Common culprits are antibiotics,[8] antiarrhythmic medications,[9] and antipsychotic medications.[10] **Fig. 2** shows an example of drug-induced polymorphic VT and torsades de pointes due to administration of Ibutilide for conversion of AF. Amiodarone can commonly cause prolongation of the QT interval; however, it rarely causes proarrhythmia. Unfortunately, when Amiodarone does cause proarrhythmia, it often manifests as electrical storm. Also, given the prolonged drug half-life with Amiodarone, patients affected with electrical storm can have multiple episodes even after the drug is discontinued. Commonly, electrical storm is related to pause-dependent early premature ventricular contractions (PVCs). Treatments that increase the heart rate and prevent pause-dependent arrhythmia such as pacing or use of isoproterenol can be helpful.

VT Storm in Patients with ICDs

Electrical storm in patients with ICDs can occur in about 10% to 20% of this population.[4] The incidence is higher in patients who receive ICDs as a secondary than primary prevention. Recipients of cardiac resynchronization therapy may present with electrical storm, especially in the early phase after implantation.[11–13] Recent advances in the management of patients with ICDs have led to recommendations for increased use of antitachycardia pacing as well as increasing the time to detect and to prevent unnecessary shocks.[14] In addition to the pain related to the ICD shocks, patients often have psychological manifestations of posttraumatic stress syndrome.

VT Storm in Inherited Channelopathies

Patients with inherited syndromes may present with electrical storm. Conditions such as the Brugada syndrome can have electrical storm with no apparent precipitating factor.[15–18] **Fig. 3** shows an example of recurrent VT in a patient with Brugada syndrome who also received an ICD.

Electrical Storm in Patients with Congestive Heart Failure

Patients with congestive heart failure (CHF) are the most common patients presenting with electrical storm. Most cases do not have an identifiable ischemic cause or clear electrolyte abnormalities. Worsening CHF can be a precipitating factor, but is not always present: many cases have not had any clinical decompensation. Electrical storm is a poor prognostic indicator in patients with CHF. **Figs. 4** and **5** shows an example of recurrent VT/VT in patients with end-stage heart failure (HF).

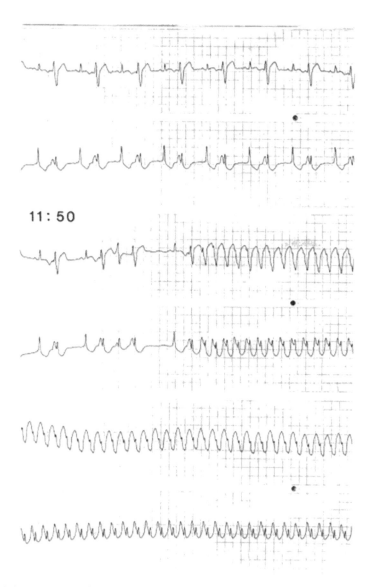

Fig. 1. Incessant VT in a patient with anterior wall myocardial infarction detected during Holter monitoring.

ECG MARKERS OF VT STORM

There are no specific ECG characteristics or predictors of VT storms. However, in some cases, ECG findings can be useful and may help lead to potential therapy. Frequent monomorphic PVCs can be seen initiating polymorphic VT. Polymorphic VT can occur in normal hearts with PVCs of usually benign morphology such as those originating from the right and left ventricular outflow tract region. In addition, PVCs initiating VF in patients with ischemic heart disease can be monomorphic and originate in a region near the Purkinje system[19] or in the peri-infract area in patients with prior infarction. Frequent episodes of nonsustained VT are also sometimes seen before an electrical storm event.

ECG manifestations of ischemia such as ST depression are commonly seen with prolongation of the QT interval and lead to dispersion of refractoriness of the QT interval, which in turn can lead to the development of recurrent ventricular arrhythmias. In severe cases, the T wave alternates in a beat-by-beat fashion resulting in visible or microvolt T-wave alternans, which is a worrisome sign and often precedes VF by only minutes.

Prolongation of the QT interval also is associated with an increase in episodes of ventricular arrhythmias. Often, this can be seen as the result

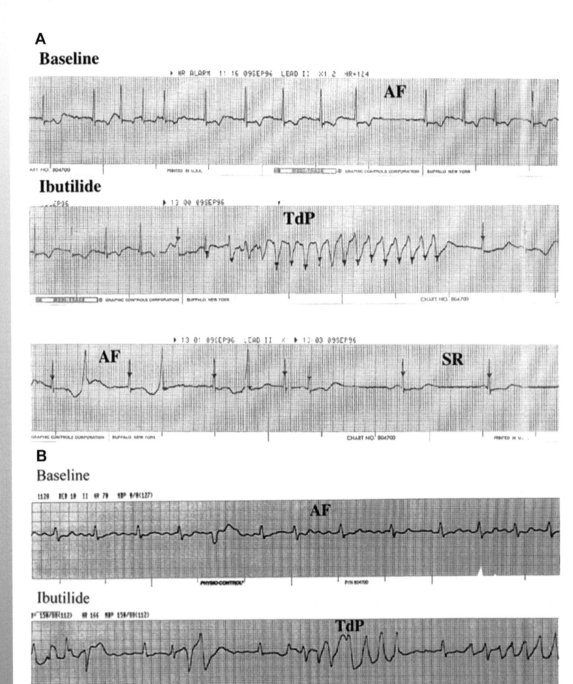

Fig. 2. (*A*) Top tracing is baseline in Atrial Fibrillation (AF). Middle tracing is after Ibutilide infusion and shows AF and torsades de pointes (TdP). Lower tracing shows conversion from AF to sinus rhythm (SR) (*B*) Ibutilide infused TdP in different patient than panel A.

A

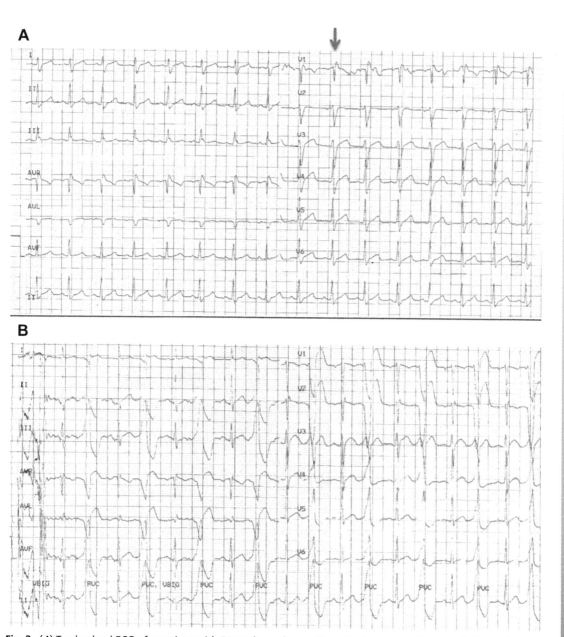

Fig. 3. (A) Twelve-lead ECG of a patient with Brugada syndrome. Note ST-elevation of V1 (arrow). (B) Twelve-lead ECG of a patient with Brugada syndrome and ventricular bigeminy.

of administration of medications that prolong the QT interval. Patients with a congenital long QT syndrome and a very long QT interval also have an increased risk of recurrent ventricular arrhythmias.

In patients with the Brugada syndrome, the ECG manifestations of an atypical right bundle branch block can often be more obvious in certain clinical states such as fever and may be associated with a higher risk of developing clinical arrhythmias.

Patients with arrhythmogenic right ventricular dysplasia (ARVD) will commonly have repolarization abnormalities as well as abnormalities of the terminal portion of the QRS. Identification of the ECG manifestations of ARVD or the Brugada syndrome in a patient with electrical storm can help correctly identify the underlying condition and can be useful in the initiation of therapy for electrical storm in these patients.

Another abnormality associated with electrical storm is the catcholaminergic polymorphic

C

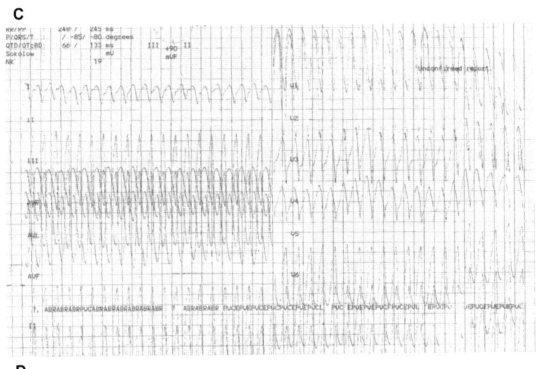

D

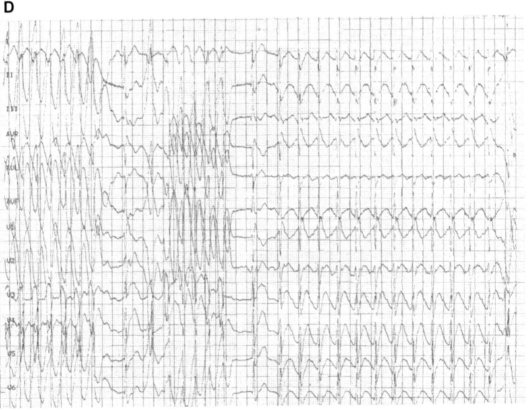

Fig. 3. (*continued*). (*C*) Rapid VT (same patient as in *A* and *B*) with a heart rate of 248 bpm. (*D*) Rapid nonsustained VT (same patient as in *A–C*).

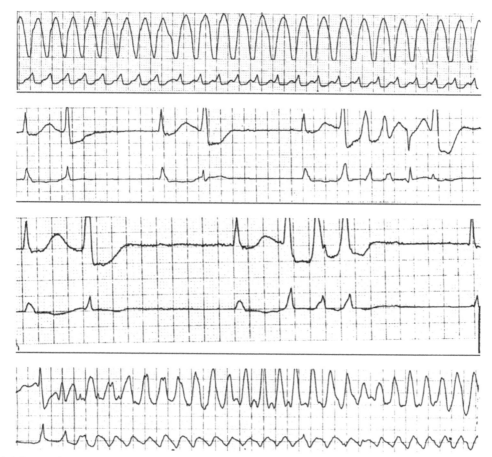

Fig. 4. VT storm in patient with CHF.

ventricular tachycardia (CPVT) syndrome. Although the baseline 12-lead ECG does not reveal any abnormalities, the ECG of the VT often shows bidirectional VT (see article by Methachittiphan and colleagues). Identification of bidirectional VT should lead to consideration of CPVT or medication toxicity such as digoxin.

Other than the ECG, because most patients with electrical storm have an ICD, the use of intracardiac ECGs can also be useful. For example, examination of the ECG preceding the shock can often reveal frequent premature ventricular beats. In addition, the morphology of these beats (at least in the near-field and far-field ECG) can occasionally be useful to identify these as monomorphic versus polymorphic beats; a repetitive beat that triggers ventricular arrhythmias can be a target for ablation.

INFARCTION ELECTRICAL STORM MANAGEMENT

Treatment of electrical storm consists of first understanding the potential cause and contributing factors that led to these individual episodes, all while stabilizing the patients often with the use of intravenous anti-arrhythmic medications. Often the use of more than one medication is needed to stabilize the patient. Occasionally, if the patient is not improved with the use of medications, sedation with the use of general anesthetics may be indicated.

Other potential contributing factors, such as electrolyte abnormalities and ischemia, should be reversed. In patients with acute HF, optimization of HF status is important. Medications that may have caused proarrhythmia should be discontinued.

RFA should be considered once the patient is stabilized. In some cases, RFA is needed because of difficulty in stabilizing the patient with medical therapy. RFA can target the initiating premature beat, if present, or can be useful to target the arrhythmia directly or via substrate modification in cases with hemodynamically intolerable episodes. Last, the use of deep sedation and mechanical support, such as ventricular assist devices, can be useful in the management of these patients. Heart transplant at specialized centers may also be considered.

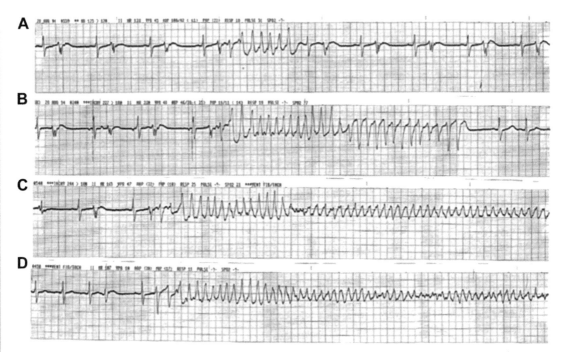

Fig. 5. From a patient with congestive heart failure with ejection fraction of 25% awaiting ICD implantation. Panels (*A-D*) shows sinus rhythm with ventricular bigeminy. Note the episodes of torsades de pointes was initiated consistently with a short long short sequence.

SUMMARY

Electrical storm is a challenging condition. The use of the ECG and intracardiac ECGs can be useful in deciding on a clinical strategy for treatment. Treating the underlying causes and contributing factors is often useful in addition to the use of medical therapy and ablation.

REFERENCES

1. Verma A, Kilicaslan F, Marrouche NF, et al. Prevalence, predictors and mortality significance of the causative arrhythmia in patients with electrical storm. J Cardiovasc Electrophysiol 2004;15:1265–70.
2. Nayyar S, Ganesan AN, Brooks AG, et al. Venturing into ventricular arrhythmias storm: a systemic review and meta-analysis. Eur Heart J 2013;34:560–9.
3. Haissaguerre M, Extramiana F, Hocini M, et al. Mapping and ablation of ventricular fibrillation storms in patients with ischemic cardiomyopathy.
4. Eifling M, Razavi M, Massumi A. The evaluation and management of electrical storm. Tex Heart Inst J 2011;38(2):111–21.
5. Carbucicchio C, Santamaria M, Trevisi N, et al. Catheter ablation for the treatment of electrical storm in patients with implantable cardioverter-defibrillators: short-and long-term outcomes in a Prospective Single-Center Study. Circulation 2008;117:462–9.
6. Remo BF, Preminger M, Bradfield J, et al. Safety and efficacy of renal denervation as a novel treatment of ventricular tachycardia storm in patients with cardiomyopathy. Heart Rhythm 2014;11:541–6.
7. Bourke T, Vaseghi M, Michowitz Y, et al. Neuraxial modulation for refractory ventricular arrhythmias: value of thoracic epidural anesthesia and surgical left cardiac sympathetic denervation. Circulation 2010;121:2255–62.
8. Huang BH, Wu CH, Hsia CP, et al. Azithromycin-induced torsade de pointes. Pacing Clin Electrophysiol 2007;31:1579–82.
9. Eckardt L, Breithardt G. Drug-induced ventricular tachycardia. In: Zipes DP, Jalife J, editors. Cardiac electrophysiology, From Cell to Bedside. 6th edition. Philadelphia: Elsevier Saunders; 2014. p. 1001–8.
10. Beach SR, Celano CM, Noseworthy PA, et al. OTc prolongation, torsades de pointes and psychotropic medications. Psychosomatics 2013;54:1–13.
11. Brigadeau F, Kouakam C, Klug D, et al. Clinical predictors and prognostic significance of electrical storm in patients with implantable cardioverter defibrillators. Eur Heart J 2006;27:700–7.
12. Arya A, Haghjoo M, Dehghani MR, et al. Prevalence and predictors of electrical storm in patients with implantable cardioverter-defibrillator. Am J Cardiol 2006;97:389–92.
13. Turitto G, El-Sherif N. Cardiac resynchronization therapy: a review of proarrhythmic and antiarrhythmic

medications. Pacing Clin Electrophysiol 2007;30: 115–22.

14. Moss AJ, Schuger C, Beck CA, et al. Reduction in inappropriate therapy and mortality through ICD programming. N Engl J Med 2012;367:2275–83.

15. Nademanee K, Taylor R, Bailey WE, et al. Treating electrical storm: sympathetic blockade versus advanced cardiac life support-guided therapy. Circulation 2000;102:742–7.

16. Veerakul G, Nademanee K. Treament of electrical storms in Brugada syndrome. Journal of Arrhythmia 2013;29:117–24.

17. Nademanee K, Veerakul G, Chandanamattha P, et al. Prevention of ventricular fibrillation episodes in Brugada syndrome by catheter ablation over the anterior right ventricular outflow tract epicardium. Circulation 2011;123:1270–9.

18. Dinckal MH, Davutoglu V, Akdemir I, et al. Incessant monomorphic ventricular tachycardia during febrile illness in a patient with Brugada syndrome: fatal electrical storm. Europace 2003;5:257–61.

19. Haissaguerre M, Shah DC, Jais P, et al. Role of Purkinje conducting system in triggering of idiopathic ventricular fibrillation. Lancet 2002;359:677–8.

Arrhythmias in Complex Congenital Heart Disease

Robert M. Hayward, MD, Zian H. Tseng, MD, MAS*

KEYWORDS

- Atrial fibrillation • Atrial flutter • Catheter ablation • Congenital heart disease
- Ventricular tachycardia

KEY POINTS

- Atrial and ventricular arrhythmias are a common cause of morbidity and mortality in the growing population of adults with congenital heart disease.
- Patients with high-risk congenital heart disease lesions such as dextro-transposition of the great arteries, levo-transposition of the great arteries, or tetralogy of Fallot should be monitored routinely for arrhythmias and associated symptoms.
- With the aid of electroanatomic mapping and newer irrigated radiofrequency energy delivery, catheter ablation is an excellent therapeutic option for a variety of arrhythmias observed in these patients when performed in experienced centers.
- Implantation of an implantable cardioverter-defibrillator is recommended for cardiac arrest survivors and congenital heart disease patients with sustained ventricular tachycardia discovered on electrophysiology study.
- In planning catheter ablation and device implantation procedures, clinicians should review specific anatomy and surgical records, obtain imaging to define possible obstructions or stenosis in vascular pathways, and be aware of associated congenital abnormalities.

INTRODUCTION

More than one million adults are living with congenital heart disease (CHD) in the United States, and this group now outnumbers children with CHD.[1,2] Late after surgical repair of complex congenital lesions, atrial arrhythmias are a major cause of morbidity, and ventricular arrhythmias and sudden cardiac death (SCD) are a major cause of mortality.[3–7] Arrhythmia mechanisms include reentry caused by substrate from previous surgeries, the long-term consequences of hemodynamic abnormalities, such as chamber enlargement and hypertrophy, and direct results of congenital abnormalities, such as the presence of accessory pathways. It has been reported that the prevalence of atrial arrhythmias is 15% in adults with CHD; for patients with complex CHD, the lifetime risk of atrial arrhythmias is more than 50%.[8] Atrial arrhythmias in these patients are associated with increased risk of stroke, heart failure, and mortality.[8] Ventricular arrhythmias are also common in CHD, especially in patients with tetralogy of Fallot (TOF), ventricular septal defect, Ebstein's anomaly, and systemic right ventricles. Drug therapy is often inadequate for these patients. Amiodarone is often avoided in younger patients because of concerns over long-term toxicity; class IC agents may have

Financial Support: This work was supported in part by National Institutes of Health/NHLBI 5R01 HL102090 (Dr Z.H. Tseng).
Disclosures: Dr Z.H. Tseng has received minor honoraria from Biotronik. Dr R.M. Hayward has received an educational travel grant from Medtronic.
Section of Cardiac Electrophysiology, Division of Cardiology, Department of Medicine, University of California, San Francisco, 500 Parnassus Avenue, San Francisco, CA 94143-1354, USA
* Corresponding author.
E-mail address: zhtseng@medicine.ucsf.edu

cardiacEP.theclinics.com

lower efficacy than in other patient groups[9] and may be contraindicated because of underlying structural heart disease. In experienced centers, catheter ablation has emerged as the preferred therapeutic option for atrial and ventricular arrhythmias in the CHD population. As increasing numbers of patients reach adulthood, the burden of arrhythmias and SCD are expected to increase even further, and the need for device implantations[10] and catheter ablation procedures will continue to grow. This review focuses on 6 cases that highlight common and important electrophysiology problems in the adult CHD population.

Case I

A 45-year-old woman with history of perimembranous ventricular septal defect after patch repair, moderate residual right ventricle (RV) enlargement, and supraventricular tachycardia (SVT) after ablation at another hospital 8 years prior was admitted with palpitations and SVT (**Fig. 1**). Electrophysiology (EP) study found 2 intra-atrial reentrant tachycardias (IARTs) involving a posterolateral right atrial scar (**Fig. 2**). Radiofrequency catheter ablation of the isthmus within the scar terminated the arrhythmias (**Fig. 3**).

The most common arrhythmia in older adults with CHD is IART. This is a macroreentrant circuit involving abnormal atrial tissue resulting from atriotomy incisions, fibrosis, or patches[11–13] and characterized by large areas of low voltage with multiple heterogeneous channels.[14] IART may be seen in any patient who has undergone atriotomy, such as this patient, but the incidence is

particularly high for patients with dextrotransposition of the great arteries (D-TGA) after Mustard[15] or Senning repair and patients with a single ventricle after Fontan. Fontan patients treated with older intra-atrial lateral tunnel operations are at higher risk than those treated with extracardiac Fontan operations.[16–20] Atrial rates in IART are typically 150 to 250 beats per minute (bpm), and 1:1 atrioventricular (AV) conduction can result in presyncope, syncope, or SCD.[21] As in this patient, multiple circuits are common.

Catheter ablation has been used with success in experienced centers. Complete procedural success is reported to be as high as 80% with the use of irrigated ablation catheters and electroanatomic mapping, but recurrence is reported in about 40% of patients. Arrhythmia recurrence is more common for those with multiple circuits, atrial fibrillation, and Fontan physiology.[22] Because IART has been associated with thromboembolism,[23] adequate anticoagulation with periprocedural transesophageal echocardiogram guidance according to standard guidelines is recommended.

Case II

A 50-year-old man with D-TGA after Mustard procedure presented with dyspnea on exertion and was found to have pulmonary venous baffle stenosis and right-to-left shunting, suggesting a systemic venous baffle leak. At the time of stent placement for the pulmonary venous baffle stenosis, he was in atrial flutter at cycle length of 280 milliseconds. Flutter waves were negative in the

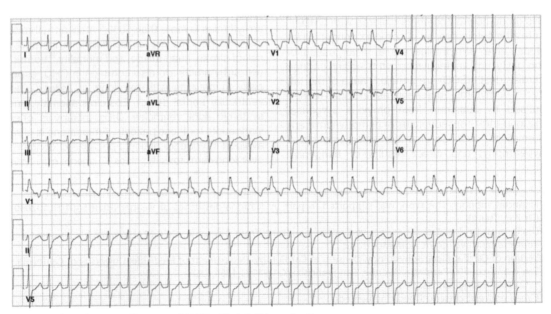

Fig. 1. Surface electrocardiogram of IART with 1:1 AV conduction.

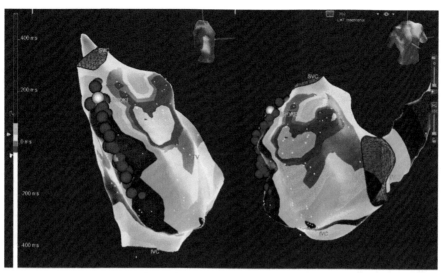

Fig. 2. Electroanatomic activation map shows slow conduction in the isthmus of the IART circuit (*purple areas*) in the posterolateral right atrium at the site of a previous atriotomy incision. Ablation through this isthmus resulted in termination of tachycardia (*white sphere*); the radiofrequency (RF) lesion set was completed by connecting the areas of low voltage in the atriotomy incision to areas of normal voltage.

inferior leads and positive in V1 suggesting typical counterclockwise flutter. During the procedure, the patient had 1:1 AV conduction in atrial flutter and became hypotensive, requiring external cardioversion. After several weeks of anticoagulation with warfarin, he underwent EP study. Typical atrial flutter was induced and dependence on the cavo-tricuspid isthmus was proven with entrainment (**Fig. 4**). Multiple radiofrequency lesions were placed in systemic venous atrium proximal to the baffle at 4 o'clock on tricuspid annulus. Because the baffle prevented access to the anterior part of the cavo-tricuspid isthmus, the ablation catheter was then advanced via the baffle leak to

the pulmonary venous (morphologic right) atrium and positioned along the cavo-tricuspid isthmus anterior and adjacent to the initial lesion set (**Fig. 5**). The ablation line was then continued anteriorly toward the tricuspid (systemic AV) valve. After ablation, atrial flutter was not inducible. Three weeks later, the patient's baffle leak was closed percutaneously using 2 vascular plugs. The patient has been free from arrhythmia symptoms and atrial flutter at follow-up.

The patient underwent a follow-up event monitor for atrial arrhythmias before stopping anticoagulation. He had no atrial flutter but was found to have nonsustained ventricular tachycardia (NSVT), up to

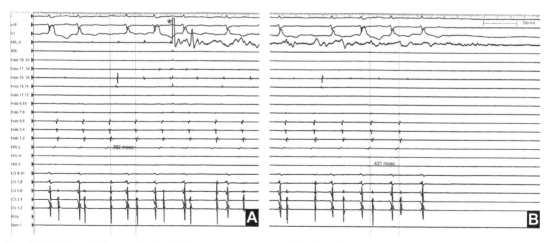

Fig. 3. (A) Prior to the onset of radiofrequency energy application (*asterisk*), intracardiac electrograms in IART show a diastolic signal on the ablation catheter representing conduction within the isthmus of the scar. (B) During radiofrequency ablation, the tachycardia cycle length increases by 50 milliseconds before termination.

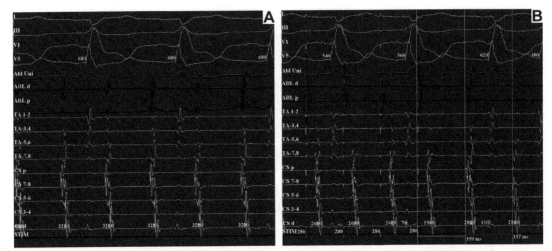

Fig. 4. (*A*) Atrial flutter. (*B*) The postpacing interval after overdrive pacing from the cavo-tricuspid isthmus (ABL d) was equal to the tachycardia cycle length.

6 beats in duration. Given moderate-to-severe systemic (RV) dysfunction, NSVT, prolonged QRS duration, and resting bradycardia, he underwent dual chamber implantable cardioverter-defibrillator (ICD) implantation.

D-TGA accounts for 3% to 7% of congenital heart defects.[24] Historically, most patients with D-TGA were treated with atrial switch operations (Mustard or Senning baffles), but since the 1980s, most patients have been treated with the arterial switch operation. However, most adults followed up with in CHD clinics underwent atrial switch repairs. These subjects are at high risk for congestive heart failure; ventricular arrhythmias and SCD are the leading cause of late mortality.[25–28] In the largest retrospective study of these

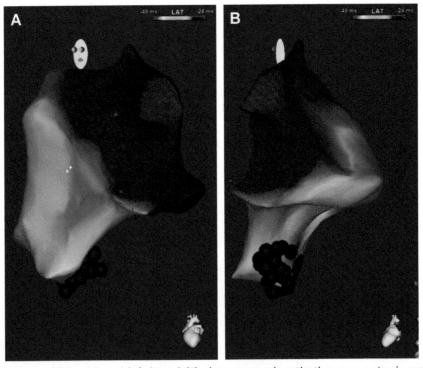

Fig. 5. Left anterior oblique (*A*) and left lateral (*B*) electroanatomic activation map systemic venous atrium. Completion of the line across the cavo-tricuspid isthmus required accessing the pulmonary venous atrium via a baffle leak (*asterisk*).

patients, ventricular tachycardia and SCD were correlated with New York Heart Association class, systolic dysfunction of the systemic ventricle, and QRS duration (hazard ratio, 13.6 for QRS duration ≥140 milliseconds) but not with supraventricular arrhythmias.[29] Another study reached different conclusions: that supraventricular arrhythmias, not QRS duration, were predictive of ventricular arrhythmias.[30] However, the decision to place an ICD in this patient is largely extrapolated from primary prevention data in patients with nonischemic cardiomyopathy (reduced function of the systemic ventricle and NSVT).[31–34]

Full access to the cavo-tricuspid isthmus via the systemic venous atrium in patients treated with older Mustard or Senning repairs is often limited by baffles. In these cases, completion of a cavo-tricuspid isthmus line often requires ablation in the systemic venous atrium followed by accessing the pulmonary venous atrium via either a retrograde approach or traversing the baffle. If there is no baffle leak present, access to the pulmonary venous atrium can be obtained through a transbaffle puncture or retrograde aortic approach.

Case III

A 76-year-old woman with levo-transposition of the great arteries (L-TGA) presented with fatigue and dyspnea on exertion. She had atrial fibrillation and atrial flutter (**Fig. 6**), and both of these arrhythmias recurred despite amiodarone and cardioversion. Because of the severe symptoms, she underwent EP study, which induced cavo-tricuspid isthmus dependent atrial flutter and a roof-dependent IART. She underwent ablation of both tachycardias and pulmonary vein isolation (**Figs. 7** and **8**).

As patients with CHD live longer, atrial fibrillation is an increasing problem.[35] In one study of pulmonary vein antrum isolation in patients with CHD, similar success rates were reported in patients without CHD, although in 60% of CHD patients, the only congenital abnormality was an atrial septal defect.[36] Accessing the pulmonary venous atrium in patients with CHD can be technically more difficult with abnormal anatomy and baffles but can be accomplished safely in most cases. Intracardiac echocardiography can be useful for transbaffle puncture and identifying important anatomic structures in CHD patients.[37,38] In patients with L-TGA, the electrophysiologist should be aware of the possibility of other abnormalities, such as ventricular septal defect and tricuspid (systemic AV valve) regurgitation. In addition, dual AV nodes have been reported, and conduction usually occurs via the anteriorly situated AV node.[39] The position of this node at the mitral-pulmonary continuity and the extended length of the His-Purkinje system are thought to render these structures susceptible to fibrosis; complete heart block is reported to occur at a rate of about 2% per year in patients with L-TGA.[40]

Case IV

A 7-year-old girl with Ebstein's anomaly of the tricuspid valve presented with palpitations. She

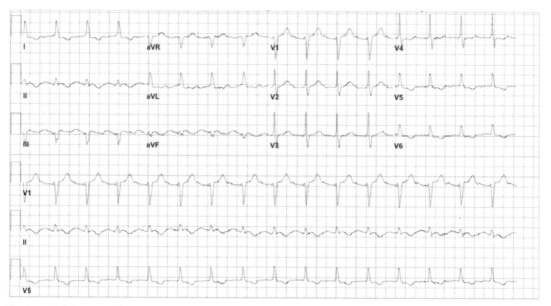

Fig. 6. Atrial flutter with 2:1 AV conduction. Note the absence of septal q-waves in the lateral precordial leads owing to right-to-left depolarization of the interventricular septum in L-TGA.

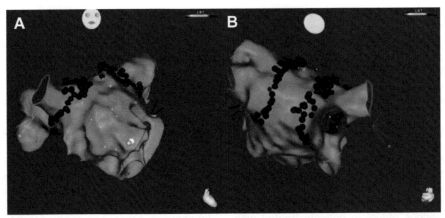

Fig. 7. (*A*) Right anterior oblique view of the normally positioned left atrium after isolation of the pulmonary veins. (*B*) Posteroanterior view of the left atrium after pulmonary vein isolation. In L-TGA, the left atrium connects to the right (systemic) ventricle via the tricuspid valve.

had supraventricular tachycardia at 2 days of age, but this was controlled with propranolol and later with propafenone. At the age of 7, she began experiencing palpitations 3 to 4 times per month and had 2 episodes of syncope while dancing. Electrocardiogram found pre-excitation (**Fig. 9**), and event monitoring found a regular, narrow-complex tachycardia at a rate of 224 bpm. Because of symptoms and syncope, she underwent EP study. During atrial overdrive pacing, there was nondecremental, eccentric AV conduction with the earliest ventricular activation on the

proximal coronary sinus catheter electrode pair. Orthodromic reciprocating tachycardia was induced with atrial extrastimulus pacing. During SVT, premature ventricular complexes introduced during His refractoriness advanced the subsequent atrial electrogram and reset the tachycardia. Based on these findings, a single manifest right posteroseptal accessory pathway was diagnosed, and radiofrequency energy application just anterior to the coronary sinus os resulted in loss of pre-excitation (**Figs. 10 and 11**). Following this lesion, there was no antegrade or retrograde accessory

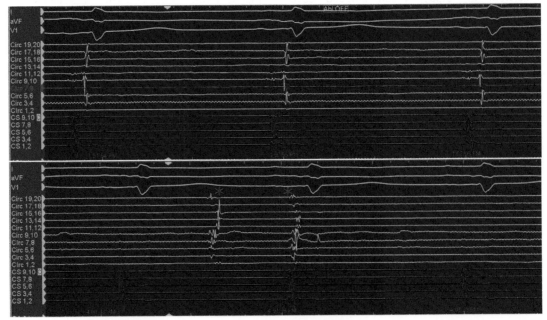

Fig. 8. Sinus rhythm with conduction into left upper pulmonary vein before ablation (*top*). Dissociation of left upper pulmonary vein potentials (*asterisk*) after pulmonary vein isolation (*bottom*).

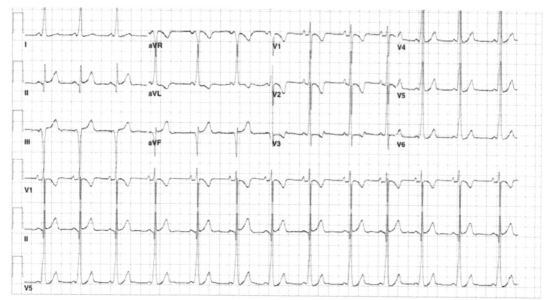

Fig. 9. Baseline electrocardiogram shows preexcitation. The V2 precordial transition with a dominant R-wave in lead I suggests a right-sided accessory pathway. As is common with posteroseptal accessory pathways, there is a pseudo inferior myocardial infarction pattern in the inferior leads.

pathway conduction observed. The patient has been free of arrhythmias at several years of follow-up.

Wolff-Parkinson-White syndrome is the most common arrhythmia in Ebstein's anomaly, but other arrhythmias, including atrial fibrillation, atrial flutter, AV nodal reentrant tachycardia, and ventricular tachycardia are seen in this patient population as well.[41,42] Radiofrequency catheter ablation is the therapy of choice for Wolff-Parkinson-White syndrome in suitable patients with Ebstein's anomaly. However, compared with catheter ablation of accessory pathways in patients without CHD, procedural success rates are

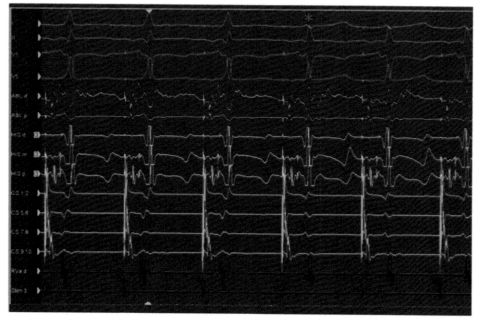

Fig. 10. During RF ablation while pacing the atrium, loss of preexcitation (*asterisk*) and delay of the earliest ventricular electrogram on the proximal coronary sinus catheter electrode (CS 9,10) were noted.

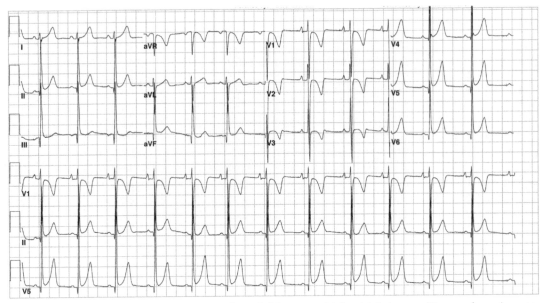

Fig. 11. Postablation electrocardiogram shows loss of delta wave. Right atrial abnormality, seen here, is a common finding in Ebstein's anomaly. Right bundle branch block is also common, although it is not seen in this case.

lower and recurrence rates are higher[43] because of the presence of multiple pathways, right-sided pathway predominance,[44] and abnormal AV node location. Because atrial septal defect and patent foramen ovale are also common, these patients may be at increased risk for paradoxical embolism during catheter ablation. Intraoperative ablation of accessory pathways can also be considered for patients undergoing tricuspid valve surgery.[42]

Case V

A 46-year-old man with TOF after repair in childhood, severe tricuspid regurgitation (caused by flail leaflet), and severe pulmonary regurgitation underwent EP study and ablation for typical atrial flutter and IART. EP study found inducible, unstable polymorphic ventricular tachycardia (PMVT) with triple extrastimuli. After tricuspid valve repair and pulmonary valve replacement, he underwent a follow-up EP study, which induced unstable monomorphic ventricular tachycardia (MMVT) at a cycle-length of 260 milliseconds with a left bundle branch block superior axis morphology. For this reason, he underwent ICD implantation. Two years later, he had an appropriate ICD discharge for MMVT.

TOF accounts for about 10% of congenital heart defects. Surgical repair has good intermediate and long-term results,[45–49] and survival has improved dramatically over the last 25 years.[50] However, ventricular arrhythmias are common, and SCD is the leading cause of late mortality.[4,51,52] Clinical sustained ventricular arrhythmias have a prevalence of approximately 15% by 35 years of age, with increased incidence in even older patients.[5,52] Arrhythmias in these patients are correlated with QRS duration (especially over 180 milliseconds), increase in QRS duration over time, number of prior surgeries, RV dilation, the presence of an right ventricular outflow tract (RVOT) patch, pulmonary regurgitation, and left ventricular diastolic dysfunction.[5,52,53] Several studies found that inducibility of ventricular arrhythmias at EP study has good sensitivity and specificity for predicting subsequent ventricular arrhythmias or SCD.[54–56] Importantly, MMVT and PMVT, both of which were induced in this patient, are found to be predictive of future events in the TOF population.[55] Because EP testing is invasive, and a positive study result alone in low-risk patients probably does not justify ICD placement,[57,58] EP study is reserved for patients with arrhythmia symptoms or abnormal results of other tests, such as rapid or frequent NSVT on Holter monitoring.

Because of areas of scar and slowed conduction in the right ventricle, TOF is the classic congenital heart defect resulting in MMVT. Because this is most commonly a macroreentrant circuit in the scar of RV free wall or near the septal patch repair, the electrocardiogram in VT typically shows a left bundle branch block pattern with an inferior axis, but other morphologies can also be seen.[59] MMVT is also seen in CHD patients with ventriculotomy incisions, ventricular septal defect patches, and Ebstein's anomaly.

ICDs, catheter ablation, and arrhythmia surgery are options for sustained VT or cardiac arrest in the CHD population. In TOF patients undergoing pulmonary valve replacement, intraoperative VT ablation has been used with success in experienced centers.[60–64] Catheter ablation of MMVT has good success rates,[65–68] but late ventricular arrhythmia recurrences are reported in the CHD population; therefore, ICDs are used as prophylaxis against sudden death.[68,69]

Case VI

A 29-year-old man with D-TGA after Mustard procedure and history of sudden cardiac arrest caused by ventricular fibrillation (VF) at 23 years of age was admitted with a transient ischemic attack manifesting as 10 minutes of numbness in his right face, right arm, and right leg. After his cardiac arrest, he underwent ICD placement. Because of lead fracture, he underwent lead revision 4 years later, and 6 months before his presentation for transient ischemic attack, he underwent lead revision at another hospital because of T-wave oversensing. Chest x-ray and transthoracic echocardiogram showed that the ICD lead was incorrectly placed in the right (systemic) ventricle via a baffle leak (**Fig. 12**). The device was extracted, and a new lead was inserted into the left

(subpulmonic) ventricle, and the patient was placed on chronic anticoagulation with no further neurologic symptoms.

Most adult CHD patients with an indication for ICD placement can undergo transvenous system implantation. Lead failure is not uncommon, especially in younger patients.[70] In addition, caution must be taken in lead placement with abnormal venous anatomy. If baffle leaks are present, decisions regarding anticoagulation are impacted, and it is possible to inadvertently place leads in the systemic ventricle, as in this case. These leaks should be closed before lead implantation to prevent systemic thromboemboli. Some patients have anatomy that precludes access to the subpulmonic ventricle (baffle obstruction or stenosis), and some patients with a single ventricle or right-to-left shunts are at risk for thromboembolism with transvenous ICD placement. In these patients, nontransvenous systems are preferred.

Additionally, patients with CHD are at risk for PMVT and VF because of pressure and volume overload, chamber enlargement, and hypoxemia. PMVT and VF are most commonly seen in congenital aortic stenosis, systemic RVs, and Eisenmenger's syndrome.[71] This patient initially underwent ICD placement because of VF in the setting of an abnormal systemic ventricle. It is important, however, to note that because of hemodynamic status and comorbidities, not all sudden deaths in high-risk patients with CHD are owing to an arrhythmic cause.[72]

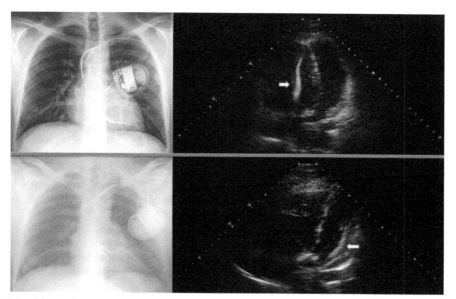

Fig. 12. ICD lead (*arrow*) in RV (systemic ventricle) via Mustard baffle leak (*top*). ICD lead (*arrow*) in left ventricle (subpulmonic ventricle) (*bottom*). Chest radiograph (*left*). Apical 4-chamber surface echocardiogram (*right*).

SUMMARY

Atrial and ventricular arrhythmias are a common cause of morbidity and mortality in the growing population of adults with CHD. Patients with high-risk CHD lesions such as D-TGA, L-TGA, or TOF should be monitored routinely for arrhythmias and associated symptoms. Catheter ablation is an excellent therapeutic option for several arrhythmias observed in these patients when performed in experienced centers by operators familiar with abnormal cardiac anatomy and associated abnormalities, such as residual shunts. ICD implantation is recommended for cardiac arrest survivors and CHD patients with sustained VTs discovered on electrophysiology study. In planning both catheter ablation and device implantation procedures, clinicians should review specific anatomy and all surgical records, and obtain detailed imaging to define possible obstructions or stenosis in vascular pathways.

ACKNOWLEDGMENTS

The authors thank Ronn Tanel, MD, for contributing the case of Wolff-Parkinson-White syndrome in Ebstein's anomaly and Edward Gerstenfeld, MD, for contributing the case of pulmonary vein isolation in L-TGA.

REFERENCES

1. Hoffman JI, Kaplan S, Liberthson RR. Prevalence of congenital heart disease. Am Heart J 2004; 147(3):425–39.
2. Warnes CA, Liberthson R, Danielson GK, et al. Task force 1: the changing profile of congenital heart disease in adult life. J Am Coll Cardiol 2001; 37(5):1170–5.
3. Oechslin EN, Harrison DA, Connelly MS, et al. Mode of death in adults with congenital heart disease. Am J Cardiol 2000;86(10):1111–6.
4. Nollert G, Fischlein T, Bouterwek S, et al. Long-term survival in patients with repair of tetralogy of Fallot: 36-year follow-up of 490 survivors of the first year after surgical repair. J Am Coll Cardiol 1997; 30(5):1374–83.
5. Gatzoulis MA, Balaji S, Webber SA, et al. Risk factors for arrhythmia and sudden cardiac death late after repair of tetralogy of fallot: a multicentre study. Lancet 2000;356(9234):975–81.
6. Abadir S, Khairy P. Electrophysiology and adult congenital heart disease: advances and options. Prog Cardiovasc Dis 2011;53(4):281–92.
7. Pillutla P, Shetty KD, Foster E. Mortality associated with adult congenital heart disease: trends in the US population from 1979 to 2005. Am Heart J 2009;158(5):874–9.
8. Bouchardy J, Therrien J, Pilote L, et al. Atrial arrhythmias in adults with congenital heart disease. Circulation 2009;120(17):1679–86.
9. Garson A Jr, Bink-Boelkens M, Hesslein PS, et al. Atrial flutter in the young: a collaborative study of 380 cases. J Am Coll Cardiol 1985;6(4):871–8.
10. Opotowsky AR, Siddiqi OK, Webb GD. Trends in hospitalizations for adults with congenital heart disease in the US. J Am Coll Cardiol 2009;54(5): 460–7.
11. Triedman JK, Bergau DM, Saul JP, et al. Efficacy of radiofrequency ablation for control of intraatrial reentrant tachycardia in patients with congenital heart disease. J Am Coll Cardiol 1997;30(4): 1032–8.
12. Kalman JM, VanHare GF, Olgin JE, et al. Ablation of 'incisional' reentrant atrial tachycardia complicating surgery for congenital heart disease. Use of entrainment to define a critical isthmus of conduction. Circulation 1996;93(3):502–12.
13. Delacretaz E, Ganz LI, Soejima K, et al. Multi atrial maco-re-entry circuits in adults with repaired congenital heart disease: entrainment mapping combined with three-dimensional electroanatomic mapping. J Am Coll Cardiol 2001;37(6):1665–76.
14. Nakagawa H, Shah N, Matsudaira K, et al. Characterization of reentrant circuit in macroreentrant right atrial tachycardia after surgical repair of congenital heart disease: isolated channels between scars allow "focal" ablation. Circulation 2001;103(5): 699–709.
15. Flinn CJ, Wolff GS, Dick M 2nd, et al. Cardiac rhythm after the Mustard operation for complete transposition of the great arteries. N Engl J Med 1984;310(25):1635–8.
16. Ghai A, Harris L, Harrison DA, et al. Outcomes of late atrial tachyarrhythmias in adults after the Fontan operation. J Am Coll Cardiol 2001;37(2): 585–92.
17. Ovroutski S, Dahnert I, Alexi-Meskishvili V, et al. Preliminary analysis of arrhythmias after the Fontan operation with extracardiac conduit compared with intra-atrial lateral tunnel. Thorac Cardiovasc Surg 2001;49(6):334–7.
18. Nurnberg JH, Ovroutski S, Alexi-Meskishvili V, et al. New onset arrhythmias after the extracardiac conduit Fontan operation compared with the intraatrial lateral tunnel procedure: early and midterm results. Ann Thorac Surg 2004;78(6):1979–88 [discussion: 1988].
19. Stamm C, Friehs I, Mayer JE Jr, et al. Long-term results of the lateral tunnel Fontan operation. J Thorac Cardiovasc Surg 2001;121(1):28–41.
20. Fishberger SB, Wernovsky G, Gentles TL, et al. Factors that influence the development of atrial flutter after the Fontan operation. J Thorac Cardiovasc Surg 1997;113(1):80–6.

21. Walsh EP. Interventional electrophysiology in patients with congenital heart disease. Circulation 2007;115(25):3224–34.

22. Triedman JK, Alexander ME, Love BA, et al. Influence of patient factors and ablative technologies on outcomes of radiofrequency ablation of intra-atrial re-entrant tachycardia in patients with congenital heart disease. J Am Coll Cardiol 2002; 39(11):1827–35.

23. Feltes TF, Friedman RA. Transesophageal echocardiographic detection of atrial thrombi in patients with nonfibrillation atrial tachyarrhythmias and congenital heart disease. J Am Coll Cardiol 1994; 24(5):1365–70.

24. Reller MD, Strickland MJ, Riehle-Colarusso T, et al. Prevalence of congenital heart defects in metropolitan Atlanta, 1998-2005. J Pediatr 2008;153(6): 807–13.

25. Puley G, Siu S, Connelly M, et al. Arrhythmia and survival in patients >18 years of age after the mustard procedure for complete transposition of the great arteries. Am J Cardiol 1999;83(7):1080–4.

26. Silka MJ, Hardy BG, Menashe VD, et al. A population-based prospective evaluation of risk of sudden cardiac death after operation for common congenital heart defects. J Am Coll Cardiol 1998;32(1):245–51.

27. Gelatt M, Hamilton RM, McCrindle BW, et al. Arrhythmia and mortality after the Mustard procedure: a 30-year single-center experience. J Am Coll Cardiol 1997;29(1):194–201.

28. Sarkar D, Bull C, Yates R, et al. Comparison of long-term outcomes of atrial repair of simple transposition with implications for a late arterial switch strategy. Circulation 1999;100(Suppl 19):II176–81.

29. Schwerzmann M, Salehian O, Harris L, et al. Ventricular arrhythmias and sudden death in adults after a Mustard operation for transposition of the great arteries. Eur Heart J 2009;30(15):1873–9.

30. Kammeraad JA, van Deurzen CH, Sreeram N, et al. Predictors of sudden cardiac death after Mustard or Senning repair for transposition of the great arteries. J Am Coll Cardiol 2004;44(5):1095–102.

31. Bardy GH, Lee KL, Mark DB, et al. Amiodarone or an implantable cardioverter-defibrillator for congestive heart failure. N Engl J Med 2005;352(3): 225–37.

32. Kadish A, Dyer A, Daubert JP, et al. Prophylactic defibrillator implantation in patients with nonischemic dilated cardiomyopathy. N Engl J Med 2004; 350(21):2151–8.

33. Epstein AE, DiMarco JP, Ellenbogen KA, et al. ACC/AHA/HRS 2008 guidelines for device-based therapy of cardiac rhythm abnormalities: a report of the American College of Cardiology/American Heart Association task force on practice guidelines (Writing Committee to Revise the ACC/AHA/NASPE 2002 guideline update for implantation of cardiac pacemakers and Antiarrhythmia devices): developed in collaboration with the American Association for Thoracic Surgery and Society of Thoracic Surgeons. Circulation 2008;117(21):e350–408.

34. Zipes DP, Camm AJ, Borggrefe M, et al. ACC/AHA/ESC 2006 guidelines for management of patients with ventricular arrhythmias and the prevention of sudden cardiac death: a report of the American College of Cardiology/American Heart Association Task Force and the European Society of Cardiology Committee for Practice Guidelines (Writing Committee to develop guidelines for management of patients with ventricular arrhythmias and the prevention of sudden cardiac Death). J Am Coll Cardiol 2006;48(5):e247–346.

35. Kirsh JA, Walsh EP, Triedman JK. Prevalence of and risk factors for atrial fibrillation and intra-atrial reentrant tachycardia among patients with congenital heart disease. Am J Cardiol 2002;90(3):338–40.

36. Philip F, Muhammad KI, Agarwal S, et al. Pulmonary vein isolation for the treatment of drug-refractory atrial fibrillation in adults with congenital heart disease. Congenit Heart Dis 2012;7(4):392–9.

37. Peichl P, Kautzner J, Gebauer R. Ablation of atrial tachycardias after correction of complex congenital heart diseases: utility of intracardiac echocardiography. Europace 2009;11(1):48–53.

38. Banchs JE, Patel P, Naccarelli GV, et al. Intracardiac echocardiography in complex cardiac catheter ablation procedures. J Interv Card Electrophysiol 2010;28(3):167–84.

39. Anderson RH, Becker AE, Arnold R, et al. The conducting tissues in congenitally corrected transposition. Circulation 1974;50(5):911–23.

40. Warnes CA. Transposition of the great arteries. Circulation 2006;114(24):2699–709.

41. Reich JD, Auld D, Hulse E, et al. The Pediatric Radiofrequency Ablation Registry's experience with Ebstein's anomaly. Pediatric Electrophysiology Society. J Cardiovasc Electrophysiol 1998;9(12):1370–7.

42. Khositseth A, Danielson GK, Dearani JA, et al. Supraventricular tachyarrhythmias in Ebstein anomaly: management and outcome. J Thorac Cardiovasc Surg 2004;128(6):826–33.

43. Chetaille P, Walsh EP, Triedman JK. Outcomes of radiofrequency catheter ablation of atrioventricular reciprocating tachycardia in patients with congenital heart disease. Heart Rhythm 2004;1(2):168–73.

44. Etheridge SP. Radiofrequency catheter ablation of left-sided accessory pathways in pediatric patients. Prog Pediatr Cardiol 2001;13(1):11–24.

45. Hennein HA, Mosca RS, Urcelay G, et al. Intermediate results after complete repair of tetralogy of Fallot in neonates. J Thorac Cardiovasc Surg 1995;109(2):332–42,. 344; [discussion: 342–3].

46. Norgaard MA, Lauridsen P, Helvind M, et al. Twenty-to-thirty-seven-year follow-up after repair for Tetralogy of Fallot. Eur J Cardiothorac Surg 1999;16(2):125–30.

47. Nakazawa M, Shinohara T, Sasaki A, et al. Arrhythmias late after repair of tetralogy of fallot: a Japanese Multicenter Study. Circ J 2004;68(2):126–30.

48. Murphy JG, Gersh BJ, Mair DD, et al. Long-term outcome in patients undergoing surgical repair of tetralogy of Fallot. N Engl J Med 1993;329(9):593–9.

49. Walsh EP, Rockenmacher S, Keane JF, et al. Late results in patients with tetralogy of Fallot repaired during infancy. Circulation 1988;77(5):1062–7.

50. Khairy P, Ionescu-Ittu R, Mackie AS, et al. Changing mortality in congenital heart disease. J Am Coll Cardiol 2010;56(14):1149–57.

51. Le Gloan L, Khairy P. Management of arrhythmias in patients with tetralogy of Fallot. Curr Opin Cardiol 2011;26(1):60–5.

52. Khairy P, Aboulhosn J, Gurvitz MZ, et al. Arrhythmia burden in adults with surgically repaired tetralogy of Fallot: a multi-institutional study. Circulation 2010;122(9):868–75.

53. Gatzoulis MA, Till JA, Somerville J, et al. Mechanoelectrical interaction in tetralogy of Fallot. QRS prolongation relates to right ventricular size and predicts malignant ventricular arrhythmias and sudden death. Circulation 1995;92(2):231–7.

54. Dietl CA, Cazzaniga ME, Dubner SJ, et al. Life-threatening arrhythmias and RV dysfunction after surgical repair of tetralogy of Fallot. Comparison between transventricular and transatrial approaches. Circulation 1994;90(5 Pt 2):II7–12.

55. Khairy P, Landzberg MJ, Gatzoulis MA, et al. Value of programmed ventricular stimulation after tetralogy of fallot repair: a multicenter study. Circulation 2004;109(16):1994–2000.

56. Alexander ME, Walsh EP, Saul JP, et al. Value of programmed ventricular stimulation in patients with congenital heart disease. J Cardiovasc Electrophysiol 1999;10(8):1033–44.

57. Khairy P. Programmed ventricular stimulation for risk stratification in patients with tetralogy of Fallot: a Bayesian perspective. Nat Clin Pract Cardiovasc Med 2007;4(6):292–3.

58. Khairy P, Dore A, Poirier N, et al. Risk stratification in surgically repaired tetralogy of Fallot. Expert Rev Cardiovasc Ther 2009;7(7):755–62.

59. Zeppenfeld K, Schalij MJ, Bartelings MM, et al. Catheter ablation of ventricular tachycardia after repair of congenital heart disease: electroanatomic identification of the critical right ventricular isthmus. Circulation 2007;116(20):2241–52.

60. Harrison DA, Harris L, Siu SC, et al. Sustained ventricular tachycardia in adult patients late after repair of tetralogy of Fallot. J Am Coll Cardiol 1997;30(5):1368–73.

61. Karamlou T, Silber I, Lao R, et al. Outcomes after late reoperation in patients with repaired tetralogy of Fallot: the impact of arrhythmia and arrhythmia surgery. Ann Thorac Surg 2006;81(5):1786–93 [discussion: 1793].

62. Oechslin EN, Harrison DA, Harris L, et al. Reoperation in adults with repair of tetralogy of fallot: indications and outcomes. J Thorac Cardiovasc Surg 1999;118(2):245–51.

63. Therrien J, Siu SC, Harris L, et al. Impact of pulmonary valve replacement on arrhythmia propensity late after repair of tetralogy of Fallot. Circulation 2001;103(20):2489–94.

64. Misaki T, Tsubota M, Watanabe G, et al. Surgical treatment of ventricular tachycardia after surgical repair of tetralogy of Fallot. Relation between intraoperative mapping and histological findings. Circulation 1994;90(1):264–71.

65. Burton ME, Leon AR. Radiofrequency catheter ablation of right ventricular outflow tract tachycardia late after complete repair of tetralogy of Fallot using the pace mapping technique. Pacing Clin Electrophysiol 1993;16(12):2319–25.

66. Goldner BG, Cooper R, Blau W, et al. Radiofrequency catheter ablation as a primary therapy for treatment of ventricular tachycardia in a patient after repair of tetralogy of Fallot. Pacing Clin Electrophysiol 1994;17(8):1441–6.

67. Gonska BD, Cao K, Raab J, et al. Radiofrequency catheter ablation of right ventricular tachycardia late after repair of congenital heart defects. Circulation 1996;94(8):1902–8.

68. Morwood JG, Triedman JK, Berul CI, et al. Radiofrequency catheter ablation of ventricular tachycardia in children and young adults with congenital heart disease. Heart Rhythm 2004;1(3):301–8.

69. Khairy P, Stevenson WG. Catheter ablation in tetralogy of Fallot. Heart Rhythm 2009;6(7):1069–74.

70. Alexander ME, Cecchin F, Walsh EP, et al. Implications of implantable cardioverter defibrillator therapy in congenital heart disease and pediatrics. J Cardiovasc Electrophysiol 2004;15(1):72–6.

71. Sherwin ED, Triedman JK, Walsh EP. Update on interventional electrophysiology in congenital heart disease: evolving solutions for complex hearts. Circ Arrhythm Electrophysiol 2013;6(5):1032–40.

72. Hayward RM, Ursell PC, Foster E, et al. Sudden death due to nonarrhythmic cause in a patient with L-TGA. Ann Noninvasive Electrocardiol 2013;19:293–7.

Electrocardiographic Analysis of Paced Rhythms
Correlation with Intracardiac Electrograms

Pugazhendhi Vijayaraman, MD, FHRS[a,b,]*,
Kenneth A. Ellenbogen, MD, FHRS[c,d]

KEYWORDS

- QRS morphology • Ventricular pacing • Biventricular pacing
- BiV responders pacemaker-mediated tachycardia • Intracardiac electrograms

KEY POINTS

- Review of the 12-lead electrocardiogram is useful for determining the site of pacing.
- A right bundle branch block pattern may rarely be seen in patients when the right ventricular pacing lead is in the right ventricle.
- The QRS morphology in V_1 is useful for determining the site of left ventricular pacing.
- A variety of device-specific, or company-specific, algorithms may be programmed on to prevent pauses, atrial fibrillation, or minimize ventricular pacing.
- Familiarity with these device-specific algorithms is necessary to avoid the mistaken diagnosis of device failure.

ELECTROGRAMS FROM IMPLANTED DEVICES

Intracardiac electrograms are produced by the movement of electrical current through the myocardium. As a wavefront of depolarization travels toward an endocardial electrode in contact with myocardium, it is manifested as a positive deflection and as the wavefront passes under the electrode, a brisk negative deflection is recorded. The intrinsic deflection recorded in the pacemaker and implantable cardioverter defibrillator (ICD) electrodes are predominantly biphasic in nature.

Whereas the surface electrocardiogram (ECG) records the electrical activity from the entire heart (smaller in amplitude), the intracardiac electrogram records only local wavefronts (larger amplitude).

Unipolar and Bipolar Electrograms

A unipolar signal is recorded from 1 electrode in contact with the myocardium (tip electrode) and the other on the pulse generator while the bipolar electrogram is recorded between the 2 electrodes

Disclosures: Dr Vijayaraman, Honoraria (Medtronic); Dr Ellenbogen, Honoraria (Medtronic), Research (Medtronic), Advisory board (Medtronic).
[a] Department of Cardiology, Geisinger Wyoming Valley Medical Center, MC 36-10, 1000 East Mountain Boulevard, Wilkes Barre, PA 18711, USA; [b] Cardiac Electrophysiology, Geisinger Heart Institute, 100 Academy Avenue, Danville, PA 17822, USA; [c] Electrophysiology Division, Virginia Commonwealth University Pauley Heart Center, Gateway Building, 1200 East Marshall Street, 3rd Floor, Room 3-223, Richmond, VA 23219, USA; [d] Division of Cardiology, Virginia Commonwealth University Pauley Heart Center, Medical College of Virginia/VCU School of Medicine, 1200 East Marshall Street, Richmond, VA 23219, USA
* Corresponding author. Geisinger Wyoming Valley Medical Center, MC 36-10, 1000 East Mountain Boulevard, Wilkes Barre, PA 18711.
E-mail address: pvijayaraman1@geisinger.edu

within the heart. Because the distance between the electrodes in the unipolar configuration is large, it may detect electrical signals that originate far from the tip electrode inside the heart (far-field R waves in an atrial lead, T waves in the ventricle) or outside the heart (local skeletal myopotentials in the pocket, diaphragmatic myopotentials). Oversensing of far-field signals are not unique to unipolar sensing and may occur in bipolar configuration, leading to altered device function. Current generation pacemakers and ICDs are capable of providing real-time, near-field, bipolar, and unipolar electrograms from the right atrium, right ventricle (RV), and left ventricle (LV), in addition to far-field electrograms from the device and the shocking coils in the RV and SVC (superior vena cava). In addition, some of these are also available as stored electrograms during an arrhythmic event, greatly improving the device's diagnostic accuracy.

In addition to sensing or pacing dysfunction leading to abnormal surface ECGs, several algorithms programmed in a device may result in what seems to be abnormal device function (autocapture, ventricular pacing avoidance algorithms, mode switch, His bundle pacing, biventricular [BiV] pacing, etc) can lead to unusual ECG findings that may confuse a casual interpreter. To correctly interpret paced ECGs, one has to be familiar with various basic functioning of cardiac implantable electronic devices (pacemaker and ICD). The appearance of the ECG in a paced patient depends on the pacing mode used, placement of pacing leads, device pacing thresholds, and the presence of native electrical activity.

EFFECT OF VENTRICULAR PACING SITE ON ECG

Typically, a ventricular pacing lead is placed in the RV apex. RV apical pacing results in left bundle branch block (LBBB) pattern with left axis deviation characterizing the ventricular activation wavefront traveling from apex to base of the heart. In contrast, if the lead is placed in the RV outflow tract, it results in a LBBB pattern with right axis deviation depicting superior to inferior spread of the activation wavefront. A right bundle branch block pattern noted during attempted RV pacing should raise concern for inadvertent LV pacing (**Box 1**). Although a RBBB pattern can occur during conventional RV apical pacing in 10% to 20% of cases,[1,2] this scenario has to be excluded by careful evaluation of ECG, echocardiogram, and radiographic images (**Fig. 1**). This pattern can also be owing to placing lead V_1 too high in the second or third intercostal space. A tall R wave in V_3 and

---

Box 1
Causes of right bundle branch block pattern on ECG during right ventricular (RV) pacing
1. RV lead placement in the middle cardiac or posterior LV branch of the coronary sinus.
2. Lead placement via the subclavian artery into the left ventricle.
3. Lead placement via patent foramen ovale or atrial septal defect into the left ventricle.
4. Possible lead perforation of the RV apex or interventricular septum.
5. Uncomplicated RV apical pacing.
6. High placement of ECG electrode V1.
Abbreviation: LV, left ventricular.

V_4 would invariably signify that the pacing lead is not in the RV.

His Bundle and Para-Hisian Pacing

Selective site pacing is currently feasible with the availability of specifically designed pacing leads and catheter delivery systems. Direct His bundle pacing can result in ventricular pacing spikes followed by isoelectric interval of 30 to 60 ms duration followed by QRS complexes similar to native morphology.[3] Differential diagnosis in this situation should include failure of capture by ventricular pacing followed by native conducted complex. Para-Hisian pacing results from capture of the His bundle with intrinsic conduction along with fusion from basal septal myocardial capture. The ECG demonstrates a slight increase in QRS amplitude with the axis concordant with the native complex and evidence for delta waves suggesting fusion.[4] Usually, no isoelectric interval is noted between pacing spike and QRS onset. In the absence of a visible pacing spike, the ECG can be mistaken for septal preexcitation (**Fig. 2**). By utilizing the His-Purkinje conduction system, pacing results in minimal or no ventricular dyssynchrony.

BiV Pacing

Electrocardiographic analysis of BiV paced rhythm is critical in the evaluation of cardiac resynchronization devices during implant and follow-up, and for troubleshooting. BiV pacing with the RV lead in the apex and LV lead in the posterior or posterolateral veins usually results in right superior axis deviation ($-90°$ to $-180°$), and the QRS complex is positive or dominant (R or Rs) in V1.[5] A negative paced QRS complex (LBBB pattern) in lead V_1

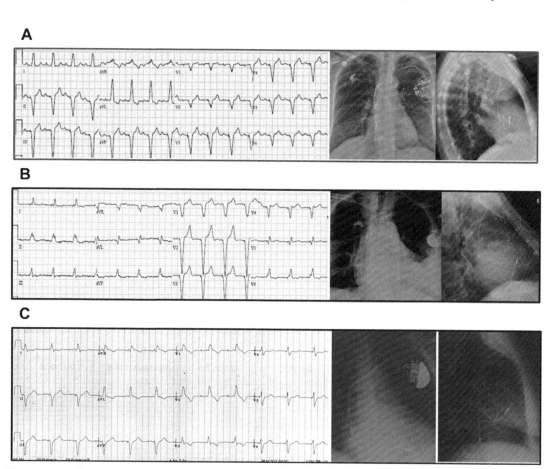

Fig. 1. Twelve-lead electrocardiogram and chest x-ray in posteroanterior (PA) and lateral views are shown. (*A*) Right ventricular (RV) apical pacing results in left bundle branch block (LBBB) pattern with left axis deviation. (*B*) RV outflow tract pacing results in LBBB pattern with right axis deviation. (*C*) Right bundle branch block pattern on ECG during attempted RV pacing. Although the chest x-ray in the PA view suggests an RV apical position, the lateral view shows the lead located posteriorly, probably in the middle cardiac vein branch of the coronary sinus.

may occur when there is no LV capture, marked LV latency,[6] marked delay in LV propagation, ventricular fusion with conducted QRS complex, or LV lead placement in the middle cardiac or anterior interventricular vein. Negative paced QRS complex in V_1 can occur in the absence of these conditions in simultaneous BiV pacing and may reflect different activation of a heterogenous BIV substrate and not necessarily indicate poor prognosis.

Observation of a LBBB pattern in V_1 during BiV pacing should lead to further evaluation (**Box 2**). If the LV lead is located in the anterior vein or middle cardiac vein, it generally leads to an LBBB pattern. If there is no clinical response to BiV pacing, alternative options for LV lead placement should be considered. If LV-only pacing clearly demonstrates a RBBB pattern in lead V_1, it is likely either there is fusion with native conduction or

significant delay in LV activation (latency or conduction delay). Optimizing AV delay (shorter) or changing LV-RV timing to allow early LV activation may offset the problem and result in ventricular synchronization (**Fig. 3**). During BiV pacing with RV lead in the apex, q waves are generally observed in lead I. Loss of q waves in lead I during BiV pacing was 100% sensitive for predicting loss of LV capture.[7]

Anodal capture is another phenomenon in which true BiV pacing may not occur. In BiV devices, pacing from any one of the LV electrodes as cathode and RV ring or coil as anode is a useful option to avoid diaphragmatic capture or improve pacing threshold. However, when pacing at high LV outputs, RV anodal capture can occur during LV-only or BiV pacing.[8,9] Although anodal capture is generally benign, it may be associated with poor outcomes.[10,11] Because anodal capture would

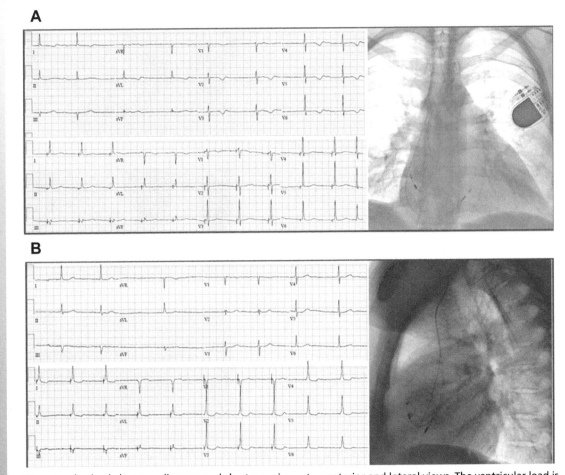

Fig. 2. Twelve-lead electrocardiogram and chest x-ray in posteroanterior and lateral views. The ventricular lead is at the level of the tricuspid annulus. (*A*) *Top panel*, High-degree atrioventricular (AV) nodal block. *Bottom panel*, His bundle pacing with ventricular pacing spike followed by an isoelectric interval and QRS morphology identical to baseline. (*B*) *Top panel*, Atrial fibrillation with slow ventricular response. *Bottom panel*, Para-Hisian pacing. The pacing spike is immediately followed by a QRS complex similar to native morphology but with a small delta wave and increased QRS amplitude.

result in simultaneous RV and LV capture, LV pacing cannot be advanced by adjusting LV-RV timing. During LV threshold testing, if LV cathode capture threshold is higher than RV anodal capture, it may result in programming an output lower than true LV threshold, resulting in loss of BiV pacing.

ELECTROCARDIOGRAPHIC CHARACTERISTICS OF BIV RESPONDERS

Cardiac resynchronization therapy (CRT) has been shown to improve cardiac function and heart failure symptoms, induce reverse myocardial remodeling, enhance quality of life, prevent heart failure admissions, and prolong survival.[12–15] It is generally accepted that greater than 30% of patients undergoing CRT do not respond to this therapy.

Several ECG criteria have been proposed to predict CRT responders (**Box 3**). Patients with LBBB morphology and QRS duration greater than 150 ms at baseline respond to CRT more favorably than patients with LBBB and QRS duration less than 150 ms and patients with non-LBBB morphology and QRS duration of greater than 150 ms.[16] A substudy of the Resynchronization–Defibrillation for Ambulatory Heart Failure Trial[17] involving 1483 patients showed that an implantable cardioverter defibrillator-CRT was associated with a significant reduction in the primary endpoint of all-cause mortality or heart failure hospitalization in patients with LBBB irrespective of QRS duration and in patients with non-LBBB and QRS duration of greater than 160 ms.

Sweeney and colleagues[18] analyzed the ECGs of 202 consecutive CRT patients and identified several ECG variables at baseline and during CRT to predict LV reverse remodeling. Greater longest baseline LV activation time ($LVAT_{max}$) was associated with a greater probability of 10% or greater reduction in end-systolic volume. Higher QRS scores for LV scar predicted reduced reverse remodeling. After CRT, dominant R wave amplitudes in V1 and V2 (baseline R $\times$ 4.5), and left-to-right frontal axis shift were positive predictors of reverse remodeling (**Fig. 4**).

Several studies have shown a correlation between the degree of QR shortening after CRT and hemodynamic benefit and/or clinical response but the degree of shortening is generally small.[19–21] In the Resynchronization Reverses Remodeling in Systolic Left Ventricular Dysfunction (REVERSE) trial of CRT among 610 patients with mild heart failure, the change in QRS duration with CRT pacing was not an independent predictor of any outcome.[22]

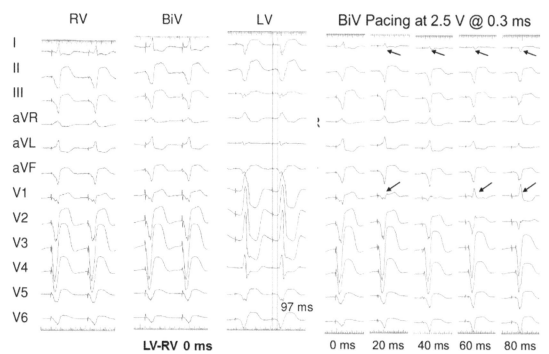

Fig. 3. Comparison of QRS morphology in 12-lead ECGs during right ventricular (RV), biventricular (BiV), and left ventricular (LV) pacing in the VVI mode at 80 bpm during complete AV block (excluding fusion with the spontaneous QRS complex). During BiV pacing (V-V delay = 0) the QRS morphology is identical to that of RV pacing (no evidence of BiV fusion). During LV pacing, the stimulus to QRS latency interval measures 97 ms. Impact of LV latency on QRS morphology during BiV pacing (80 bpm) at incremental left to right ventricular (V-V) delay at 2.5 V at 0.3 ms is shown on the right. There is subtle evidence of BiV fusion at a V-V delay of 20 ms (*arrows*). At 80 ms V-V delay, the ECG pattern suggests a greater LV contribution to the QRS complex. (*From* Herweg B, Ilercil A, Madramootoo C, et al. Latency during left ventricular pacing from the lateral cardiac veins: a cause of ineffectual biventricular pacing. Pacing Clin Electrophysiol 2006;29:578; with permission.)

Box 3
Electrocardiographic (ECG) predictors of response to cardiac resynchronization therapy (CRT)

Baseline

1. LBBB with QRS duration of greater than 150 ms.

2. Greater left ventricular activation time ($LVAT_{max}$).

3. Lower QRS score (smaller LV scar volume).

Post CRT

1. Dominant R wave amplitude in V1-V2 (baseline R in V1 × 4.5).

2. Left → right frontal axis shift.

3. Evidence for ventricular activation fusion (change of R in I, L to qR, QR, QS; QS in V1 → rS, RS, Rs, R, etc).

4. Post CRT QRS duration (poor specificity).

Abbreviation: LBBB, left bundle branch block.

DDD PACING ALGORITHMS
Ventricular Pacing Avoidance Algorithms

Several clinical trials have demonstrated increased risk of heart failure hospitalization and atrial fibrillation (AF), as well as higher mortality with RV apical pacing.[23,24] Because of concerns about the potential deleterious effects of frequent RV pacing, several algorithms are currently available in dual chamber pacemakers and ICDs to minimize ventricular pacing. These include managed ventricular pacing (MVP), AAIsafeR mode, search AV hysteresis, and ventricular intrinsic pacing. In MVP and AAIsafeR algorithms, the device can switch from DDD (R) to AAI (R) mode, but continue to monitor AV conduction. If a critical number of P waves are not followed by a QRS complex, the pacemaker can automatically switch to DDD mode without sacrificing AV synchrony. In MVP, the device functions in AAI (R) mode and, if AV conduction fails for 1 beat, a ventricular backup stimulus is delivered 80 ms after the next atrial beat. If AV conduction fails for 2 of 4 successive atrial events (sensed or paced), the device switches to DDD (R) mode. To a casual observer, the telemetry rhythm strips would raise the possibility of device malfunction (**Fig. 5**). The device performs periodic 1-cycle checks for AV conduction and the opportunity to resume AAI (R) therapy. The first check for AV conduction occurs after 1 minute. Subsequent checks occur at progressively longer intervals (2, 4, 8 ... min) up to 16 hours and then occur every 16 hours thereafter. Depending on the patient's intrinsic

rhythm and conduction, MVP allows V-V cycle variations and occasional pauses of up to twice the lower rate interval. In addition, the minimal ventricular pacing algorithms can result in long PR intervals of up to 600 ms and may result in pacemaker syndrome owing to loss of AV synchrony. These algorithms have significantly reduced the amount of ventricular pacing from 90% to 1% in select patient populations.[24,25]

AUTOCAPTURE

Most pacemaker and ICDs currently have automatic capture verification algorithms for RV capture. These algorithms monitor cardiac capture on a beat to beat analysis and deliver an output just above the capture threshold while providing a high-output backup safety pulse in the event of noncapture. This feature has been shown to increase device longevity, improve device follow-up, and enhance patient safety.[26] All ventricular autocapture algorithms rely on sensing the evoked response to the test pulse. Capture is confirmed by the presence or absence of the evoked response. Some algorithms (Autocapture, St Jude Medical; Capture control, Biotronik; Automatic capture, Boston Scientific) confirm capture on a beat to beat basis. Others (capture management; Medtronic, Minneapolis, MN, USA) can perform a pacing threshold search at programmable or fixed intervals. After automatic confirmation of beat–beat capture or periodic threshold determination, the pacemaker regulates the output to provide a small safety margin above the pacing threshold and thereby decreasing the energy consumption. In the event of noncapture, the device delivers a backup pulse at high output approximately at 100 ms after the primary pulse. Spontaneous autocapture threshold measurement by the device on a patient in the hospital setting can create a confusing rhythm on telemetry ECG (loss of capture, double stimuli at 100-ms intervals) and cause concern of a pacing system malfunction.

Automatic algorithms for pacing capture management for atrial and LV are currently available in both pacemaker and ICD platforms. Atrial capture management determines capture by evoked response or the timing of the conducted response. LV capture management determines capture by applying a test pulse to the LV lead and comparing the timing of a conducted response in the RV to a predetermined A-RV and LV-RV conduction times. The LV capture management (Medtronic) test occurs every day at 1:00 AM if the patient's rhythm is stable enough to support a pacing threshold search (ie, programmed LV output >6 V, unstable patient rhythm [R-R

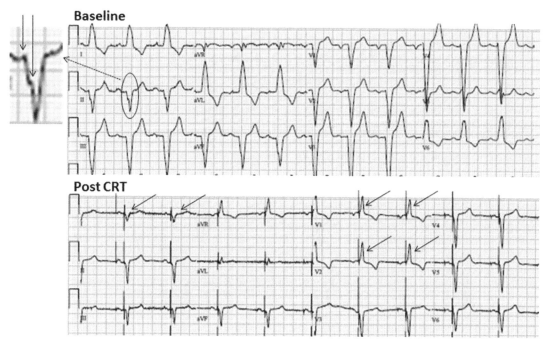

Fig. 4. Twelve-lead ECG in a patient with severe nonischemic cardiomyopathy, left ventricular (LV) ejection fraction (EF) of 20% and baseline QRS duration of 170 ms. First downward arrow in the inset shows the QRS onset in lead II, and the second arrow shows the first QRS notch, which represents the transition from RV to LV activation. The time difference between the 2 arrows is the right ventricular activation time (RVAT), which is measured in multiple anatomic regions with QRS notching. $QRSd - RVAT_{min} = LVAT_{max}$ (170 – 45 = 125 ms). Left bundle branch block (LBBB) morphology with baseline QRSd of 170 ms in nonischemic cardiomyopathy and $LVAT_{max}$ of 125 ms suggest a greater probability of response to biventricular (BiV) pacing. Bottom panel, ECG during BiV pacing. Emergence of QS complex in I (*arrows*) suggesting left → right activation reversal and prominent R waves in V_1 and V_2 (>5 × baseline R) post cardiac resynchronization therapy (CRT) would also favor response to BiV pacing. The paced QRS duration is 120 ms. Patient's functional status improved from New York Heart Association class III/IV to class I with normalization of LVEF to 65% after 3 months of BiV pacing. $LVAT_{max}$, LV activation time; QRSd, QRS duration; $RVAT_{min}$, RV activation time.

variability >200 ms] or arrhythmia; heart rate >90 bpm). If stability checks are unsuccessful, the device automatically continues to schedule searches every 30 minutes. Automatic threshold measurements of RV and LV leads can lead to different paced QRS morphologies in a patient with BiV device and cause a confusing rhythm pattern on telemetry (**Fig. 6**).

Ventricular Safety Pacing

In dual chamber pacemakers, there is potential for inhibition of ventricular channel owing to oversensing of atrial output (cross-talk), leading to the possibility of catastrophic ventricular asystole in patients with complete heart block. To prevent this, the AV interval has a ventricular blanking period of 12 to 120 ms after an atrial paced event. Immediately after this interval is a cross-talk sensing window during which, if any ventricular-sensed event (premature ventricular contraction [PVC], oversensing of leading edge of atrial output)

occurs, leads to a ventricular pacing stimulus at a shorter AV interval of 100 to 120 ms. On surface ECG, if PVC occurs during the cross-talk sensing window of the AV interval, this may lead to a ventricular pacing artifact at a shorter AV delay and appear as a sensing failure. In reality, this represents appropriate pacing response to a sensed event.

Atrial Fibrillation Suppression Algorithms

Several pacing algorithms (dynamic atrial overdrive, atrial preference pacing, continuous atrial pacing) have been studied in randomized trials for decreasing AF burden.[27,28] Atrial preference pacing (Medtronic) responds to changes in the atrial rate by accelerating the pacing rate until it reaches a steady paced rhythm that is slightly faster than the intrinsic rate, up to a programmed maximum rate. After each nonrefractory atrial sensed event, the device decreases the atrial pacing interval by the programmed interval decrement

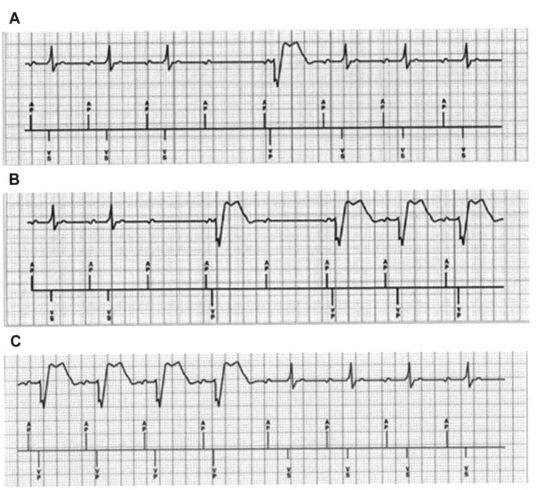

Fig. 5. Rhythm strips during managed ventricular pacing mode are shown. (*A*) While operating in AAI (R) mode, atrioventricular (AV) conduction fails after an atrial-paced event and is followed by a ventricular rescue pacing stimulus delivered 80 ms after the next programmed atrial beat, so that long pauses are avoided. (*B*) AAI (R) pacing with first-degree AV block followed by AV conduction failure. Ventricular rescue pacing stimulus is delivered 80 ms after the next programmed atrial beat and, because 2 of 4 A-A intervals without AV conduction, mode switch to DDD (R) occurs. (*C*) AV conduction search occurs for 1 beat and, if present, mode switches back to AAI (R). (*Courtesy of* Medtronic, Minneapolis, MN.)

value. Beats continue at this elevated rate until the pacing rate exceeds the intrinsic rate, resulting in an atrial paced rhythm. The increased rate is sustained for the number of beats programmed as the search beats parameter. Atrial preference pacing then decreases the pacing rate slightly (by 20 ms; nonprogrammable) to search for the next intrinsic beat. This results in a dynamic, controlled, stair-step increase or decrease in the pacing interval, maintaining a pacing rate slightly above the intrinsic rate. On ECG, after a few sensed atrial beats (sinus or premature atrial contractions [PACs]), the atrial pacing rate increases to a higher rate compared with the programmed sensor driven lower rate limit.

Rate Drop Response

This algorithm is designed to recognize a sudden decline in heart rate and initiate dual chamber pacing at 100 to 120 bpm and is intended to provide backup pacing and prevent associated symptoms in patients who experience occasional episodes of significant drop in heart rate (eg, syncope from cardioinhibitory and mixed forms of carotid sinus syndrome). On surface ECG, this may present as sudden and unexpected increase in pacing rates to 100 to 120 bpm. During sleep, a patient's sinus rate may fall below the programmed lower rate, thereby triggering intervention pacing at an inappropriate time. This can be

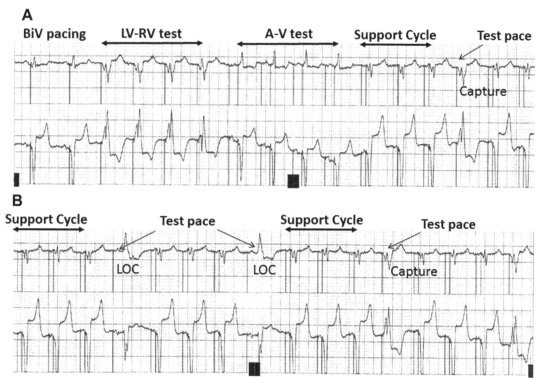

Fig. 6. Left ventricular (LV) capture management. Rhythm strips of ECG lead I and II are shown during spontaneous LV capture management test. (*A*) Atrial sensed biventricular (BiV) pacing is seen for first 2 beats followed by LV-right ventricular (RV) conduction check for 4 beats and atrioventricular (AV) conduction check. A sequence of pacing support cycles precedes the LV pacing threshold search (LVPTS). The first 3 beats in support cycle are in BiV pacing mode followed by the LV test pace at 2 V at 0.5 ms in LV, resulting in capture. (*B*) The first 3 beats in support cycles in BiV pacing mode is followed by LV test pace at 0.5 V at 0.5 ms, which is ineffectual, resulting in loss of capture (LOC) with spontaneous conducted beat with change in morphology. This is followed by a pacing support cycle and another ineffectual LV test pace. The third LV test pace is effective at 1 V at 0.5 ms. Because of the short paced AV delay (PAV) (30 ms) and low-output voltage (0.5 V) during LVPTS, only the atrial pacing stimulus is visible. Note multiple morphology of paced QRS complexes (BiV, LV only), test pace with conducted beat, varying AV (sensed and paced) delays and pacing rates. Typically, LV capture management (Medtronic) test occurs at 1:00 AM if the patient's rhythm is stable enough to support a pacing threshold search.

avoided by programming sleep function on, during which time rate drop response is disabled.

Rate Smoothing

Rate smoothing algorithms (rate smoothing, atrial rate stabilization, ventricular rate stabilization, ventricular rate regularization) are designed to prevent sudden changes in heart rates. In cases of sinus arrest, the atrial rate may decrease from 80 to 90 bpm to the lower rate limit of 50 bpm. Rate smoothing would result in more gradual decrease in heart rate by the programmable rate-smoothing percentage of 3% to 24%. When a patient experiences a PVC, it is often followed by a long pause in the cardiac cycle. This pause is sometimes associated with the onset of pause-dependent ventricular tachyarrhythmias. Ventricular rate stabilization is a programmable feature designed to eliminate

the long pause that commonly follows a PVC. Ventricular rate stabilization responds to a PVC by increasing the pacing rate, then gradually slowing it back to the programmed pacing rate or intrinsic rate. Irregularities in ventricular rate during atrial fibrillation may result in significant symptoms. VRR is an algorithm specifically designed to stabilize ventricular rate during AF. Ventricular pacing with VRR is based on a weighted average of the last 32 sensed and paced R-R intervals, pacing close to the mean ventricular rate and after its mean fluctuations over time and adjusting the pacing rates accordingly.

Noncompetitive Atrial Pacing

If a PAC occurs in the PVARP, it is not sensed (AR) and a new atrial pacing event can occur in the atrial vulnerable period and possibly trigger an atrial tachyarrhythmia. Noncompetitive atrial pacing (NCAP) stops delivery of an atrial pace during the atrial refractory period. When NCAP is programmed, a refractory sensed atrial event falling in the PVARP starts a 300-ms NCAP period, during which no atrial pacing occurs. If a sensor-driven or lower rate pacing stimulus is scheduled to occur during the NCAP period, the ventriculoatrial (VA) interval is extended until the NCAP period expires. When an atrial pacing stimulus is delayed by the NCAP operation, the pacemaker attempts to maintain a stable ventricular rate by shortening the PAV interval that follows. It will not, however, shorten the PAV interval to less than 30 ms. When a relatively high lower rate and long PVARP are programmed, NCAP operation may result in ventricular pacing slightly below the lower rate.

Fusion and Pseudofusion

A cardiac event may be sensed in the atrial or ventricular channel well beyond the onset of P or QRS on the surface ECG. In the setting of RBBB, a ventricular event will be sensed by the RV lead very late in the timing of the QRS complex. This can lead to pacing artifact in a native QRS, leading to fusion or pseudofusion. If the pacing stimulus does not alter the morphology of native QRS, it is called a pseudofusion beat. If the resulting QRS morphology is intermediate between the native QRS and fully paced complex, it is called a fusion beat. This does not represent undersensing; rather, it is normal sensing occurring late in the chamber owing to a conduction delay. Appropriate programming of a longer AV delay avoids unnecessary pacing.

PACEMAKER-MEDIATED ARRHYTHMIAS

Pacemaker-mediated tachycardia is a general term that encompasses several conditions in which in any undesired rapid pacing rate is caused by the device or by the interaction of the pacing system with the patient. These include endless loop tachycardia (ELT), sensor-driven tachycardia, ventricular tracking in atrial arrhythmias, myopotential tracking, runaway pacemaker, and pacemaker-facilitated ventricular tachycardia (VT)/ventricular fibrillation (VF; **Box 4**).

The most common form of pacemaker-mediated tachycardia is ELT, which results from a repetitive sequence of a sensed retrograde P wave triggering a ventricular pacing event at maximum tracking rate (MTR). The onset of this tachycardia requires at least transient AV dissociation allowing retrograde VA conduction to occur. Only patients capable of conducting retrogradely through the AV node or an accessory pathway can support

---

Box 4
Pacemaker-mediated arrhythmias

1. Endless loop tachycardia
2. Sensor driven tachycardia
3. Ventricular tracking in atrial arrhythmias (upper rate behavior)
4. Myopotential tracking
5. Runaway pacemaker
6. AF suppression algorithm driven atrial overdrive pacing
7. Repetitive non-reentrant ventriculoatrial synchronous rhythm
8. Device-induced pro-arrhythmia
   a. Pacemaker-facilitated VT/VF
   b. VT/VF-induced by inappropriate ATP (SVT, far-field atrial oversensing, T wave oversensing, double counting RV-LV in BiV devices)
   c. VF-induced by acceleration of VT from appropriate ATP
   d. Pacemaker-facilitated atrial arrhythmias

Abbreviations: AF, atrial fibrillation; ATP, antitachycardia pacing; BiV, biventricular; LV, left ventricular; RV, right ventricular; VF, ventricular fibrillation; VT, ventricular tachycardia.

---

this rhythm in dual chamber or BiV devices. Whenever there is atrial sensed ventricular pacing at or close to MTR, ELT has to be suspected. Occasionally, when the bipolar pacing artifact is small and not visible on ECG, this may be interpreted as a wide-complex tachycardia. Atrial-sensed ventricular pacing at MTR can also occur in sinus or atrial tachycardia at those rates. The causes for ELT include frequent PVCs, atrial undersensing, atrial oversensing, loss of atrial capture, or magnet application to the pacemaker. Once initiated, ELT continues until there is spontaneous VA block or loss of atrial sensing. Pacemaker algorithms have been developed to prevent ELT by extending the postventricular atrial refractory period (PVARP) or initiating a DVI cycle (during which atrial channel is refractory), after a premature ventricular event (defined as a ventricular-sensed event not preceded by an atrial event). Programming a longer PVARP may prevent ELT, but will limit the MTR. Once pacemaker-mediated tachycardia is detected (typically P wave tracking at or slightly below MTR) for a certain number of beats (fixed or programmable), the device can automatically initiate a termination algorithm (PVARP extension, DVI cycle, or atrial pace; **Fig. 7**A).

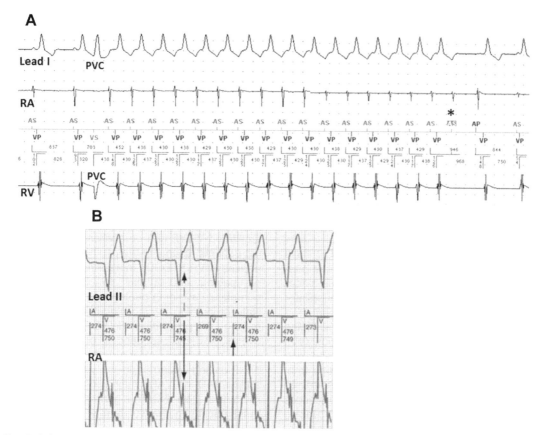

Fig. 7. (*A*) A premature ventricular complex (PVC) results in retrograde conduction. Because the retrograde P wave (AS) occurs after the postventricular atrial refractory period (PVARP), it is tracked resulting in ventricular paced event (VP) with retrograde conduction to the atrium, which is tracked again. This results in classic endless loop tachycardia (ELT). This ELT is automatically terminated by extending the PVARP for 1 cycle (*asterisk*) after tracking at or near the upper rate limit for a number of cycles. (*B*) An example of repetitive non-reentrant ventriculoatrial (VA) synchronous rhythm is shown. Paced ventricular event is associated with a retrograde P wave falling in the PVARP (functional undersensing), allowing delivery of an atrial-paced event (AP), which fails to capture (functional noncapture). This is followed by a ventricular paced event that again results in retrograde conduction. This pattern occurs repetitively. ([*B*] *Adapted from* Love CJ. Pacemaker troubleshooting and follow-up. In: Ellenbogen KA, Kay GN, Lau CP, et al, editors. Clinical cardiac pacing, defibrillation and resynchronization therapy. 4th edition. Philadelphia: Elsevier; 2011. p. 884; with permission.)

Repetitive Nonreentrant VA Synchronous Rhythm

Repetitive nonreentrant VA synchronous rhythm occurs in the setting of DDD or DDI mode with a long PVARP. The trigger for this rhythm is identical to the factors initiating ELT that allow retrograde conduction to occur. Because of long PVARP, the retrograde P wave falls in the refractory period and is not sensed, allowing the atrial escape interval to complete, resulting in atrial pacing output. This output does not result in atrial capture (atrial myocardium is still refractory), but is followed by ventricular pacing at the completion of the AV interval. This pattern is repetitive (VP-AR-AP), resulting in loss of AV synchrony but with the ventriculoatrial synchrony similar to pacemaker

syndrome occurring in VVI pacing. This can lead to significant symptoms of palpitations, dizziness, and dyspnea. This rhythm can be prevented by programming to AAI (R) mode in patients with intact AV conduction or by programming PVARP extension algorithm in patients with frequent PVCs triggering this rhythm (see **Fig. 7**B).

Sensor-driven tachycardia is a rapid atrial or ventricular pacing at high heart rates occurring in single, dual, or BiV rate-modulated devices. An inappropriate increase in sensor-driven heart rates can occur owing to a threshold setting that is too low or a slope setting that is too high. Depending on the sensor used in the device (vibration, minute ventilation, QT interval), variety of stimuli (pressure on device, bumpy ride, hyperventilation, cautery, electromagnetic interference, sympathomimetic drugs, etc) can cause higher pacing rates. Myopotential tracking occurs when muscle potentials are sensed in the atrial channel, leading to sequential ventricular pacing and is more common in unipolar sensing mode. Runaway pacemaker is a rare malfunction of pacemaker or ICD owing to component failure, resulting in rapid pacing and has the potential for inducing VT or fibrillation. Emergent surgical intervention to replace the device may be necessary.

DEVICE-INDUCED PROARRHYTHMIA
Pacemaker-Facilitated VT/VF

Many patients with pacemakers or ICD have tachycardias where the relationship to the pacing stimulus is unclear. VT/VF in some pacemaker/implantable cardioverter-defibrillator patients might be initiated by short-long-short (S-L-S) sequences that are actively facilitated by normal bradycardia pacing operation (VVI, DDD, or MVP mode).[29,30] Sweeney and colleagues[31] reviewed 1356 VT/VF episodes from 1055 patients in 2 ICD trials and determined that pacing facilitated VT/VF (S-L-S sequences actively facilitated by ventricular pacing including the terminal beat after a pause) accounted for 8% to 15% of all VT/VF episodes.[32] Pacing facilitated VT/VF was the only onset

sequence in 4% to 10% of patients with VT/VF (**Fig. 8**). This type of VT is common to all modes of pacing, but least common with MVP mode. Most pacing-facilitated S-L-S episodes were monomorphic VT occurring in patients with coronary artery disease, suggesting scar-related reentry as the mechanism. The incidence of S-L-S VT/VF is very low compared with the overall frequency of triggers (VPDs, isolated VPs) causing S-L-S sequences in patients with pacemakers and ICDs. It is likely that S-L-S VT/VF can occur only in a setting of additional factors promoting electrical instability (eg, ischemia, electrolyte imbalance, influence of the autonomic nervous system). Managing pacing-facilitated VT/VF can be challenging. In individual patients, changing the pacing mode to avoid pauses (MVP to DDD), increasing the lower rate of pacing (40–50/min to 60–70/min), or completely avoiding pacing may be helpful.[33,34] Rate smoothing pacing algorithms may be effecting in preventing S-L-S related VT/VF events.[35] S-L-S sequences occurring in the atrium can trigger similar atrial tachyarrhythmias. Atrial pacing occurring in the vulnerable period after a PAC in PVARP may also trigger atrial arrhythmias. The NCAP algorithm may prevent atrial pacing in the vulnerable period in such situations.

Supraventricular arrhythmias (atrial fibrillation, atrial tachycardia, or sinus tachycardia) incorrectly

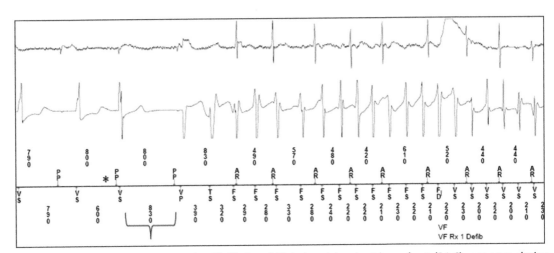

Fig. 8. Pacemaker-facilitated ventricular fibrillation (VF) induced by short-long-short (S-L-S) sequence during managed ventricular pacing. For pacing facilitated S-L-S, a premature ventricular complex (PVC; 600-ms interval, *asterisk*; "short") occurs almost simultaneously with an atrial pace (AP; 800-ms interval). The PVC is marked as a sensed event but, because it falls in the 80-ms cross-talk window, is not considered a true ventricular event. The next AP (800 ms) fulfills the criteria for an A-A interval without an intervening ventricular sense (VS) event, and a single ventricular pacing (VP) is delivered ("long"). The pause (bracket) is only 830 ms, because of rate modulation. An early-coupled PVC (390 ms; "short") anticipates onset of VF. (*Adapted from* Sweeney MO, Ruetz LL, Belk P, et al. Bradycardia pacing-induced short-long-short sequences at the onset of ventricular tachyarrhythmias: a possible mechanism of proarrhythmia? J Am Coll Cardiol 2007;50:614–22.)

diagnosed as VT by ICD may lead to inappropriate therapy in the form of antitachycardia pacing (ATP), which may in turn induce VT or VF, leading to further ICD therapies or shocks. Fine-tuning SVT discrimination algorithms (onset, stability, morphology, AV relationship, etc) may reduce inappropriate ICD therapies. Oversensing of T wave, far-field atrial electrograms, or double counting of RV-LV bipolar electrograms can also lead to inappropriate ATP therapy, resulting in device-induced ventricular arrhythmias (**Fig. 9**). Appropriate ATP therapy for VT can also accelerate into VF.

Diagnosis of Arrhythmias by Device Electrograms

Intracardiac electrograms stored by cardiac rhythm devices can be valuable in the diagnosis of cardiac arrhythmias. Real-time intracardiac electrograms can be helpful in the immediate diagnosis of ongoing arrhythmias (**Fig. 10**). Several characteristics such as onset, stability,

and morphology can be helpful in differentiating atrial and ventricular arrhythmias in single chamber devices. In addition to these characteristics in dual chamber devices, VA relationship can often clinch the diagnosis. V>A would confirm VT, whereas A>V might suggest supraventricular arrhythmia. If the AV relationship is 1:1, then onset (initiated by PAC), change in AA preceding change in VV intervals might point toward the diagnosis of SVT (see **Fig. 10B**). In ICDs, response to ATP may also help in the discrimination of VT from SVT. Both SVT and VT may terminate with ATP. If there is no termination and no change in the AA interval during ATP, atrial tachycardia may be confirmed. If no termination but atria is entrained, the post pacing response to ATP may provide additional clues. If VAAV response is noted post pacing, this may confirm atrial tachycardia. Alternately VAV response may point to atrioventricular nodal reentrant tachycardia, atrioventricular reentrant tachycardia, or VT. VVA response to post pacing would point to VT.

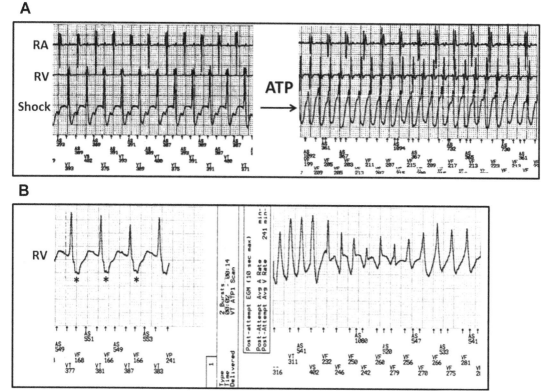

Fig. 9. Ventricular fibrillation induced by inappropriate antitachycardia pacing (ATP). (*A*) Right atrial (RA), right ventricular (RV), and shock electrograms from a dual chamber implantable cardioverter defibrillator (ICD) are shown. Sinus tachycardia (cycle length of 380 ms) is detected as ventricular tachycardia by the device, resulting in ATP therapy, which induced ventricular fibrillation. (*B*) T wave oversensing (*asterisk*) occurs, resulting in inappropriate diagnosis of ventricular tachycardia. Ensuing ATP induces ventricular fibrillation.

A

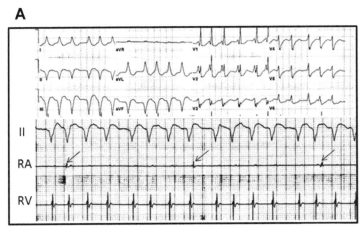

B

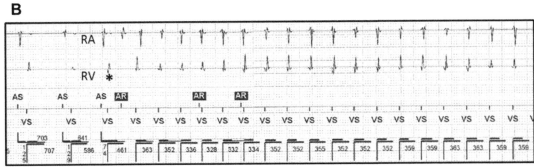

Fig. 10. (*A*) Twelve-lead ECG in a 70-year-old man who presented with an irregular wide complex tachycardia. The electrocardiogram (ECG) was suggestive of atrial fibrillation (AF) with aberrant conduction, except for wide R wave in V_2, which pointed toward ventricular tachycardia. Intracardic electrograms from his dual chamber pacemaker confirm ventricular tachycardia with underlying sinus bradycardia (*arrow*). (*B*) Intracardiac electrograms from a patient's pacemaker with recurrent sustained palpitations. The third atrial beat (sinus) is followed by a PVC (*asterisk*), which results in retrograde atrial conduction followed by a regular tachycardia with 1:1 atrioventricular (AV) conduction with simultaneous atrial and ventricular activation suggestive of possible AV node reentrant tachycardia. He was diagnosed with atrioventricular nodal reentrant tachycardia (AVNRT) and underwent successful ablation during a subsequent electrophysiology study.

SUMMARY

The ECG may be useful in evaluating patients with CRT therapy and in particular may help to determine the site of LV pacing and whether a patient is likely to respond to CRT therapy. Other electrocardiographic features of a wide variety of pacing algorithms are discussed. Knowledge of these specific pacing algorithms may avoid unnecessary evaluation for pacing system malfunction. Many of these algorithms are carefully described in the manufacturers' manuals.

REFERENCES

1. Barold SS, Falkoff MD, Ong LS, et al. Electrocardiographic analysis of normal and abnormal pacemaker function. Cardiovasc Clin 1983;14:97–134.

2. Klein HO, Beker B, Sareli P, et al. Unusual QRS morphology associated with transvenous pacemakers. The pseudo RBBB pattern. Chest 1985;87:517–21.

3. Deshmukh P, Casavant D, Romanyshyn M, et al. Permanent direct His bundle pacing: a novel approach to cardiac pacing in patients with normal His-Purkinje activation. Circulation 2000;101:869–77.

4. Zanon F, Barol SS. Direct His bundle and parahisian cardiac pacing. Ann Noninvasive Electrocardiol 2012;17:70–8.

5. Barold SS, Herwed B, Giudici M. Electrocardiographic follow-up of biventricular pacemakers. Ann Noninvasive Electrocardiol 2005;10:231–55.

6. Herweg B, Ilercil A, Madramootoo C, et al. Latency during left ventricular pacing from the lateral cardiac veins: a cause of ineffectual biventricular pacing. Pacing Clin Electrophysiol 2006;29:574–81.

7. Georger F, Scavee C, Collet B. Specific electrocardiographic patterns may assess left ventricular capture during biventricular pacing [abstract]. Pacing Clin Electrophysiol 2002;25:56.

8. van Gelder BM, Bracke FA, Meijer A, et al. The effect of anodal stimulation on V-V timing at varying V-V intervals. Pacing Clin Electrophysiol 2005;28:771–6.

9. Thibault B, Roy D, Guerra PG, et al. Anodal right ventricular capture during left ventricular stimulation in CRT-implantable cardioverter defibrillators. Pacing Clin Electrophysiol 2005;28:613–9.

10. Champagne J, Healey JS, Krahn AD, et al, ELECTION Investigators. The effect of electronic repositioning on left ventricular pacing and phrenic nerve stimulation. Europace 2011;13:409–15.

11. Dendy KF, Powell BD, Cha YM, et al. Anodal stimulation: an under recognized cause of nonresponders to cardiac resynchronization therapy. Indian Pacing Electrophysiol J 2011;11:64–72.

12. Bristow MR, Saxon LA, Boehmer J, et al. Cardiac-resynchronization therapy with or without an implantable defibrillator in advanced chronic heart failure. N Engl J Med 2004;350:2140–50.

13. Cleland JG, Daubert JC, Erdmann E, et al. The effect of cardiac resynchronization on morbidity and mortality in heart failure. N Engl J Med 2005;352:1539–49.

14. Abraham WT, Fisher WG, Smith AL, et al. Cardiac resynchronization in chronic heart failure. N Engl J Med 2002;346:1845–53.

15. Yu CM, Chau E, Sanderson JE, et al. Tissue Doppler echocardiographic evidence of reverse remodeling and improved synchronicity by simultaneously delaying regional contraction after biventricular pacing therapy in heart failure. Circulation 2002;105:438–45.

16. Dupont M, Rickard J, Baranowski B, et al. Differential response to cardiac resynchronization therapy and clinical outcomes according to QRS morphology and QRS duration. J Am Coll Cardiol 2012;60(7): 592–8.

17. Birnie DH, Ha A, Higginson L, et al. Impact of QRS morphology and duration on outcomes after cardiac resynchronization therapy: results from the resynchronization-defibrillation for ambulatory heart failure trial (RAFT). Circ Heart Fail 2013;6(6):1190–8.

18. Sweeney MO, van Bommel RJ, Schalij MJ, et al. Analysis of ventricular activation using surface electrocardiography to predict left ventricular reverse volumetric remodeling during cardiac resynchronization therapy. Circulation 2010;121:626–34.

19. Molhoek SG, Van Erven L, Bootsma M, et al. QRS duration and shortening to predict clinical response to cardiac resynchronization therapy in patients with end-stage heart failure. Pacing Clin Electrophysiol 2004;27:308–13.

20. Lecoq G, Leclercq C, Leray E, et al. Clinical and electrocardiographic predictors of a positive response to cardiac resynchronization therapy in advanced heart failure. Eur Heart J 2005;26:1094–100.

21. Iler MA, Hu T, Ayyagari S, et al. Prognostic value of electrocardiographic measurements before and after cardiac resynchronization device implantation in patients with heart failure due to ischemic or non ischemic cardiomyopathy. Am J Cardiol 2008;101: 359–63.

22. Gold MR, Thébault C, Linde C, et al. Effect of QRS duration and morphology on cardiac resynchronization therapy outcomes in mild heart failure: results from the resynchronization reverses remodeling in systolic left ventricular dysfunction (REVERSE) study. Circulation 2012;126:822–9.

23. Sweeney MO, Hellkamp AS, Ellenbogen KA, et al, Mode Selection Trial Investigators. Adverse effect of ventricular pacing on heart failure and atrial fibrillation among patients with normal baseline QRS duration in a clinical trial of pacemaker therapy for sinus node dysfunction. Circulation 2003;107:2932–7.

24. Wilkoff BL, Cook JR, Epstein AE, et al, DAVID Trial Investigators. Dual-chamber pacing or ventricular backup pacing in patients with an implantable defibrillator: the dual chamber and VVI implantable defibrillator (DAVID) trial. JAMA 2002;288:3115–23.

25. Murakami Y, Tsuboi N, Inden Y, et al. Difference in percentage of ventricular pacing between two algorithms for minimizing ventricular pacing: results of the IDEAL RVP (identify the best algorithm for reducing unnecessary right ventricular pacing) study. Europace 2010;12:96–102.

26. Biffi M, Bertini M, Saporito D, et al. Actual pacemaker longevity: the benefit of stimulation by automatic capture verification. Pacing Clin Electrophysiol 2010;33:873–81.

27. Ward KJ, Willett JE, Bucknall C, et al. Atrial arrhythmia suppression by atrial overdrive pacing: pacemaker Holter assessment. Europace 2001;3:108–14.

28. Israel CW, Gronefeld G, Ehrlich JR, et al. Prevention of immediate reinitiation of atrial tachyarrhythmias by high-rate overdrive pacing: results from a prospective randomized trial. J Cardiovasc Electrophysiol 2003;14:954–9.

29. Vavasis C, Slotwiner DJ, Goldner BG, et al. Frequent recurrent polymorphic ventricular tachycardia during sleep due to managed ventricular pacing. Pacing Clin Electrophysiol 2010;33:641–4.

30. Vlay LC, Vlay SC. Pacing induced ventricular fibrillation in implantable cardioverter defibrillator patients: a new form of proarrhythmia. Pacing Clin Electrophysiol 1997;20:132–3.

31. Sweeney MO, Ruetz LL, Belk P, et al. Bradycardia pacing-induced short-long-short sequences at the onset of ventricular tachyarrhythmias: a possible mechanism of proarrhythmia? J Am Coll Cardiol 2007;50:614–22.

32. Fisher JD. Pacemaker pro-arrhythmia: beyond spike-on-T and endless loop tachycardia. J Am Coll Cardiol 2007;50:623–5.

33. Mansour F, Khairy P. Electrical storm due to managed ventricular pacing. Heart Rhythm 2012;9: 842–3.

34. Himmrich E, Przibille O, Zellerhoff C, et al. Proarrhythmic effect of pacemaker stimulation in patients with implanted cardioverter defibrillators. Circulation 2003;108:192–7.

35. Wietholt D, Kuehlkamp V, Meisel E, et al. Prevention of sustained ventricular tachyarrhythmias in patients with implantable cardioverter defibrillators—The PREVENT Study. J Interv Card Electrophysiol 2003;9:383–9.

Index

Note: Page numbers of article titles are in **boldface** type.

cardiacEP.theclinics.com

Printed and bound by CPI Group (UK) Ltd, Croydon, CR0 4YY

03/10/2024

01040379-0003